Self-Assessment in Dermatopathology

Meera Mahalingam

VA Consolidated Laboratories, New England

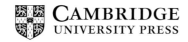

CAMBRIDGE
UNIVERSITY PRESS

CAMBRIDGE
UNIVERSITY PRESS

University Printing House, Cambridge CB2 8BS, United Kingdom

One Liberty Plaza, 20th Floor, New York, NY 10006, USA

477 Williamstown Road, Port Melbourne, VIC 3207, Australia

314–321, 3rd Floor, Plot 3, Splendor Forum, Jasola District Centre,
New Delhi – 110025, India

79 Anson Road, #06–04/06, Singapore 079906

Cambridge University Press is part of the University of Cambridge.

It furthers the University's mission by disseminating knowledge in the pursuit
of education, learning, and research at the highest international levels of
excellence.

www.cambridge.org
Information on this title: www.cambridge.org/9781316622872
DOI: 10.1017/9781316761540

© Meera Mahalingam 2018

First published 2018

Printed and bound in Great Britain by Clays Ltd, Elcograf S.p.A.

A catalog record for this publication is available from the British Library.

Library of Congress Cataloging-in-Publication Data
Names: Mahalingam, Meera, author.
Title: Self-assessment in dermatopathology / Meera Mahalingam.
Description: Cambridge, United Kingdom ; New York, NY : Cambridge
    University Press, 2018. | Includes bibliographical references and index.
Identifiers: LCCN 2018034164 | ISBN 9781316622872 (paperback : alk. paper)
Subjects: | MESH: Skin Diseases–diagnosis | Skin–pathology | Histological
    Techniques | Study Guide
Classification: LCC RL105 | NLM WR 18.2 | DDC 616.5/075–dc23
LC record available at https://lccn.loc.gov/2018034164

ISBN 978-1-316-62287-2 Paperback

Self-Assessment in Dermatopathology

An essential examination resource for anyone sitting their primary or maintenance of certification examinations in dermatology, pathology or dermatopathology, *Self-Assessment in Dermatopathology* uses histopathology as a catalyst for constructive and critical thinking and to trigger relevant clinical, genetic and syndromic associations.

Concise explanations at the end of each chapter give short answers to each question and expand on each answer choice. Each chapter consists of an increasingly difficult selection of questions, allowing the reader to develop and self-test their knowledge. Tables relevant to the section covered have also been incorporated in the answer section. Using this practical approach, the reader will become familiar with the pathologic basis of clinically relevant dermatoses and cutaneous tumors.

The question and answer format make this book the first resource of its kind. Thinking about information in a new way is the foundation of this book, making it an invaluable addition for any trainee.

For Acca, with love, always

Contents

Tables

Foreword

For those trying to learn dermatopathology, the subject too often seems like an enigmatic maze of terminological difficulties, diagnostic conundrums and controversies involving an endless list of entities. Although several textbooks and monographs have tried to deal with this formidable challenge over the years with varying levels of success, there has been little attempt to publish a self-assessment tool in a textbook format which allows the reader to both review and acquire core competence skills in dermatopathology. *Self-Assessment in Dermatopathology* by Dr. Mahalingam is a timely addition to the dermatopathology repertoire whose primary and novel objective is to assist trainees and experienced practitioners in preparing for either primary or maintenance of certification examinations respectively, in dermatology, pathology and dermatopathology.

Covering a wide range of cutaneous infections, non-infectious inflammatory dermatoses, skin tumors and other conditions including pigmentary disorders and genodermatoses, *Self-Assessment in Dermatopathology* incorporates the clinicopathologic and basic science aspects of most of the common conditions one is likely to encounter in routine dermatopathology practice. It uses the time tested multiple choice question format, challenging the reader with a question (accompanied by a high quality representative photomicrograph where appropriate) and a set of options. The layout of the corresponding answer section is unique as it starts with a general summary list of relevant entities, key histopathologic features and helpful clues in a richly illustrated and user friendly tabular layout. This is followed by a discussion centered on the correct answer which also touches upon how the incorrect options were excluded. I believe this format of providing a summary of the core issues at the outset and then following it up with a brief discourse on individual conditions succeeds in reinforcing key information in a persuasive manner.

It did not take me long to convince myself that *Self-Assessment in Dermatopathology* is much more than simply an essential examination resource. Numerous tables and explanatory comments pertinent to the answers of the multiple choice questions provide a treasure of information which educates, inspires and encourages the reader not only to learn but also to think critically about specific conditions and beyond. Some of these "gems" flagged up in sections with headings like "short guide," "cheat sheet," "at a glance" and "quick recap" will no doubt catch the reader's attention and imagination. Given the wide range of entities covered, I will not be surprised if trainees find additional use of this volume as an easy reference to look up practical queries during daily sign outs.

Those like me who have had the good fortune of knowing Dr. Mahalingam as their mentor or colleague will be able to establish a connection between the underlying spirit of this book and her indomitable energy as an enthusiastic, passionate and inspirational teacher. Through a systematic, logical and morphologically sound approach, she has successfully created a resource which is not only an excellent learning and self-assessment tool but also a delight to read. No matter how far up the learning curve a student is, one is sure to learn something new by reading *Self-Assessment in Dermatopathology*. I look forward to the publication of this text and wish it all the success it truly deserves.

Dr. Asok Biswas MD, FRCPath, Dip RCPath
President, British Society of Dermatopathology, 2018–2020
Consultant Dermatopathologist and Honorary Senior Lecturer
Department of Pathology
Western General Hospital and the University of Edinburgh
Edinburgh, UK

Assessment is defined as "an appraisal or evaluation (as of merit)."* To assess the self occurs when one looks inward to evaluate his or her knowledge and to determine whether he or she is fit for the challenges now and in the future. It is an intensely personal evaluation.

It is no secret that dermatopathology is one of the most challenging fields in all of pathology if not all of medicine. Its roots are in general medicine, dermatology, and pathology; however, it has evolved into an exacting discipline in its own right. Those who practice it are inundated daily with scores of conditions – common and rare – that must be accessible immediately by dint of one's experience or by one's ability to access the information in journals or books (or both). If one is fortunate, one has access to an experienced colleague to facilitate the connections.

Having known Dr. Mahalingam for close to two decades, having worked with her in committees in the American Society of Dermatopathology, as well as discussing ideas in dermatopathology with her, she's the real thing. She knows the field, and knows how to teach it to others, which – you might be surprised to learn – are two rare abilities made rarer, still, when they occur in the same person.

As challenging as the discipline is, there is something for everyone here, from medical students, to residents, to fellows, and to seasoned dermatopathologists. This is a book of vignettes on related themes, of questions followed by tables (which are extremely useful; look at tables G8 and H11 for just two of many practical examples), with relevant high quality photomicrographs, and with answers that include some exposition. It is not necessary to begin at the beginning, although it enhances the experience by moving through it in sequence. Yet, conversely, part of the fun of this work consists in discovering, serendipitously, "gems" within the tables and the explanations of the correct answers to the questions. I have no doubts that some will disagree with some of the conclusions presented here; this is not an impediment but a valuable aspect of the book. This book is a tool for thought and is one of many reasons why Dr. Mahalingam's work is so important.

Why, then, are you considering any longer what *I* have to say about this book? You have it in your hands; all you need to do is open your mind to its many "pearls." *You* can now decide for *yourself* how useful it is.

Mark A. Hurt, MD
President, WCP Pathology, Cutaneous Pathology, & Laboratories
Maryland Heights (St. Louis County), Missouri
(Past President, American Society of Dermatopathology)

* "Assessment." *Webster's Third New International Dictionary, Unabridged*. Web. Accessed May 2, 2018.

Preface

Through a style emulating the traditional style of standardized examinations, this book uses histopathology as a tool to trigger associations. The questions are not meant to be actual examination questions but to serve as tools for study as well as a catalyst for constructive and critical thinking about topics covered. The reader is not supposed to know all the answers (or else there would be no need for this book!). The concise explanations at the end of each chapter give short answers to each question and expand on each answer choice. Tables relevant to the section covered have also been incorporated in the answer sections. Using this approach, the reader will become familiar with the pathologic basis of most clinically relevant dermatoses and cutaneous tumors.

Author Credentials

Meera Mahalingam MD, PhD, FRCPath.
www.meeramahalingam.com

Meera Mahalingam is a board certified pathologist and dermatopathologist. Her training in pathology in both the UK and USA enable her to have the unique perspective of what is required of trainees across continents.

She currently serves as the Section Chief of Dermatopathology for VA Consolidated Laboratories, New England.

Acknowledgements are due to the following:

Neil Ryan and his team at Cambridge University Press, for executing my design for the cover to perfection

Anna Whiting of Cambridge University Press, for streamlining my efforts so seamlessly

Stephen Broecher, PhD, Huma Fatima, MD, Rajiv M Patel, MD, Vijaya Reddy, MD, Adam I Rubin, MD, Rajendra Singh, MD (www.pathpresenter.com) and Claudia I Vidal, MD, PhD, for contributing select image/s

My parents, J, and my children, with love and gratitude, for their unending support of all I endeavor to do

My students, for making me learn every time I teach

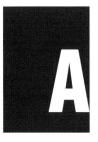

General Clues Questions

1. This is likely a consequence of:

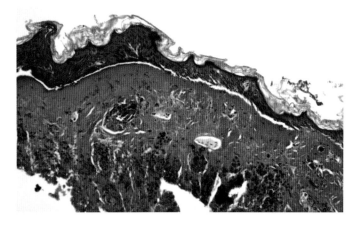

A. Embedding
B. Autolysis
C. Fixation
D. Cautery
E. Grossing

2. The most likely diagnosis is:

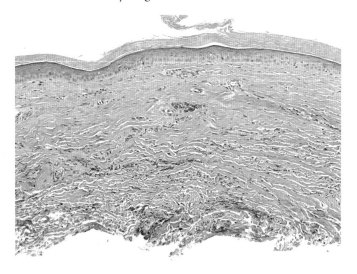

A. Dermatofibroma
B. Cautery artefact

C. Microvenular hemangioma
D. Monsel's tattoo
E. Stasis dermatitis

3. This is typically associated with:

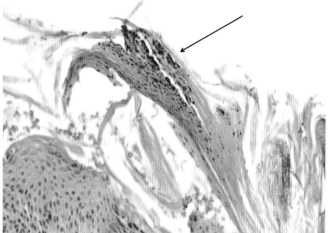

A. Contact dermatitis
B. Lupus erythematosus
C. Seborrheic dermatitis
D. Hartnup disease
E. Stasis dermatitis

4. This is typically associated with:

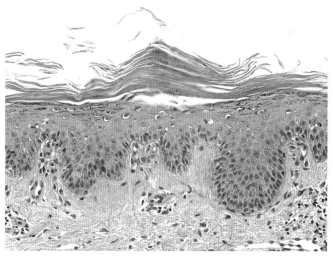

A. Pityriasis rosea
B. Pityriasis rubra pilaris
C. Pityriasis lichenoides chronica
D. Pityriasis lichenoides et varioliformis acuta
E. Transient acantholytic dermatosis

5. Which of the following is NOT a clue to a deficiency state:
   A. Vertically oriented collagen
   B. Confluent parakeratosis
   C. Superficial epidermal pallor
   D. Psoriasiform epidermal hyperplasia
   E. Hemorrhage

6. Which of the following is NOT a paraneoplastic dermatosis:
   A. Acanthosis nigricans
   B. Basex's syndrome
   C. Acquired icthyosis
   D. Scleromyxedema
   E. Scleroderma

7. An absent stratum corneum may be associated with:
   A. Reticular erythematous mucinosis
   B. Interstitial granulomatous disease
   C. Cutaneous T-cell lymphoma
   D. Staphylococcal scalded skin syndrome
   E. Acrodermatitis enteropathica

8. Intraluminal giant cells may be seen in:
   A. Juvenile xanthogranuloma
   B. Rosai-Dorfman disease
   C. Wells's syndrome
   D. Erythema nodosum leprosum
   E. Lichen nitidus

9. Which of the following is an INCORRECT association:
   A. Tricholemmoma and Brooke-Spiegler syndrome
   B. Sebaceous adenoma and Muir-Torre syndrome
   C. Cutaneous myxoma and Carney's complex
   D. Fibrofolliculoma and Birt-Hogg-Dubé syndrome
   E. Leiomyomas and Reed's syndrome

10. Which of the following is NOT a proto-oncogene:
    A. RAS
    B. MYC
    C. ERK
    D. RAF
    E. MSH2

11. Which of the following is a tumor suppressor:
    A. GNAQ
    B. NRAS
    C. MLH1
    D. PTEN
    E. BRAF

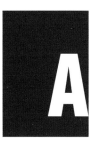

General Clues Answers

Table A1 Special stains commonly used in dermatopathology

Stain	Color	Utility
Alcian blue	Bluish green	Identification of nature of mucin pH 2.5 – Sulfated and carboxlyated acid mucopolysaccharides and sialomucins positive pH 5 – Only sulfated mucopolysaccharides positive
Alizarin red	Reddish orange	Identification of calcium
Bodian	Black	Identification of reticulum and nerve fibers
Chloroacetate esterase (Leder's stain)	Pinkish orange	Identification of granulocytes and mast cells *Negative in immature granulocytes and/or significant monocytic expression*
Colloidal iron	Bright blue	Demonstration of carboxylated and sulfated mucopolysaccharides and glycoproteins
Congo red	Red with apple-green birefringence	Identification of amyloid *More yellow than apple-green in localized cutaneous amyloidosis*
Fite	Red (acid-fast bacilli), blue-gray (nuclei)	Better for the identification of *Mycobacterium leprae* as it is much less acid-fast and alcohol-fast than the tubercle bacillus
Fontana-Masson	Black	Identification of melanin *False positive staining with nerves and reticulum fibers*
Giemsa	Purple	Identification of mast cells, leishmania
Gram	Red (Gram-negative), purple (Gram-positive)	Identification of bacteria
Hematoxylin and eosin (H&E)	Pink (cytoplasm), blue/black (nuclei/calcium), red-pink (cytoplasm, collagen, muscle, nerve, fibrin)	Identification of most neoplastic and inflammatory dermatoses *Most commonly used stain in dermatopathology*
Masson-trichrome	Red (muscle, keratin), blue/green (collagen), black (nuclei)	Identification of smooth muscle differentiation, inclusion bodies in digital fibromatosis
Oil Red O	Red	Identification of fat *Requires fresh tissue*
Perls's Prussian blue	Bright blue	Identification of iron-containing decomposition products
Periodic acid-Schiff (PAS)	Deep pink (fungus, fibrin)	Identification of fungi, fibrin
PAS with diastase (PASD)	Pink	Identification of neutral mucopolysaccharides (diastase resistant) Identification of glycogen (diastase labile)
Toluidine blue	Dark blue (nuclei), violet (mast cell granules)	Identification of mast cells
Thioflavine T	Yellow	Identification of amyloid *Fades rapidly with time*

Table A1 Special stains commonly used in dermatopathology (*cont.*)

Stain	Color	Utility
Verhoff-von Gieson (VVG/EVG)	Black	Identification of elastic fibers
Von Kossa	Black	Identification of calcium
Ziehl-Neelsen	Red (acid-fast bacilli)	Identification of mycobacteria

Table A2 Immunohistochemical stains commonly used in dermatopathology

Stain	What it picks up	Uses specific to dermatopathology
Actin (SMA, MSA)	Smooth muscle, myofibroblasts	Myofibroblastic and smooth muscle proliferations Positive in PEComa *Not a definitive marker of smooth muscle differentiation* *SMA is more specific than MSA*
Adipophilin	Mature sebocytes	Identification of sebaceous differentiation in clear cell neoplasms *Can be positive in renal cell carcinoma*
Androgen receptor (AR)	Apocrine and sebaceous glands	Differentiating sclerosing neoplasms (positive in basal cell carcinoma, infiltrating type) Apocrine marker Positive in Paget's disease Supports sebaceous differentiation
Bcl-2	B lymphocytes (mantle zone), T lymphocytes	Cutaneous B-cell lymphoproliferative disease
Bcl-6	Germinal center cells, intrafollicular CD4+ T lymphocytes	Cutaneous B-cell lymphoproliferative disease
BerEp4	Basolateral surface of epithelial cells	Basal cell carcinoma
BRAF	*BRAFV600E* mutation	Does *not* differentiate benign from malignant melanocytic proliferations *Nevi as well as melanomas can be positive*
Caldesmon	Smooth muscle	Smooth muscle neoplasms *Definitive marker of smooth muscle differentiation*
CD1a	Langerhans cells	Langerhans cell histiocytosis (LCH) *Select cases of LCH can be CD1a negative* Negative in cutaneous Rosai-Dorfman disease
CD2	Pan T lymphocyte marker	Cutaneous T-cell lymphoproliferative disease
CD3	Pan T lymphocyte marker	Cutaneous T-cell lymphoproliferative disease
CD4	T helper lymphocytes, monocytes, dendritic cells	Cutaneous T-cell lymphoproliferative disease
CD5	Pan T lymphocyte marker	Cutaneous T-cell lymphoproliferative disease
CD7	Pan T lymphocyte marker	Cutaneous T-cell lymphoproliferative disease
CD8	Cytotoxic/suppressor T lymphocytes	Cutaneous T-cell lymphoproliferative disease
CD10 (CALLA)	Germinal center cells	Cutaneous lymphoproliferative disease Identification of renal primary in cutaneous metastasis Positive in atypical fibroxanthoma (not specific though)
CD15	Neutrophils, Reed-Sternberg cells	Positive in cutaneous Hodgkin disease Positive in histiocytoid Sweet's syndrome
CD19	B lymphocytes	Cutaneous B-cell lymphoproliferative disease
CD20	B lymphocytes	Cutaneous B-cell lymphoproliferative disease
CD21	B lymphocytes	Cutaneous B-cell lymphoproliferative disease
CD22	B lymphocytes	Cutaneous B-cell lymphoproliferative disease

Table A2 Immunohistochemical stains commonly used in dermatopathology (*cont.*)

Stain	What it picks up	Uses specific to dermatopathology
CD23	B lymphocytes, follicular dendritic cells	Cutaneous B-cell lymphoproliferative disease
CD30	Activated T and B lymphocytes	Cutaneous T-cell lymphoproliferative disease, Lyp, ALCL
CD31	Endothelial cells	Vascular neoplasms *Histiocytes can be CD31 positive*
CD34	Progenitor cells	Positive in several non-lineage related entities (*summarized in section on cutaneous mucinoses*)
CD43	Pan T lymphocyte marker	Cutaneous B-cell lymphoproliferative disease
CD45/leukocyte common antigen (LCA)	Leukocytes	Identification of leukocytes in a mixed inflammatory cell infiltrate *Not helpful in differentiating benign from malignant lymphoproliferative disease*
CD45RO	Pan T lymphocyte marker, specifically picks up memory T lymphocytes	Cutaneous T-cell lymphoproliferative disease
CD56	NK cells	Cutaneous B-cell lymphoproliferative disease
CD57	NK cells	Cutaneous lymphoproliferative disease Positive in nerve sheath myxoma[+]
CD68	Histiocytes, macrophages	Identifying a reactive process
CD79a	B lymphocytes	Cutaneous lymphoproliferative disease
CD117	Mast cells	Mast cell dyscrasia
CD138	Plasma cells	Nodular amyloidosis
CD163	Monocytes/macrophages	Positive in histiocytoid lesions Positive in atypical fibroxanthoma (not specific though)
CD207 (langerin)	Langerhans cells	Langerhans cell histiocytosis (LCH) *More specific in diagnosis of LCH than CD1a*
CDX2	Intestinal epithelial cells	Identification of intestinal primary in cutaneous metastasis
CEA	Tumor marker for adenocarcinoma	Identification of intestinal primary in cutaneous metastasis
CK5/6, high molecular weight cytokeratin	Squamous epithelium	Positive in squamous epithelial-derived malignancies Identification of amyloid in localized cutaneous amyloidosis
CK7, low molecular weight cytokeratin	Non-squamous epithelium, adnexal epithelium, Toker cells	Differentiating MCC from non-cutaneous neuroendocrine carcinoma (negative in MCC) Differentiating atypical intraepidermal pagetoid proliferations (positive in EMPD)
CK15	Follicular bulge stem cells	Differentiation of PCAT from cutaneous metastasis (positive in PCAT) Lost from bulge region in all scarring alopecias
CK20, low molecular weight cytokeratin	Non-squamous epithelium, adnexal epithelium	Differentiating MCC from non-cutaneous neuroendocrine carcinoma (positive in MCC) *Select MCC can be CK20 negative* Differentiating sclerosing neoplasms (positive in desmoplastic trichoepithelioma)
CK903, high molecular weight cytokeratin	Squamous epithelium	Squamous epithelial-derived malignancies Identification of amyloid in localized cutaneous amyloidosis
D2–40	Lymphatic endothelium	Vascular neoplasms Differentiation of PCAT from cutaneous metastasis (positive in PCAT)

Table A2 Immunohistochemical stains commonly used in dermatopathology (*cont.*)

Stain	What it picks up	Uses specific to dermatopathology
Desmin	Smooth muscle	Smooth muscle proliferations *Definitive marker of smooth muscle differentiation*
EMA (CD227, MUC1)	Glandular, ductal epithelia, mature sebocytes, perineural tissue	Helpful in differentiating BCC from a basaloid SCC (negative in former) Highlights sebaceous differentiation Positive in epithelioid sarcoma (vimentin and LMW keratin also positive) Positive in perineurioma
HMB45	Melanocytes	Positive in benign and malignant lesions derived from melanocytes Loss of gradient used by some to differentiate benign from malignant spitzoid proliferations Positive in PEComa
Ki-67	Proliferation index	Increased in malignant proliferations irrespective of lineage
MART-1	Melanocytes	Not useful in identification of actual density of basal melanocytes in sun-damaged skin (overestimates) Low sensitivity in spindled melanocytic neoplasms Positive in PEComa *Macrophages can be positive*
MITF	Melanocytes	Useful in identification of the actual density of basal melanocytes in sun-damaged skin Low sensitivity in spindled melanocytic neoplasms Positive in neurothekeoma* Positive in PEComa *Scars can be positive*
MLH1	Mismatch repair proteins	Lost in sebaceous neoplasms associated with Muir-Torre syndrome
MSH2	Mismatch repair proteins	Lost in sebaceous neoplasms associated with Muir-Torre syndrome
MSH6	Mismatch repair proteins	Lost in sebaceous neoplasms associated with Muir-Torre syndrome
MPO	Myeloid cells	Myeloid leukemia cutis
MUM1/IRF4	Lymphocytes	Cutaneous B-cell lymphoproliferative disease
NKI/C3 (CD63)	Diverse distribution in cell types including lymphoid, myeloid, endothelial cells and melanoma	Positive in neurothekeoma* *Sensitive but not specific for neurothekeoma*
PGP9.5	Neural and neuroendocrine-derived tissue	Positive in neurothekeoma* *Sensitive but entirely non-specific neural/nerve sheath marker*
p40	Squamous epithelium, adnexal basal/myoepithelial cells	Differentiation of PCAT from cutaneous metastasis (positive in PCAT)
p63	Squamous epithelium, adnexal basal/myoepithelial cells	Differentiation of PCAT from cutaneous metastasis (positive in PCAT)
p75NGFR	Neural tissue	Useful in screening spindled melanocytic neoplasms (which can be negative for other routinely used melanocytic markers including S100) *Scars can be positive*
Procollagen	Fibroblasts	Positive in atypical fibroxanthoma (not specific though)
RCC	Renal tissue	Identification of renal primary in cutaneous metastasis Sensitive and specific for primary renal cell *Select cases of renal metastasis can be RCC negative*

Table A2 Immunohistochemical stains commonly used in dermatopathology (*cont.*)

Stain	What it picks up	Uses specific to dermatopathology
S100	Neural crest-derived cells, chondrocytes, adipocytes, myoepithelial cells, macrophages, Langerhans cells, dendritic cells	Positive in melanocytic proliferations Particularly useful in screening spindled melanocytic neoplasms (which can be negative for other routinely used melanocytic markers) Positive in select eccrine neoplasms Positive in granular cell tumors Positive in cutaneous Rosai-Dorfman disease Positive in nerve sheath myxoma[+] Positive in interdigitating dendritic cell sarcoma *Promiscuous antigen (sensitive but not specific)*
S100A6	Neural crest-derived cells	Positive in nerve sheath myxoma[+] Positive in neurothekeoma[*]
SOX10	Melanocytes	Particularly useful in spindled melanocytic neoplasms (which can be negative for other routinely used melanocytic markers including S100) *Scars can be positive*
TdT	Pre-B, pre-T lymphoid cells, and acute lymphoblastic leukemia/lymphoma cells	Cutaneous lymphoproliferative disease
TTF-1	Thyroid, epithelia from upper respiratory tract	Differentiating MCC from non-cutaneous neuroendocrine carcinoma (negative in MCC)
Vimentin	Endothelial cells, fibroblastic reticulum cells, fibroblasts, interdigitating dendritic cells, Langerhans cells, vascular smooth muscle	Positive in mesenchymal proliferations Positive in melanoma *Not a specific marker for anything*

ALCL = Anaplastic large cell lymphoma; CALLA = Common acute lymphoblastic leukemia antigen; EMPD = Extramammary Paget's disease; IRF4 = Interferon regulatory factor 4; Lyp = Lymphomatoid papulosis; MCC = Merkel cell carcinoma; MSA = Muscle specific actin; MUM1 = Multiple myeloma oncogene 1; PCAT = Primary cutaneous adnexal tumors; PEComa = Tumors derived from perivascular epithelioid cells; RCC = Renal cell carcinoma marker; SMA = Smooth muscle actin
* Previously called cellular neurothekeoma; [+]Previously called myxoid neurothekeoma

---

1. D. Image shown is the consequence of a cautery artefact.

   In polypoid lesions, the base of the lesion is typically clinically cauterized to minimize or stop bleeding. This results in unrecognizable cytomorphology and artefactual separation of the epidermis from the dermis.

2. D. Image shown is that of a Monsel's tattoo.

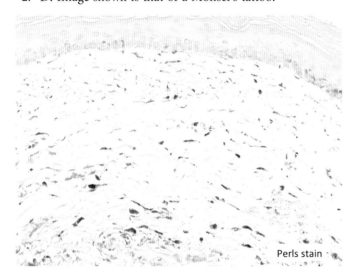

Perls stain

Monsel's solution (ferric subsulfate) is a chemical hemostatic agent that is used to stop and/or prevent bleeding. The use of this agent is associated with deposition of dark brown/black pigment (stains positive for iron with Perls's stain). The presence of admixed multinucleate giant cells is a helpful clue in differentiating this from a nevomelanocytic proliferation.

3. C. Shoulder parakeratosis is typically associated with seborrheic dermatitis.

   Other entities that can exhibit shoulder parakeratosis or parakeratotic follicular lipping include:
   - Pityriasis rubra pilaris (follicular lesion)
   - Spongiotic processes or psoriasis involving the face (likely a function of the increased density of follicles in this area)

   Other patterns of parakeratosis useful as a clue to the underlying disease include the following:

   "Mound-like" parakeratosis – Pityriasis rosea, pityriasiform drug reaction

   Parakeratosis with neutrophils but no serum – Psoriasis, psoriasiform drug reaction

   Parakeratosis with neutrophils and serum – Fungal infection

   Parakeratosis in tiers – Porokeratosis, palmoplantar psoriasis

7

"Capped" parakeratosis – Verruca vulgaris
Horizontally oriented alternating parakeratosis and orthokeratosis – Actinic keratosis, ILVEN
Horizontally and vertically oriented alternating parakeratosis and orthokeratosis – Pityriasis rubra pilaris
Parakeratosis with overlying orthokeratosis – Resolving dermatosis, NOS
"Thick" parakeratosis – Glucagonoma, deficiency states, granular parakeratosis, pityriasis lichenoides

4. **B.** Vertically and horizontally oriented alternating orthokeratosis and parakeratosis is typically seen in pityriasis rubra pilaris.

   Primarily horizontally oriented alternating orthokeratosis and parakeratosis are seen in:
   - ILVEN
   - Actinic keratosis

5. **A.** Vertically oriented collagen bundles in the reticular dermis are associated with digital fibromatosis and acral fibrokeratoma, NOT a deficiency state.

   Clues to deficiency states include:
   - Confluent parakeratosis
   - Superficial epidermal pallor
   - Superficial epidermal necrosis
   - Psoriasiform epidermal hyperplasia with spongiosis
   - Hemorrhage (in pellagra primarily)

6. **E.** Scleroderma is NOT a paraneoplastic dermatosis.

   The most common paraneoplastic dermatoses include:
   - Acanthosis nigricans
   - Acquired icthyosis
   - Basex's syndrome
   - Cutaneous amyloidosis
   - Dermatomyositis
   - Erythema gyratum repens
   - Granuloma annulare
   - Hypertrichosis languinose acquisita
   - Leser-Trélat sign
   - Multicentric reticulohistiocytosis
   - Necrobiotic xanthogranuloma
   - Necrolytic migratory erythema
   - Paraneoplastic pemphigus
   - Pyoderma gangrenosum
   - Scleromyxedema
   - Sweet's syndrome
   - Tripe palms

7. **D.** Staphylococcal scalded skin syndrome may be associated with an absent stratum corneum.

   Other entities associated with absence of the stratum corneum include:
   - Pemphigus foliaceus
   - Psoriatic erythroderma
   - Artefactual

8. **B.** Intraluminal giant cells may be seen in cutaneous Rosai-Dorfman disease.

   Other entities associated with intraluminal giant cells include:
   - Melkersson-Rosenthal syndrome
   - Angioendotheliomatosis
   - Recurrent genitocrural infections

9. **A.** Trichilemmomas are a feature of Cowden syndrome NOT Brooke-Spiegler syndrome.

   Cowden syndrome is associated with mutations in *PTEN*, a tumor suppressor gene, that cause the PTEN protein not to work properly leading to hyperactivity of the mTOR pathway. These mutations lead to characteristic features including macrocephaly, intestinal hamartomatous polyps, benign skin tumors (multiple trichilemmomas, papillomatous papules, and acral keratoses) and dysplastic gangliocytoma of the cerebellum (Lhermitte-Duclos disease). In addition, there is a predisposition to breast carcinoma, follicular carcinoma of the thyroid, and endometrial carcinoma.

10. **E.** MSH2 is a mismatch repair protein, NOT a proto-oncogene.

    MSH2 is a protein that in humans is encoded by the *MSH2* gene, which is located on chromosome 2. *MSH2* is a tumor suppressor gene and more specifically a caretaker gene that codes for a DNA mismatch repair (MMR) protein MSH2, which forms a heterodimer with MSH6 to make the human MutSα mismatch repair complex. MSH2 is involved in many different forms of DNA repair, including transcription-coupled repair, homologous recombination, and base excision repair. Mutations in *MSH2* are associated with microsatellite instability.

11. **D.** PTEN is a tumor suppressor.

    Phosphatase and tensin homolog (PTEN) is a protein that, in humans, is encoded by the *PTEN* gene. This gene has been identified as a tumor suppressor that is mutated in a large number of cancers at high frequency. Mutations in the *PTEN* gene are associated with Cowden syndrome. Mutations in the *PTEN* gene cause several other disorders that, like Cowden syndrome, are characterized by the development of non-cancerous tumors called hamartomas. These disorders include Bannayan-Riley-Ruvalcaba syndrome and Proteus-like syndrome. Together, the disorders caused by *PTEN* mutations are called PTEN hamartoma tumor syndromes, or PHTS.

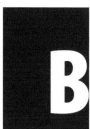

B Genodermatoses and Epidermal Disorders Questions

1. Icthyosis vulgaris is characterized by all of the following EXCEPT:
   A. Autosomal dominant mode of inheritance
   B. Hyperkeratosis
   C. Hypergranulosis
   D. Defective synthesis of filaggrin
   E. Sparing of flexural creases

2. X-linked icthyosis is characterized by all of the following EXCEPT:
   A. Dominant mode of inheritance
   B. Hyperkeratosis
   C. Hypergranulosis
   D. Absent steroid sulfatase activity
   E. Involvement of flexural creases

3. Bullous congenital icthyosiform erythroderma is associated with defects in:
   A. Keratins 3 and 12
   B. Keratins 6 and 12
   C. Keratins 8 and 18
   D. Keratins 1 and 10
   E. Keratins 5 and 14

4. The underlying metabolic defect in Refsum's disease is:
   A. Accumulation of lactic acid
   B. Loss of lactic acid
   C. Accumulation of phytanic acid
   D. Loss of phytanic acid
   E. Loss of ascorbic acid

5. Which of the following is correct regarding the image shown:

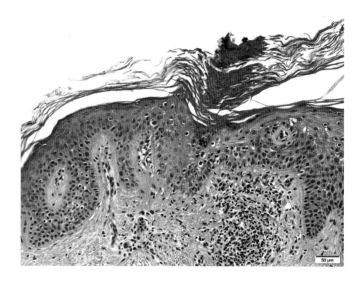

   A. Is a genodermatosis
   B. Is associated with defects in keratins 1 and 10
   C. Has a predilection for intertriginous areas
   D. Is not specific to porokeratosis
   E. The underlying granular cell layer is typically increased

6. Darier's disease has a predilection for:
   A. Sun-exposed areas
   B. Intertriginous areas
   C. Seborrheic areas
   D. Extremities

7. Galli-Galli disease is an acantholytic variant of:
   A. Grover's disease
   B. Goltz-Gorlin syndrome
   C. Darier's disease
   D. Dowling-Degos disease
   E. Brooke-Spiegler syndrome

8. A 48-year-old male presents with sudden-onset, extremely itchy, papulovesicular lesions on the trunk. The best-fit diagnosis for this is:

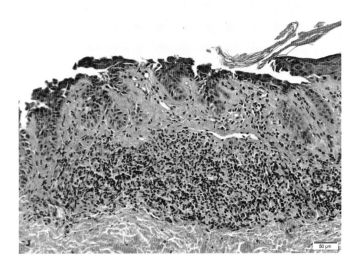

   A. Hailey-Hailey disease
   B. Grover's disease
   C. Pemphigus vulgaris
   D. Bullous pemphigoid
   E. Warty dyskeratoma

9. Hailey-Hailey disease is characterized by mutations involving:
   A. *ATP2A2* gene
   B. Type VII collagen
   C. *ATP2C1* gene
   D. *LAMA3* gene
   E. Keratins 5 and 14

10. The characteristic triad of Netherton's syndrome includes:
    A. Icthyosis, vitiligo, trichostasis spinulosa
    B. Icthyosis, trichorrhexis invaginata, atopic diathesis
    C. Icthyosis, alopecia, bony deformities
    D. Icthyosis, palmoplantar hyperkeratosis, acro-osteolysis
    E. Icthyosis, peridodontitis, alopecia

11. Focal dermal hypoplasia:
    A. Is inherited as an autosomal dominant trait
    B. Is associated with adenomatous polyps
    C. Is associated with pseudoainhum constricting bands
    D. Is caused by mutations in *PORCN*
    E. Is associated with an atopic diathesis

12. Flegel's disease:
    A. Manifests at birth
    B. Presents as hypopigmented macules
    C. Is due to faulty keratinization
    D. Has a predilection for the trunk
    E. Is characterized by cornoid lamellae

13. Granular parakeratosis:
    A. Is an inherited abnormality of keratinization
    B. Clinically manifests as flaccid blisters
    C. Only occurs in the axilla
    D. Is the result of defective processing of profilaggrin
    E. Is characterized by eosinophilic inclusions within the stratum basalis

14. Histopathology of nevoid hyperkeratosis of the nipple is identical to that of:
    A. Granular parakeratosis
    B. Kyrle's disease
    C. Seborrheic keratosis
    D. Warty dyskeratoma
    E. Hailey-Hailey disease

15. Acrokeratosis verruciformis:
    A. Is X-linked
    B. Manifests at birth
    C. Manifests clinically as papules on extremities
    D. Is associated with Kyrle's disease
    E. Is histopathologically characterized by epidermolytic hyperkeratosis

16. The histopathology of Kyrle's disease is best characterized by:
    A. A cup-shaped invagination filled with suprabasal clefting
    B. A keratin plug overlying an invaginated atrophic epidermis
    C. Elongation of rete ridges and acantholytic dyskeratosis
    D. A parakeratotic column involving follicular infundibulae
    E. Densely compacted, orthokeratosis arising from an epidermal elevation

17. Bullae in epidermolysis bullosa:
    A. Are trauma induced
    B. Manifest at birth
    C. Are associated with antibodies to desmogleins 1 and 3

18. The target antigen in epidermolysis bullosa acquisita is:
    A. Dsg1
    B. Dsg3
    C. BPAg1
    D. BPAg2
    E. Type VII collagen

19. Pauci-inflammatory subepidermal blisters include all of the following EXCEPT:
    A. Epidermolysis bullosa
    B. Paraneoplastic pemphigus
    C. Porphyria cutanea tarda
    D. Kindler's syndrome
    E. Bullous solar elastosis

A. Pemphigus foliaceus
B. Acantholytic acanthoma
C. Warty dyskeratoma
D. Grover's disease
E. Pemphigus erythematosus

20. The most likely diagnosis is:

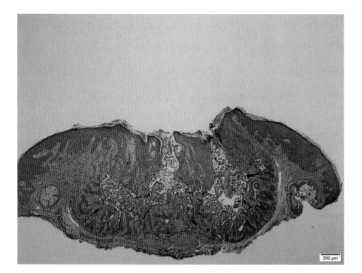

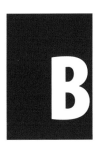

Genodermatoses and Epidermal Disorders Answers

Table B1 Keratins and associated diseases

Type	Number	Disease
Epithelial keratins	**K1**	Bullous congenital icthyosiform erythroderma
		Epidermolytic palmoplantar keratoderma
		Striate palmoplantar keratoderma
		Icthyosis hystrix, Curth-Macklin type
	K2	Icthyosis bullosa of Siemens
	K3	Meesmann's epithelial corneal dystrophy
	K4	White sponge nevus
	K5	Epidermolysis bullosa simplex
		Dowling-Degos disease
	K6a/6b	Pachyonychia congenita
	K6c	Focal palmoplantar keratoderma
	K9	Epidermolytic palmoplantar keratoderma
	K10	Bullous congenital icthyosiform erythroderma
	K12	Meesmann's epithelial corneal dystrophy
	K13	White sponge nevus
	K14	Epidermolysis bullosa simplex
		Nageli-Franchesetti-Jadassohn disease
	K16	Pachyonychia congenital
		Non-epidermolytic palmoplantar keratoderma
	K17	Pachyonychia congenital
		Steatocystoma multiplex
	K74	Autosomal dominant wooly hair
	K75	Pseudofolliculitis barbae
Hair and nail keratins	**K81**	Monilethrix
	K83	Monilethrix
	K85	Hair-nail ectodermal dysplasia
	K86	Monilethrix

Table B2 Genes and target proteins in inherited epidermolysis bullosa (EB)

EB type	Gene defect/s	Target protein/s involved
Simplex	*DSP, PKP1*, Keratins 5, 14, *PLEC1, ITGA6, ITGB4*	Desmoplakin, plakophilin-1, K5, K14, plectin, $\alpha_6\beta_4$ integrin
Junctional	*LAMA3, LAMB3, LAMC2, COL17A1, ITG176, ITGB4*	Laminin 5, type XVII collagen, $\alpha_6\beta_4$ integrin, laminin 332
Dystrophic	*COL7A1*	Type VII collagen

1. C. The granular cell layer in icthyosis vulgaris is diminished or absent and NOT increased.

    Icthyosis vulgaris is inherited in an autosomal dominant manner and is clinically characterized by scales that are large and adherent ("fish scales") on the extremities with sparing of flexural creases. Keratosis pilaris is often present and typically flexural creases are spared. Characteristic histopathologic features include hyperkeratosis with a *reduced or absent granular cell layer.* The disease is believed to be a retention keratosis, due to a defect in the synthesis of filaggrin – a histidine-rich protein located at 10*q*21.

2. **A.** X-linked icthyosis is recessively inherited (with gene deletion in >90% of cases) and does NOT have a dominant mode of inheritance.

   In contrast to icthyosis vulgaris, the flexural creases are involved and the granular cell layer is normal or increased. Like icthyosis vulgaris, hyperkeratosis is a feature and the disease is believed to be a retention hyperkeratosis due to absence of steroid sulfatase activity – located on X*p*22.3.

3. **D.** Bullous congenital icthyosiform erythroderma is associated with defects in keratins 1 and 10.

   Bullous congenital icthyosiform erythroderma is an autosomal dominant inherited disease that is clinically characterized by generalized erythroderma and vesicles and bullae in the first few years of life. Flexural surfaces show marked involvement. Histopathologic features include epidermolytic hyperkeratosis and a markedly thickened granular cell layer.

4. **C.** The metabolic defect in Refsum's disease is an accumulation of phytanic acid (due to deficiency of alpha-phytanic acid alpha-hydroxylase).

   Refsum's disease is an autosomal recessive disease that is characterized by icthyosis, cerebellar ataxia, progressive paresis of the extremities and retinitis pigmentosa. Histopathologic features include acanthosis with hyperkeratosis and hypergranulosis.

5. **D.** Image shown is that of a cornoid lamella. Cornoid lamellation is NOT specific to porokeratosis.

   Although the key histologic feature of porokeratosis, cornoid lamellation has been noted in several other entities as a "tissue reaction" pattern. The cornoid lamella, characterized by a column of parakeratosis with an underlying decreased or absent granular cell layer and individually necrotic, dyskeratotic keratinocytes, is believed to represent a localized area of faulty keratinization and has been regarded as a clonal disease. Clinically it manifests as a raised keratotic plaque.

   Historically, porokeratosis is a misnomer in that it was erroneously coined on the assumptions that cornoid lamellae emerged from pores of the sweat glands. There are several clinical types of porokeratosis and a given patient may develop more than one type of porokeratosis simultaneously or consecutively.

6. **C.** Darier's disease involves the head, neck and trunk ("seborrheic distribution") areas.

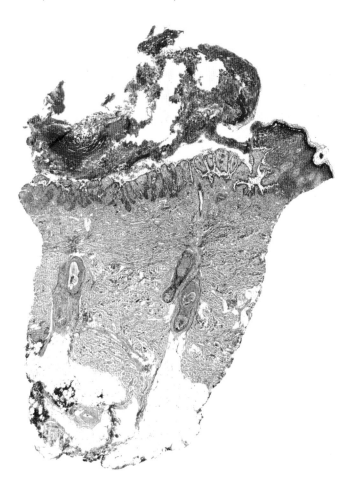

   Areas devoid of follicles such as palms, soles and oral mucosa may also be involved. Darier's disease is an uncommon autosomal dominant genodermatosis that is clinically characterized by greasy, yellow/brown crusted lesions. The mechanisms underlying the acantholysis are still a subject of debate although most believe that it is due to a defect in the synthesis or maturation of the tonofilament-desmosome complex. Histopathologic features of Darier's disease, shown above, include suprabasal acantholysis with lacune formation and corps ronds (solitary or groups of dyskeratotic cells in the stratum malphigian and corneum layers) and corps grains (small cells with elongate nuclei in the superficial epidermal layers).

7. **D.** Galli-Galli disease is an autosomal dominant acantholytic variant of Dowling-Degos disease.

   Galli-Galli disease is characterized by progressive pigmented lesions involving large body folds and flexural areas. Histopathologic features include elongate rete ridges with increased pigmentation of the basal layer and suprabasal lacunae.

8. **B.** In conjunction with the clinical presentation, the best-fit diagnosis for the image shown is that of Grover's disease.

   Grover's disease, clinically characterized by a pruritic papulovesicular rash, typically develops in the trunks of older men. Despite the histopathologic similarity to Darier's disease, Grover's disease does not share an abnormality in the *ATP2A2* gene. Histopathologic features of Grover's disease vary with the age of the lesion but typically include acantholysis, dyskeratotic keratinocytes and a dermal infiltrate containing eosinophils. Older lesions may have pronounced acanthosis and only subtle acantholysis.

9. **C.** The responsible gene in Hailey-Hailey disease (familial benign chronic pemphigus) is *ATP2C1* mapped to *3q21–q24*.

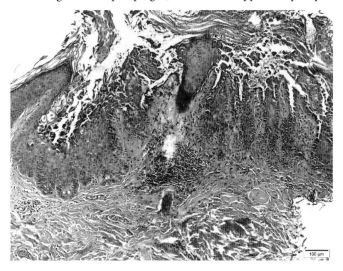

   Hailey-Hailey disease is inherited as an autosomal dominant condition and is clinically characterized by a chronic course with spontaneous remission and subsequent exacerbation. Vesicular plaques progress to flaccid bullae with a predilection for the neck and intertriginous areas.

   Histopathologic features of Hailey-Hailey disease, shown above, include acanthosis and acantholytic dyskeratosis and vary with the age of the lesion.

   Early lesions: Lacunae formed by suprabasilar clefting containing acantholytic dyskeratotic keratinocytes either singly or in clusters

   Late lesions: Lacunae progress to form broad acantholytic vesicles and bullae, intercellular edema leads to acantholysis ("dilapidated brick wall" appearance)

10. **B.** The triad of Netherton's syndrome consists of icthyosis, trichorrhexis invaginata (bamboo hair) and an atopic diathesis.

    Netherton's syndrome is a rare autosomal dominant disease characterized by elevated IgE levels. It is due to mutations in *SPINK5*, encoding a serine protease inhibitor that plays a crucial role in epidermal growth and differentiation, located on chromosome *5q32*.

11. **D.** Focal dermal hypoplasia is caused by mutations in *PORCN* (an endoplasmic reticulum protein involved in the secretion of Wnt proteins).

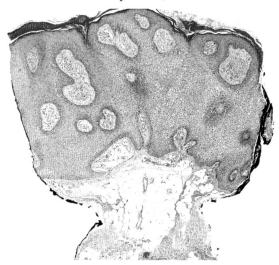

    Focal dermal hypoplasia, an X-linked dominant trait, also known as Goltz-Gorlin syndrome, is a rare syndrome associated with multiple congenital malformations of mesoderm and ectoderm. Clinical manifestations include widely distributed linear areas of hypoplasia, lack of a digit ("lobster claw deformity"), and colobomata of the eyes. Radiographic evidence of osteopathic striata is a reliable diagnostic marker of Goltz-Gorlin syndrome.

    Histopathologic features of focal dermal hypoplasia include dermal atrophy and attenuation of collagen with extension of subcutaneous fat upwards into the superficial dermis.

12. **C.** Flegel's disease is the result of faulty keratinization.

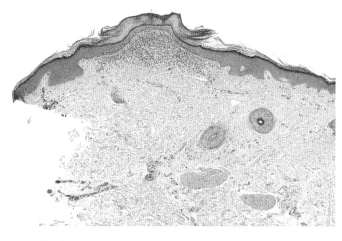

    Also known as hyperkeratosis lenticularis perstans,

Flegel's disease is a late-onset genodermatosis that presents in adults and is clinically characterized by the development of discrete, multiple keratoses that are most prominent on the dorsum of the feet and anterior aspect of the legs.

A distinctive histopathologic feature of Flegel's disease is the presence of a discrete zone of thickened, compact, deeply eosinophilic hyperkeratosis.

13. **D.** Granular parakeratosis is the result of a defect in the processing of profilaggrin to filaggrin.

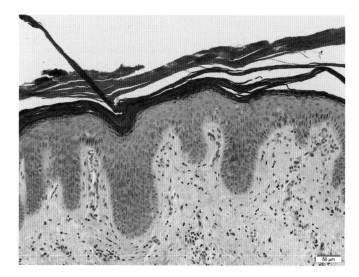

Granular parakeratosis, an acquired abnormality of keratinization, a benign condition, was first described in 1991 as a skin disease manifesting with erythematous hyperpigmented and hyperkeratotic papules and plaques of the cutaneous folds. Since its initial description in the axilla, it has been described in other intertriginous areas as well as the trunk and extremities. Clinical course is spontaneous resolution after months.

Histopathologic findings, shown above, include a thick layer of parakeratosis with retention of keratohyaline granules. The underlying epidermis may be normal, atrophic or acanthotic.

14. **C.** Histopathologic findings of nevoid hyperkeratosis bear a superficial resemblance to seborrheic keratosis.

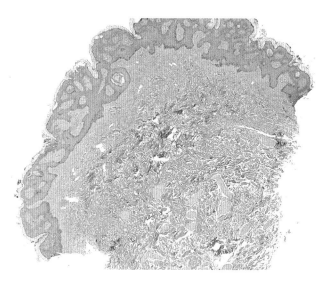

Nevoid hyperkeratosis of the nipple manifests clinically by hyperpigmentation of the nipple accompanied by verrucous thickening.

Histopathologic features, shown above, include hyperkeratosis, papillomatosis and acanthosis with elongation of rete ridges.

15. **C.** Acrokeratosis verruciformis is characterized clinically by multiple papules on the hands and fingers.

Acrokeratosis verruciformis is an autosomal dominant genodermatosis. Onset is usually before puberty. Similar lesions have been noted in a significant number of patients with Darier's disease. Histopathologic findings include hyperkeratosis, acanthosis and low papillomatosis ("church spire" appearance).

16. **B.** Kyrle's disease is histopathologically characterized by a keratin plug overlying an invaginated and atrophic epidermis.

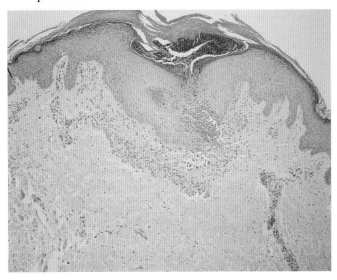

Kyrle's disease is a perforating skin condition characterized by the presence of large keratotic papules distributed widely throughout the body and in particular on the extremities and the trunk. The papules contain a central keratotic plug, which histologically correlates with keratin and necrotic debris. The disease is most closely associated with diabetes mellitus and renal failure.

17. **A.** Bullae in epidermolysis bullosa (EB) are trauma induced.

    EB encompasses a heterogeneous group of disorders inherited in an autosomal dominant or recessive form. The 3 types include: EB simplex (intraepidermal), junctional EB (intralamina lucida) and dystrophic EB (sublamina densa). Target proteins in each subtype are summarized in Table B2. In EB simplex, the plane of

cleavage is so low that in routine H&E stained sections, it appears as a cell-poor subepidermal blister. Electron microscopy is the gold standard for diagnosis.

18. **E.** The target antigen in EBA is type VII collagen with a molecular weight of 290 kDa.

    Epidermolysis bullosa acquisita (EBA) is a non-hereditary subepidermal bullous disorder in which blisters develop at the site of trauma. Involvement of the mucous membranes occurs in 30–50% of cases. Serology using ELISA is diagnostic.

19. **B.** Paraneoplastic pemphigus is characterized by a suprabasilar NOT a subepidermal blister.

    Entities characterized by a pauci-inflammatory subepidermal blister include:
    - Epidermolysis bullosa
    - Porphyria cutanea tarda
    - Bullous pemphigoid (cell-poor variant)
    - Burns
    - Toxic epidermal necrolysis
    - Suction blister
    - Bullous elastosis
    - Bullous amyloidosis
    - Waldenström's macroglobulinemia
    - Kindler's syndrome

20. **C.** Image shown is that of warty dyskeratoma.

    Defining histopathologic features of warty dyskeratoma are a cup-shaped epidermal invagination filled with a plug of keratinaceous material. The epidermal component shows suprabasal clefting with numerous dyskeratotic and acantholytic cells within the lacuna. Clinically, they present as a solitary nodule with an umbilicated center.

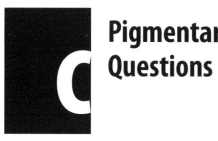

Pigmentary Disorders
Questions

1. The best-fit diagnosis is:

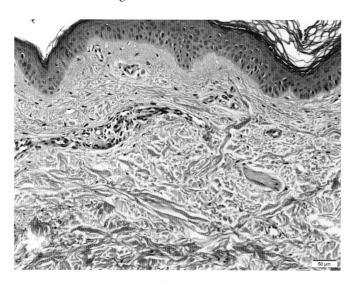

   A. Nevus depigmentosus
   B. Oculocutaneous albinism
   C. Chediak-Higashi syndrome
   D. Vitiligo
   E. Pityriasis alba

2. The key enzyme in melanin biosynthesis is:
   A. Tyrosinase
   B. Tyrosine hydroxylase
   C. DOPA oxidase
   D. Phenylalanine hydroxylase
   E. Dihydroxyindole oxidase

3. Tuberous sclerosis is characterized by:
   A. Epilepsy, piebaldism and angiofibromas
   B. Epilepsy, angiokeratomas and mucosal lentigines
   C. Epilepsy, mental retardation and adenoma sebaceum
   D. Epilepsy, oculocutaneous albinism and pyogenic infections
   E. Epilepsy, acromelanosis and sebaceomas

4. Hyperpigmentation is not a feature of:
   A. Chediak-Higashi syndrome
   B. Dowling-Degos disease
   C. Peutz-Jeghers syndrome
   D. Laugier-Hunziker syndrome
   E. Macules of Albright's syndrome

5. Café-au-lait spots are not seen in:
   A. Bloom's syndrome
   B. Neurofibromatosis
   C. Muir-Torre syndrome
   D. Cowden's disease
   E. Fanconi's anemia

6. Which of the following is not a feature of Laugier-Hunziker syndrome:
   A. Labial lentigo
   B. Longitudinal melanonychia
   C. Dysplastic nevi

7. The most likely diagnosis for this shoulder lesion is:

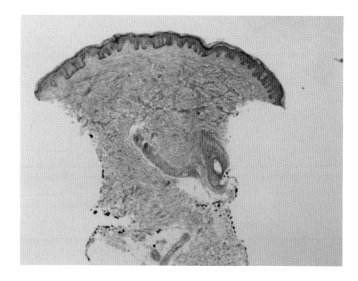

   A. Labial lentigo
   B. Seborrheic keratosis
   C. Café-au-lait macule

D. Becker's nevus

E. Nevus spilus

8. Pigmentation in Dowling-Degos disease is best characterized by which of the following:

A. Diffuse

B. Localized

C. Reticulate

D. Dyschromatosis

9. Which of the following is NOT a feature of Peutz-Jeghers syndrome:

A. Sebaceous neoplasms

B. Gastrointestinal polyps

C. Labial lentigos

D. Predisposition to cancers

E. Digital pigmented macules

Pigmentary Disorders Answers

Table C1 Entities/disorders commonly characterized by hypopigmentation

Entity		Mutation/s, etiopathogenesis	Clinical features	Histopathologic features
Piebaldism		*KIT, PAX3, MITF, SOX10*	AD, non-progressive discrete patches of leukoderma present since birth	Melanin and melanocytes are completely absent in the leukodermic area
Vitiligo		Melanocyte destruction by a neurochemical mediator (*neural theory*) or "self" (*autocytotoxicity*) or due to an *inherent defect* or *autoimmune mediated*	Acquired, idiopathic disorder, predilection for face, back of hands, axillae, groin, umbilicus and genitalia, 20–30% have an associated autoimmune disease	*Lesional area* – complete loss of melanin and melanocytes, superficial lymphocytic infiltrate *Advancing border* – melanocytes may be increased in size with increased dendrites
Oculocutaneous albinism	Type 1A[#]	11q14 (tyrosinase activity absent)	Photophobia, nystagmus, strabismus and reduced visual acuity	Complete loss of melanin in skin and hair bulbs, *melanocytes are normal in number and morphology*
	Type 1B[#]	11q14 (tyrosinase activity reduced)	Hypopigmentation at birth and yellow/blonde hair	
	Type 2[#]	15q11 (*P* gene deleted)	Hypopigmentation of skin, hair and eyes	
	Type 3	9p23, mutations in *TYRP1*	Found predominantly in Africans	
	Type 4	5p13	Hypopigmentation, most common type in Japan	
Hermansky-Pudlak syndrome		10q23, 5q14.1	AR, OCA	Complete loss of melanin in skin and hair bulbs, melanocytes are normal in number and morphology
Chediak-Higashi syndrome			AR, partial OCA, frequent pyogenic infections, abnormal large granules in leukocytes	Reduction or complete absence of melanin in skin and hair bulbs
Tuberous sclerosis		Wide spectrum involving 9q34 (TSC1) and 16p13 (TSC2)	Epilepsy, mental retardation and multiple angiofibromas, "ash leaf spots" (macules of hypopigmentation)	Reduced *but not absent* melanin
Idiopathic guttate hypomelanosis			Multiple hypochromic/achromic macules on sun-exposed extremities	Reduced melanin and reduced *but not completely absent* dopa-positive melanocytes

Table C1 Entities/disorders commonly characterized by hypopigmentation (*cont.*)

Entity	Mutation/s, etiopathogenesis	Clinical features	Histopathologic features
Hypomelanosis of Ito	Mosaicism	Onset at birth/infancy, sharply demarcated hypopigmented lesions in a blaschkoid distribution	Mild reduction in basal layer pigmentation, weak tyrosinase immunoreactivity in melanocytes
Nevus depigmentosus/ achromicus		Isolated hypopigmented macules	Decreased melanin, normal melanocyte density
Pityriasis alba		Variably hypopigmented patches on the face, neck and shoulders	Decreased melanin, normal melanocyte density

AD = Autosomal dominant; # Most common types; TYRP1 = Tyrosinase-related protein-1; AR = Autosomal recessive; OCA = Oculocutaneous albinism; TSC = Tuberous sclerosis

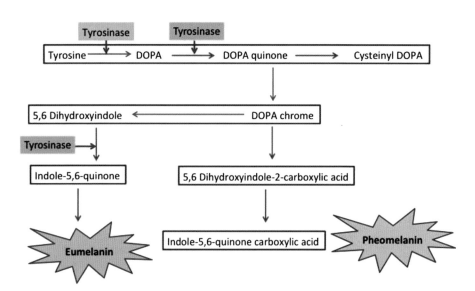

Figure C1 Melanin biosynthetic pathway

Table C2 Entities commonly characterized by hyperpigmentation

Pattern of hyperpigmentation	Entity	Histopathologic features
Diffuse	Scleroderma	Basal layer hyperpigmentation
	Addison's disease	Basal layer hyperpigmentation
	Myxedema	Basal layer hyperpigmentation
	Graves's disease	Basal layer hyperpigmentation
	Malnutrition (pellagra, chronic liver disease, hemochromatosis, Wilson's disease)	Basal layer hyperpigmentation
	Universal acquired melanosis	Basal layer hyperpigmentation
Localized/patchy	Freckle	Basal layer hyperpigmentation
	Café-au-lait spots	Basal layer hyperpigmentation
	Albright's syndrome	Basal layer hyperpigmentation
	Laugier-Hunziker syndrome	Basal layer hyperpigmentation
	Peutz-Jeghers syndrome	Basal layer hyperpigmentation
	Becker's nevus	Basal layer hyperpigmentation

Table C2 Entities commonly characterized by hyperpigmentation (*cont.*)

Pattern of hyperpigmentation	Entity	Histopathologic features
	Acromelanosis	Basal layer hyperpigmentation
	Melasma	Basal layer hyperpigmentation
	Fixed drug eruption	Lichenoid infiltrate with pigment incontinence (depth varies with age of lesion) and interface change
	Frictional melanosis	Patchy interface change with pigment incontinence
	Notalgia paresthetica	Pigment incontinence, epidermal atrophy and/or dyskeratotic cells
Punctate/reticulate	Dowling-Degos disease	Epidermal change resembling lentigo
	Kitamura's disease	Epidermal change resembling lentigo plus intervening epidermal atrophy
	Naegeli-Francesschetti-Jadassohn syndrome	Pigment incontinence
	Macular amyloidosis	Pigment incontinence and amyloid deposits
	Dermatopathia pigmentosa	Pigment incontinence
	Confluent and reticulated papillomatosis	Epidermal change in the form of papillomatosis
Dyschromatosis (hyper and hypo pigmentation)	Dyskeratosis congenita	Pigment incontinence, epidermal atrophy and/or dyskeratotic cells
	Dyschromatosis Universalis hereditaria	Basal layer hyperpigmentation
	Fanconi's anemia	Basal layer hyperpigmentation

Table C3 Syndromic associations of lentigines

Pattern	Entity	Specific comments
Generalized	LEOPARD syndrome	*L*entigines, *E*KG changes, *o*cular hypertelorism, *p*ulmonary stenosis, *a*bnormal genitalia, growth *r*etardation, *d*eafness Lentigines occur early in childhood, AD
	Carney complex (NAME/LAMB syndrome)	Multiple diffuse mucocutaneous lentigines, cardiac/subcutaneous myxomas, endocrine abnormalities, AD
Localized	Peutz-Jeghers syndrome	Lentigines involving perioral region, oral mucosa and hands, melanonychia striata, multiple hamartomatous gastrointestinal polyps and a predisposition to pancreatic and ovarian/testicular cancers, AD
	Bandler syndrome	Lentigines involving perioral region, oral mucosa and hands, gastrointestinal bleeding with small intestine hemangiomas
	Laugier-Hunziker syndrome	Lentigines involving perioral region, oral mucosa, hands and digits, longitudinal melanonychia, genital melanosis
	Cowden's disease	Periorificial and acral pigmented macules, AD
	Xeroderma pigmentosum	Lentigines in sun-exposed sites predominantly, multiple cutaneous malignancies, AR

AD = Autosomal dominant; AR = Autosomal recessive

Table C4 Disorders associated with café-au-lait macules (CALM)

Entity	Specifics
NF1	6 or more CALM, AD
NF2	6 or more CALM (seen only in a minority of patients though), AD
NF3/NF4	Patients with type 4 do not have CALM
NF5	CALM only in affected segment

Table C4 Disorders associated with café-au-lait macules (CALM) *(cont.)*

Entity	Specifics
NF6	Only have CALM, may have axillary and inguinal freckling and Lisch nodules, AD
Noonan syndrome	Also have keratosis pilaris atrophicans, nevi, AD
McCune-Albright syndrome	CALM respect midline, also have polyostotic fibrous dysplasia
Tuberous sclerosis	Hypopigmented and hyperpigmented macules, infantile spasms, seizure disorders, multiple hamartomas, AD
Piebaldism	Congenital leukoderma of skin, poliosis, CALM in involved as well as uninvolved skin, AD
Bannayan-Riley-Ruvacaba syndrome	Penile lentigines, verrucae, vascular malformations, lipomas, acanthosis nigricans, macrocephaly, CNS abnormalities, mutations in *PTEN*, AD
Cowden's disease	Multiple trichilemmomas, oral mucosal cobblestoning, palmoplantar keratosis, sclerotic fibromas, perioral lentigines, hamartomas, carcinomas (breast, thyroid, colon), mutations in *PTEN*, AD
Fanconi's anemia	Generalized hyperpigmentation, guttate hypopigmented macules, pancytopenia, AR

AD = Autosomal dominant; AR = Autosomal recessive

1. **D.** The best-fit diagnosis for the image which shows complete absence of melanin in the basal layer and loss of basal melanocytes is vitiligo.

   Oculocutaneous albinism and Chediak-Higashi syndrome are characterized histopathologically by complete loss of melanin in the basal layer as well as the hair bulbs but by a normal density and morphology of basal melanocytes. Nevus depigmentosus and pityriasis alba are characterized by decreased melanin but a normal density of basal melanocytes (Table C1).

2. **A.** The key enzyme in melanin biosynthesis is tyrosinase.

   The first step of the biosynthetic pathway for both eumelanins and pheomelanins (found in skin and hair) is catalyzed by tyrosinase: **Tyrosine → DOPA → dopaquinone.** Other steps catalyzed by tyrosinase are detailed in Figure C1.

3. **C.** Tuberous sclerosis is characterized by the triad of epilepsy, mental retardation and angiofibroma ("adenoma sebaceum").

   Tuberous sclerosis (TS) is an autosomal dominant condition. While the principal genes involved are located in chromosomes 9q34 (*TSC1*) and 16p13 (*TSC2*), no identifiable mutations have been observed in up to 20% of affected patients. Over 95% of patients have skin lesion which occur in the form of *hypopigmented macules* (present at birth or appear in infancy, >5 highly suggestive of TS), *angiofibromas* (50% occur by the age of 3), *plaques representing connective tissue nevi* ("shagreen" patch, present in up to 40%) and/or *periungual papules* or nodules (Koenen's tumors, present in 20%).

4. **A.** Hyperpigmentation is not a feature of Chediak-Higashi syndrome (CHS).

   CHS is a variant of oculocutaneous albinism (OCA) (Table C1). Other features of CHS include frequent pyogenic infections and the presence of abnormal large granules in leukocytes and other cells. All other entities listed are characterized by hyperpigmentation (Table C2). The hyperpigmentation is patchy or localized in Peutz-Jeghers syndrome, macules of Albright's syndrome and Laugier-Hunziker syndrome, and reticulate in Dowling-Degos disease.

5. **C.** Café-au-lait spots are NOT a feature of Muir-Torre syndrome (MTS).

   MTS is part of the cancer family syndrome and characterized by sebaceous neoplasms (adenomas, epitheliomas and carcinomas) outside of the head and neck area and/or keratoacanthomas and internal malignancies involving varied organ systems.

   Café-au-lait spots are uniformly pigmented tan/brown macules with considerable variation in size (freckle-like lesions to lesions >20 cm). They may be present at birth or appear soon after. They are found in up to 15% of normal individuals and are not increased in individuals with tuberous sclerosis. Multiple café-au-lait spots are seen in neurofibromatosis, Bloom's syndrome, Fanconi's anemia, Cowden's disease, ataxia telangiectasia, nevoid BCC syndrome and Noonan's syndrome (Table C4).

6. **C.** Dysplastic nevi are not a feature of Laugier-Hunziker syndrome.

   Features of Laugier-Hunziker syndrome include lentigines involving perioral region, oral mucosa and hands, longitudinal melanonychia and genital melanosis.

7. **D.** The best-fit diagnosis for the image shown is Becker's nevus.

   Becker's nevus or melanosis is typically found in the shoulder region of adolescent young men and presents clinically as a hyperpigmented area of "thickened" skin. Hypertrichosis may develop but is not inevitable. Histopathologic features include epidermal change in the form of acanthosis and mild papillomatosis with elongate rete ridges and pigmentation of basal keratinocytes, pigment incontinence and an increase in size and number of sebaceous glands and follicle/s. Hypertrophy of the arrectores pilorum as well as smooth muscle bundles in the dermis have been reported – leading some to contend that this is one end of the spectrum of developmental abnormalities involving hamartomatous changes to the pilar unit and arrectores pilorum. Smooth muscle hamartoma typically has a congenital onset and involves the extremities in addition to the trunk.

8. **C.** Pigmentation in Dowling-Degos disease is best characterized as reticulate or punctate.

   Other entities characterized by reticulate pigmentation include Kitamura's disease, Naegeli-Francesschetti-Jadassohn syndrome, macular amyloidosis, dermatopathia pigmentosa and confluent and reticulated papillomatosis (Table C2).

9. **A.** Sebaceous neoplasms are NOT a feature of Peutz-Jeghers syndrome but are a feature of Muir-Torre syndrome.

   Features of Peutz-Jeghers syndrome, an autosomal dominant entity, include lentigines involving perioral region, oral mucosa and hands, melanonychia striata, multiple hamartomatous gastrointestinal polyps and a predisposition to pancreatic and ovarian/testicular cancers (Table C3).

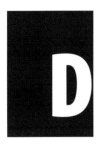

Tissue Reaction Patterns

D1 Psoriasiform Reaction Patterns Questions

1. Which of the following entities would NOT be expected to exhibit this histopathologic reaction pattern:

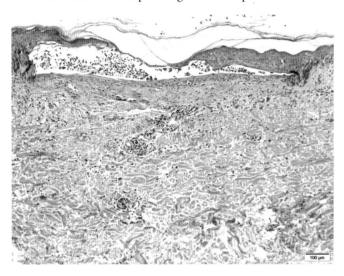

   A. Sneddon-Wilkinson disease
   B. Bullous pemphigoid
   C. IgA pemphigus
   D. Superficial folliculitis
   E. Impetigo

2. Which of the following entities is NOT characterized by this histopathologic reaction pattern:

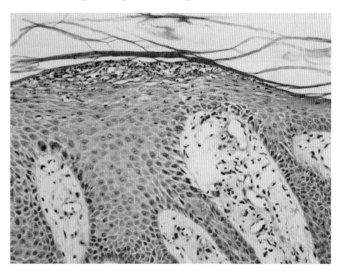

   A. Seborrheic dermatitis
   B. Psoriasis
   C. Reiter's syndrome
   D. Acrodermatitis enteropathica
   E. Glucagonoma syndrome

3. Which of the following is NOT a step in the pathogenetic cascade of psoriasis:
   A. T-cell activation
   B. T-cell differentiation
   C. T-cell trafficking
   D. Keratinocyte proliferation
   E. Cellular senescence

4. Keratinocyte proliferation in psoriasis results in upregulation of:
   A. K1
   B. K2
   C. K10
   D. K17
   E. K19

5. Which of the following is NOT a histopathologic feature of psoriasis:
   A. Munro microabscesses
   B. Pautrier microabscesses
   C. Spongiform pustules of Kogoj
   D. Increased basal layer mitoses
   E. Suprapapillary attenuation

6. A useful diagnostic clue to AIDS-associated psoriasiform dermatitis is the presence of:
   A. Neutrophils in the horn
   B. Psoriasiform epidermal hyperplasia
   C. Hypogranulosis
   D. Plasma cells
   E. Papillary dermal telangiectases

7. The triad of Reiter's syndrome includes:
   A. Gonococcal urethritis, colitis and arthritis
   B. Gonococcal urethritis, conjunctivitis and arthritis
   C. Non-gonococcal urethritis, conjunctivitis and arthritis
   D. Non-gonococcal urethritis, colitis and arthritis

8. Histocompatibility antigens most commonly associated with Reiter's syndrome include:
   A. HLA-A1
   B. HLA-B6
   C. HLA-B27
   D. HLA-DR3
   E. HLA-DQ

9. The best-fit diagnosis is:

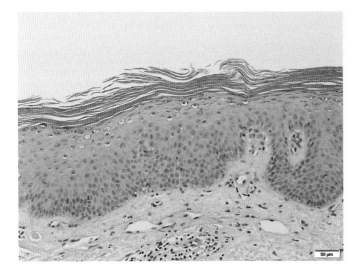

   A. Subcorneal pustular dermatosis
   B. Reiter's syndrome
   C. Pityriasis rosea
   D. Pityriasis rubra pilaris
   E. Seborrheic dermatitis

10. A useful clinical clue to erythroderma secondary to pityriasis rubra pilaris is:
    A. Photodistribution of lesions
    B. Nappes claires
    C. Congenital onset
    D. Pre-existing plaques
    E. Severe pruritus

11. Perifollicular keratotic papules are characteristic of:
    A. Psoriasis
    B. Atopic dermatitis
    C. Cutaneous T-cell lymphoma
    D. Pityriasis rubra pilaris
    E. Chronic actinic dermatitis

12. A useful clinical clue to erythroderma secondary to psoriasis is:
    A. Photodistribution of lesions
    B. Nappes claires
    C. Congenital onset
    D. Presence of pre-existing plaques
    E. Severe pruritus

13. The best-fit diagnosis is:

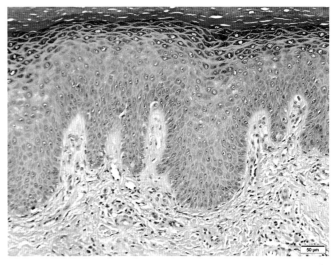

    A. Lichen planus
    B. Lichen striatus
    C. Lichen simplex chronicus
    D. Lichen nitidus
    E. Lichen amyloidosus

14. The best-fit diagnosis for this biopsy of a pruritic linear eruption on the lower extremities is:

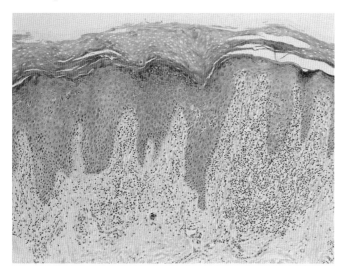

    A. Verruca vulgaris
    B. Pityriasis rubra pilaris
    C. Inflammatory linear verrucous epidermal nevus
    D. AIDS-associated psoriasiform dermatitis
    E. Acrodermatitis enteropathica

15. The clinical correlate of this is:

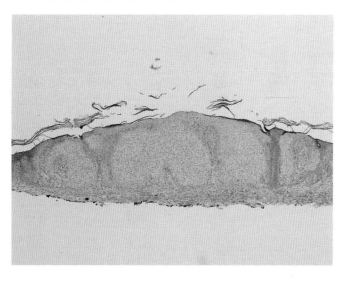

    A. A plaque with associated nail changes
    B. A "stuck on" plaque on the lower extremity
    C. A perifollicular keratotic papule
    D. An urticarial plaque in the axilla
    E. A melanoerythrodermic plaque

16. The clinical correlate of this is:

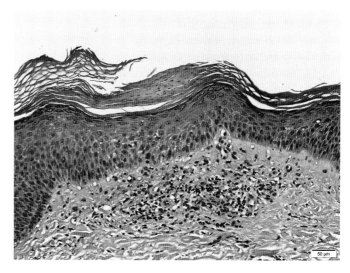

    A. An exanthematous eruption with a preceding erythematous plaque
    B. An erythrodermic eruption with preceding nail changes
    C. A photodistributed eruption with preceding mucosal lesions

17. A histopathologic clue to pityriasis rosea is presence of:
    A. Patchy parakeratosis
    B. Acantholytic dyskeratosis
    C. Subepidermal blister
    D. Epidermolytic hyperkeratosis
    E. Leukocytoclastic vasculitis

18. Pellagra is secondary to deficiency of:
    A. Ascorbic acid
    B. Retinol
    C. Vitamin D
    D. Vitamin K
    E. Nicotinic acid

19. Which of the following is NOT a clinical manifestation of pellagra:
    A. Dizziness
    B. Diarrhea
    C. Dementia
    D. Dermatitis

20. The best-fit diagnosis is:

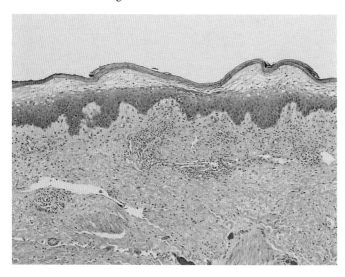

   A. Clear cell acanthoma
   B. Seborrheic dermatitis
   C. Pustular psoriasis
   D. Granular parakeratosis
   E. Acrodermatitis enteropathica

21. The typical clinical correlate of this (based on the image shown above) is:
   A. Diarrhea, dementia and dermatitis
   B. Diarrhea, dementia and alopecia
   C. Diarrhea, dermatitis and alopecia

22. Acrodermatitis enteropathica is due to:
   A. Deficiency of the lysosomal enzyme fucosidase
   B. Deficiency of acid ceramidase
   C. Defect in the zinc transporter protein ZIP4
   D. Absence of sphingomyelinase
   E. Absence of galactosylceramidase

23. Necrolytic migratory erythema is a feature of:
   A. Hartnup's disease
   B. Glucagonoma syndrome
   C. Secondary syphilis
   D. Reiter's syndrome
   E. Lamellar ichthyosis

24. Histopathologic features specific to secondary syphilis include:
   A. Psoriasiform epidermal hyperplasia
   B. Plasma cell-rich infiltrate
   C. Periadnexal inflammatory infiltrate
   D. Scattered CD30 positive lymphocytes
   E. None of the above

D1 Psoriasiform Reaction Patterns Answers

Table D1.1 Histopathologic features and clues to entities/diseases commonly exhibiting the psoriasiform reaction pattern

Entity	Key histopathologic features	Helpful clue/s	Image
Psoriasis	Confluent scale crust with neutrophils Psoriasiform epidermal hyperplasia with hypogranulosis Basal keratinocyte atypia Suprapapillary attenuation Papillary dermal telangiectases	Munro's microabscess Spongiform pustule of Kogoj	

Table D1.1 Histopathologic features and clues to entities/diseases commonly exhibiting the psoriasiform reaction pattern (*cont.*)

Entity	Key histopathologic features	Helpful clue/s	Image
AIDS-associated psoriasiform dermatitis	Confluent scale crust with neutrophils Psoriasiform epidermal hyperplasia with hypogranulosis Basal keratinocyte atypia	Differentiating features from psoriasis: Presence of dyskeratotic keratinocytes Absence of thinning of suprapapillary plate Presence of plasma cells	
Pustular psoriasis	Numerous spongiform pustules Psoriasiform epidermal hyperplasia with hypogranulosis Basal keratinocyte atypia Suprapapillary attenuation Papillary dermal telangiectases	Spongiform pustules more prominent than psoriasiform epidermal hyperplasia	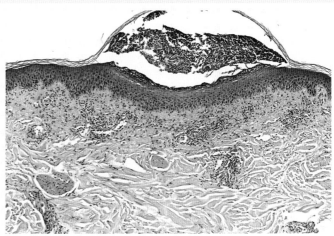

Table D1.1 Histopathologic features and clues to entities/diseases commonly exhibiting the psoriasiform reaction pattern (*cont.*)

Entity	Key histopathologic features	Helpful clue/s	Image
Reiter's syndrome	Identical to pustular psoriasis	Thick scale crust	
Pityriasis rubra pilaris	Alternating orthokeratosis and parakeratosis Perinuclear vacuolization of Malpighian layer Follicular plugging with "shoulder" parakeratosis	Differentiating features from psoriasis: Preservation of granular cell layer Paucity of neutrophils	
Small plaque parapsoriasis/ chronic superficial dermatitis/ digitate dermatosis	Irregular to psoriasiform epidermal hyperplasia, +/− spongiosis Variable lymphocyte exocytosis Mild superficial perivascular lymphoid cell infiltrate	None	

Table D1.1 Histopathologic features and clues to entities/diseases commonly exhibiting the psoriasiform reaction pattern (*cont.*)

Entity	Key histopathologic features	Helpful clue/s	Image
Lichen simplex chronicus	Irregular to psoriasiform epidermal hyperplasia with hypergranulosis Thickened suprapapillary plates Vertical fibrosis	None	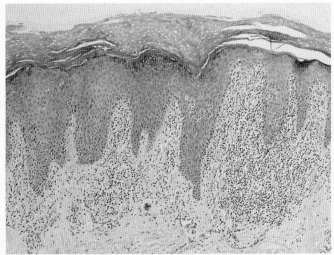
ILVEN	Papillomatosis Alternating orthokeratosis and parakeratosis Irregular to psoriasiform epidermal hyperplasia	Parakeratosis overlying hypogranulosis	
Clear cell acanthoma	Psoriasiform epidermal hyperplasia Neutrophil exocytosis Full-thickness keratinocyte pallor	Clues to differentiate this from psoriasis: Absence of scale crust with neutrophils Sharply demarcated epidermal pallor	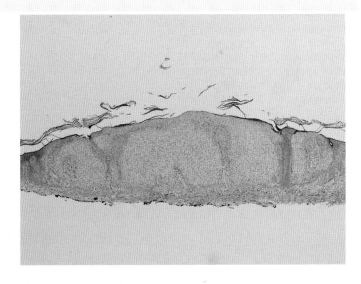

Table D1.1 Histopathologic features and clues to entities/diseases commonly exhibiting the psoriasiform reaction pattern (*cont.*)

Entity	Key histopathologic features	Helpful clue/s	Image
Pityriasis rosea	Patch parakeratosis Minimal psoriasiform epidermal hyperplasia Mild superficial perivascular lymphoid cell infiltrate Extravasated erythrocytes	"Mound-like" parakeratosis	
Acrodermatitis enteropathica	Confluent parakeratosis Psoriasiform epidermal hyperplasia with spongiosis Superficial epidermal pallor	Psoriasiform epidermal hyperplasia with spongiosis Superficial epidermal pallor	

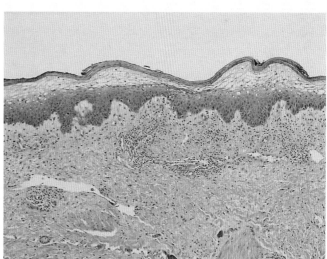

Table D1.2 Histopathologic features and clues to entities/diseases commonly exhibiting a subcorneal/intraepidermal pustule

Entity	Key histopathologic features	Helpful clue/s	Image
Impetigo	Gram-positive cocci within the bullous cavity	Acantholytic keratinocytes within the bullous cavity	

Table D1.2 Histopathologic features and clues to entities/diseases commonly exhibiting a subcorneal/intraepidermal pustule (*cont.*)

Entity		Key histopathologic features	Helpful clue/s	Image
Superficial fungal infection		Hyphae and pseudophyphae (latter only for superficial candidiasis)	Scale crust with neutrophils	
Superficial folliculitis		Pustule overlying the follicle	Perifollicular inflammation particularly around the infundibulum	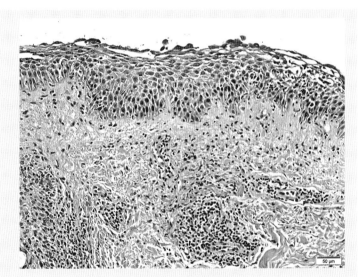
Autoimmune bullous disease	**Pemphigus foliaceus**	Superficial acantholysis	Dyskeratotic cells within the granular cell layer	
	IgA pemphigus	Suprabasal acantholysis	Mixed inflammatory infiltrate	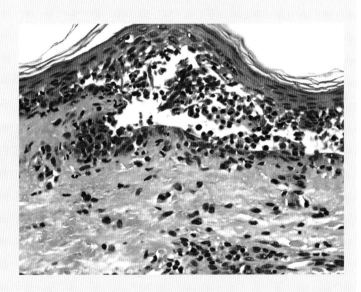

Table D1.2 Histopathologic features and clues to entities/diseases commonly exhibiting a subcorneal/intraepidermal pustule (*cont.*)

Entity	Key histopathologic features	Helpful clue/s	Image
Pustular psoriasis	Numerous spongiform pustules Psoriasiform epidermal hyperplasia with hypogranulosis Basal keratinocyte atypia Suprapapillary attenuation Papillary dermal telangiectases	Spongiform pustules more prominent than psoriasiform epidermal hyperplasia	
Acute generalized exanthematous pustulosis	Spongiform pustule	Underlying eosinophil-rich inflammatory infiltrate	

1. **B.** Bullous pemphigoid is NOT characterized by a subcorneal pustule.

   Entities commonly associated with a subcorneal and/or intraepidermal pustule include impetigo, superficial fungal infection including candidiasis, superficial folliculitis, select autoimmune bullous disease (pemphigus foliaceus and IgA pemphigus), Sneddon-Wilkinson disease, pustular psoriasis, Reiter's syndrome and acute generalized exanthematous pustulosis. Uncommon entities include transient neonatal pustular melanosis and acropustulosis of infancy (Table D1.2).

2. **A.** Seborrheic dermatitis is NOT characterized by an intraepidermal pustule.

Histopathologic features of seborrheic dermatitis vary with age of the lesion and to varying degrees involve both the epidermis and dermis.

Epidermal changes: Shoulder parakeratosis, mild epidermal hyperplasia with spongiosis

Dermal changes: A mild superficial perivascular infiltrate with occasional neutrophils

Acute lesions: Scale crust centered around the follicle, papillary dermal edema and telangiectases and a mild superficial perivascular lymphoid infiltrate with occasional neutrophils

Subacute lesion: Psoriasiform epidermal hyperplasia plus changes seen in an acute lesion

Chronic lesion: More pronounced psoriasiform epidermal hyperplasia and spongiosis

AIDS-related seborrheic dermatitis: Demonstrates individually necrotic, dyskeratotic keratinocytes in addition to changes observed in an acute lesion.

Entities commonly associated with an intraepidermal pustule include psoriasis, pustular psoriasis, Reiter's syndrome, AIDS-associated psoriasiform dermatitis, acrodermatitis enteropathica and glucagonoma syndrome (Table D1.1 and Table D1.2).

3. **E.** Induction of cellular senescence is NOT a step in the pathogenetic cascade of psoriasis.

The proposed psoriatic cascade is as follows:

Step 1: Langerhans cells capture and process antigens and migrate from the epidermis through the dermis to the draining lymph nodes.

Step 2: Langerhans cells then show enhanced expression of cell-surface molecules for antigen presentation known as costimulatory molecules. In the lymph nodes, mature dendritic cells present antigen to naïve CD4+ and CD8+ T-cells.

Step 3: T-cells are activated and clonally expand giving rise to antigen-specific effector and memory T-cells, which emigrate from the lymph nodes and migrate to blood.

Step 4: T-cells acquire a cell surface marker, cutaneous lymphocyte-associated antigen, which allows them to home to the skin.

Step 5: Upon encountering the initiating antigen, there is activation of antigen-specific cutaneous lymphocyte-associated antigen positive memory-effector T-cells, which have been induced in the lymph nodes.

Step 6: The subsequent release of T-cell cytokines accounts for keratinocyte proliferation and inflammation.

4. **D.** Aberrant expression of K17 by proliferating keratinocytes plays a key role in the pathogenesis of psoriasis.

Keratin 17 (K17) is an intermediate filament protein present in the basal cells of complex epithelia, such as nails, hair follicles, sebaceous glands, and eccrine sweat glands. K17 is also closely associated with the immune system and plays an important role in the pathogenesis of psoriasis. High levels of expression of K17 in psoriatic lesions contribute to local abnormal immune reactions by forming a K17/T-cell/cytokine autoimmune positive feedback loop. There is evidence to suggest that select interleukins such as IL-17A can upregulate K17 expression in keratinocytes in a dose-dependent manner through STAT1- and STAT3-dependent mechanisms. The results indicate that IL-17A

might be an important cytokine in the K17/T-cell/cytokine autoimmune loop associated with psoriasis.

5. **B.** Pautrier microabscesses are a feature of cutaneous T-cell lymphoma and NOT psoriasis.

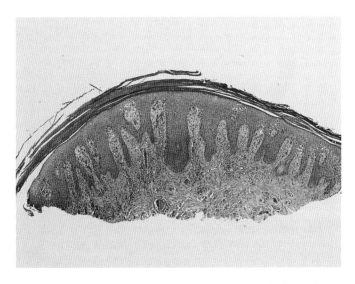

Psoriasis is a dynamic dermatosis with morphological changes during the evolution of an individual lesion.

Papular stage: In lesions that are <24 hours old, elongation and dilatation of blood vessels of the papillary derma, with associated edema and a mild perivascular lymphocytic infiltrate (perivascular cuffing) may be noted. Papillary dermal vessels may be dilated and tortuous. Rare erythrocytes extravasated may be found. *Epidermis during this phase is quite normal*. After 24 hours, there is increased basal layer keratinocyte mitotic activity, mild psoriasiform epidermal hyperplasia, papillary dermal vessels are still dilated and tortuous and their lumen may contain neutrophils and extravasated erythrocytes.

Plaque stage: This is characterized by mound-like parakeratosis with neutrophils superficially, intracorneal (Munro microabscesses) and intraspinous (spongiform pustule of Kogoj) neutrophilic aggregates, prominent psoriasiform epidermal hyperplasia with hypogranulosis, papillary dermal telangiectases and extravasated erythrocytes (more abundant within the dermal papillae).

Partially treated lesions: These may or may not show features typically associated with psoriasis. Depending on the length of the treatment, the granular cell layer may be retained.

6. **D.** The presence of plasma cells is a useful clue to the diagnosis of AIDS-associated psoriasiform dermatitis.

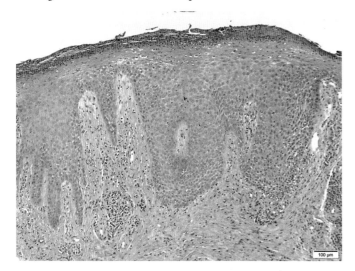

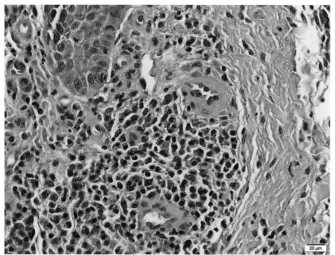

Histopathologic features of AIDS-associated psoriasiform dermatitis are difficult to distinguish from those of psoriasis as both entities exhibit confluent scale crust with neutrophils, psoriasiform epidermal hyperplasia with hypogranulosis, basal keratinocyte atypia and papillary dermal telangiectases. Differentiating features from psoriasis include:

- Presence of dyskeratotic keratinocytes (absent in psoriasis)
- Absence of thinning of the suprapapillary plate (typical of psoriasis)
- Presence of plasma cells (usually absent in psoriasis) (Table D1.1)

7. **C.** The triad of Reiter's syndrome (RS) includes non-gonococcal urethritis, conjunctivitis and arthritis.

Reiter's syndrome has been defined as a peripheral arthritis lasting longer than 1 month, associated with urethritis, cervicitis, or diarrhea. Symptoms generally appear within 1–3 weeks but can range from 4–35 days from onset of inciting episode of urethritis/ cervicitis or diarrhea. Signs and symptoms usually remit within 6 months. However, a significant percentage of patients have recurrent episodes of arthritis (15–50%), and some patients develop chronic arthritis (15–30%).

RS is triggered by bacterial infection that enters *via* mucosal surfaces, usually (but not always) associated with human leukocyte antigen (HLA)-B27. Non-gonococcal venereal disease (most often chlamydia) and infectious diarrhea usually precede RS. These include infections with: *Shigella flexneri, Shigella dysenteriae, Salmonella typhimurium, Salmonella enteritidis, Streptococcus viridans, Mycoplasma pneumonia, Cyclospora, Chlamydia trachomatis, Yersinia enterocolitica* and *Yersinia pseudotuberculosis,* and *Campylobacter jejuni.* Of note, RS was the first rheumatologic disease noted in association with HIV. RS is most common in individuals aged between 15–35 years. It is more common in men with a male-to-female ratio of 5–10:1. The incidence is estimated at 3.5 per 100,000, and it is uncommon among black people.

All patients with newly diagnosed RS should be tested for HIV as the association between these two entities is quite strong. HLA-B27 antigen may be present in the HIV-infected patients.

8. **C.** The histocompatibility antigen most commonly associated with Reiter's syndrome is HLA-B27.

Other entities that are part of the HLA-B27 syndrome include the following:

- Acute anterior uveitis
- Ankylosing spondylitis
- Reactive arthritis (including Reiter's syndrome)
- Inflammatory bowel disease
- Psoriatic arthritis

9. **D.** The best-fit diagnosis for the image shown is pityriasis rubra pilaris (PRP).

Histopathologic features of PRP are not pathognomonic but are distinctive in the context of the clinical presentation. These include hyperkeratosis with alternating orthokeratosis and parakeratosis ("checkerboard pattern" in the stratum corneum), focal or confluent hypergranulosis, follicular plugging with perifollicular parakeratosis ("shoulder" parakeratosis) effect, thick suprapapillary plates, broad rete ridges, narrow dermal papillae, and a sparse superficial dermal lymphocytic perivascular infiltrate. An unusual feature is the presence of perinuclear vacuolization of cells in malphigian layer. Acantholysis has been reported as an additional histologic finding in pityriasis rubra pilaris and may be restricted to adnexal epithelium. *The presence of acantholysis, hypergranulosis, follicular plugging, and the absence of dilated capillaries and epidermal pustulation help distinguish pityriasis rubra pilaris from psoriasis.*

Ultrastructural features include a decreased number of keratin filaments and desmosomes, enlarged intercellular spaces, parakeratosis with lipid-like vacuoles, large numbers of lamellar granules, and a focal split in the basal lamina at the dermoepidermal junction.

10. **B.** Nappes claires is a useful clinical clue to the diagnosis of PRP.

    Clinically, PRP is characterized by orange-red or salmon-colored scaly plaques with sharp borders, which may expand to involve the entire body. Often, areas of uninvolved skin, referred to as *islands of sparing (nappes claires)*, are present. Palmoplantar keratoderma occurs in most patients and tends to have an orange hue. Painful fissures may develop in patients with palmoplantar keratoderma.

11. **D.** Perifollicular keratotic papules are characteristic of PRP.

    Follicular hyperkeratosis in the form of perifollicular keratotic papules is commonly seen on the dorsal aspects of the proximal phalanges, the elbows, and the wrists. This pattern is often referred to as *nutmeg grater papules*.

12. **D.** The presence of pre-existing plaques is a useful clinical clue to the diagnosis of erythroderma secondary to psoriasis.

    Multiple types of psoriasis are identified, with plaque-type psoriasis, also known as discoid psoriasis, *being the most common type*. Plaque psoriasis usually presents with plaques on the scalp, trunk, and limbs. These plaques appear as focal, raised, inflamed, edematous lesions covered with silvery-white "micaceous" scales.

    Other clinical types of psoriasis include:

    Chronic stationary psoriasis (psoriasis vulgaris): Most common type of psoriasis; involves the scalp, extensor surfaces, genitals, umbilicus, and lumbosacral and retroauricular regions
    Plaque psoriasis: Most commonly affects the extensor surfaces of the knees, elbows, scalp, and trunk
    Guttate psoriasis: Presents predominantly on the trunk; frequently appears suddenly, 2–3 weeks after an upper respiratory tract infection with group A β-hemolytic streptococci; this variant is more likely to itch, sometimes severely
    Inverse psoriasis: Occurs on the flexural surfaces, armpit, and groin, under the breast, and in the skin folds; this is often misdiagnosed as a fungal infection
    Pustular psoriasis: Presents on the palms and soles or diffusely over the body
    Erythrodermic psoriasis: Typically encompasses nearly the entire body surface area with red skin and a diffuse, fine, peeling scale
    Scalp psoriasis: Affects approximately 50% of patients and may present as a scarring alopecia
    Nail psoriasis: May be indistinguishable from, and more prone to developing, onychomycosis

Psoriatic arthritis: Affects approximately 10–30% of those with skin symptoms; usually in the hands and feet and, occasionally, the large joints
Oral psoriasis: May present as severe cheilosis, with extension onto the surrounding skin, crossing the vermillion border
Eruptive psoriasis: Involves the upper trunk and upper extremities; most often seen in younger patients

13. **C.** The best-fit diagnosis for the image shown is lichen simplex chronicus (LSC).

    Histopathologic features commonly observed in LSC include:
    - Hyperkeratosis and compact orthokeratosis (resembling acral skin)
    - Patchy parakeratosis
    - Irregular to psoriasiform epidermal hyperplasia with hypergranulosis
    - Thickened papillary dermis
    - Vertically oriented collagen
    Uncommon features include:
    - Montgomery giant cell (believed to represent clumped endothelial cells)
    - Excoriation

14. **C.** In the context of the clinical presentation, the best-fit diagnosis for the image shown is inflammatory linear verrucous epidermal nevus (ILVEN).

    Clinically, ILVEN presents as a linear, persistent, pruritic plaque, usually first noted on a limb in early childhood. ILVEN is believed to be a clinical and histopathologic type of linear verrucous nevus that is often inflammatory or psoriasiform. Unlike the other types of epidermal nevi, ILVEN demonstrates erythema and sometimes pruritus. Inflammatory linear verrucous epidermal nevus accounts for approximately 5% of patients with epidermal nevi and has been described in a mother and daughter.

    While ILVEN is distinct from psoriasis, shared select common pathogenic pathways are those mediated by interleukin 1, interleukin 6, tumor necrosis factor-alpha, and intercellular adhesion molecule-1. *Of note, involucrin expression in psoriasis is confined to the suprabasilar keratinocytes whereas in ILVEN it is confined to the area of orthokeratosis.*

    Commonly observed histopathologic features of ILVEN include:
    - Alternating parakeratosis without a granular layer, and orthokeratosis with a thickened granular layer
    - Psoriasiform epidermal hyperplasia

15. **B.** Image shown is that of clear cell acanthoma (CCA) which clinically presents as a "stuck-on" plaque on the lower extremity.

Also known as "acanthome cellules claires of Degos and Civatte," "Degos acanthoma," and "pale cell acanthoma," CCA is a benign tumor (although there are still some who regard it as a reactive dermatosis). It typically presents as a moist solitary firm, brown-red, well-circumscribed, 5 mm to 2 cm "stuck-on" nodule or plaque on the lower extremities of middle-aged to elderly individuals The lesion has a crusted, scaly peripheral collarette and vascular puncta on the surface. It is characterized by slow growth, and may persist for years.

Histopathologically, CCA is characterized by a sharply demarcated psoriasiform epidermal hyperplasia composed of a proliferation of slightly enlarged keratinocytes, and basal cells with pale-staining glycogen-rich cytoplasm with neutrophil exocytosis.

Differentiating features from psoriasis include:
- Absence of scale crust with neutrophils
- Sharp demarcation of epidermal pallor laterally (Table D1.1)

16. **A.** Image shown is that of pityriasis rosea (PR) which clinically presents as an exanthematous eruption with a preceding erythematous plaque.

Pityriasis rosea (PR) is a benign rash and a common skin disorder observed in otherwise healthy people, most frequently children and young adults. The name means "fine pink scale." PR manifests as an acute, self-limiting, exanthematous, papulosquamous eruption. It evolves rapidly, usually beginning with a patch that heralds the eruption, the so-called "herald patch" and has an average duration of 6–8 weeks. The primary plaque is seen on the skin in 50–90% of cases a week or more before the onset of the eruption of smaller lesions. This secondary eruption occurs 2–21 days later in crops following the lines of cleavage of the skin. On the back, this eruption produces a "Christmas tree" pattern. Prognosis is excellent and the recurrence rate is low (approximately 2%). PR usually lasts for 6–8 weeks, but can last as long as 3–6 months. Protracted cases of severe eczematous or drug-induced PR are referred to as pityriasis rosea perstans.

Approximately 20% of patients present with *atypical or variant forms of PR*. These variations may involve differences in the lesions themselves, differences in how they are distributed, or both. Photosensitivity may occur. In 10–50% of cases, the herald patch may be absent, a finding that is more frequently observed in drug-induced PR. Alternatively, the herald patch may occur as multiple lesions or in atypical locations, such as the soles or the scalp. Sometimes, it is the only manifestation of the disease and is not followed by the typical rash. An inverse pityriasis rosea may be seen, in which the generalized rash spreads to areas it usually does not affect, such as the face, hands, and feet. The face may be more commonly affected in young children, pregnant women, and black people. A morphologic variant characterized by atypical large patches that tend to be fewer in number and coalescent has been described. In this variant, commonly referred to as *pityriasis circinata et marginata* of Vidal or limb-girdle PR, the eruption generally appears in the axillae, the groin, or both, with the trunk and extremities usually spared. Individual patches are 3–6 cm in diameter, exhibiting the characteristic central clearing and collarette of scale with surrounding erythema.

In terms of etiopathogenesis, PR has often been considered to be a viral exanthem, a view supported by the condition's seasonal occurrence, its clinical course, the possibility of epidemic occurrence, the presence of occasional prodromal symptoms, and the low rate of recurrence. PR-like eruptions can also occur in association with many drugs. These typically include:
- Acetylsalicylic acid
- Anti-tumor necrosis factor (TNF)-α agents (adalimumab and etanercept)
- Barbiturates
- Bismuth
- Captopril
- Clonidine
- Clozapine
- Gold
- Imatinib
- Isotretinoin
- Ketotifen
- Levamisole
- Metronidazole
- Nortryptiline
- Omeprazole
- D-penicillamine
- Rituximab
- Terbinafine

It may also occur in association with select vaccines (e.g., bacille Calmette-Guérin (BCG), human papilloma virus, and diphtheria).

While PR-like drug eruptions may be difficult to distinguish from non-drug-induced cases, the former often last longer than non-drug-induced pityriasis rosea.

17. **A.** Patchy parakeratosis in "mounds" is a diagnostic histopathologic clue to pityriasis rosea (PR).

In terms of histopathology, features of PR include patchy parakeratosis (in "mounds"), spongiotic vesicles with aggregates of lymphocytes (*quite characteristic*), a mild superficial perivascular dermatitis with occasional eosinophils and extravasated erythrocytes. Biopsy of the "herald patch" reveals findings compatible with subacute spongiotic dermatitis (epidermal hyperplasia with mild spongiosis). *A PR-like drug eruption cannot be distinguished on histopathologic grounds from PR.*

18. **E.** Pellagra is secondary to deficiency of nicotinic acid.

Other vitamin deficiency associations include:

Vitamin A/Retinol – Phrynoderma (dry scaly skin with follicular keratotic papules)
Vitamin B₁₂ – Poikilodermatous pigmentation
Vitamin C/Ascorbic acid – Scurvy
Vitamin D – Rickets (children), osteomalacia (adults)
Vitamin K – Purpura

19. **A. Dizziness is not a feature of pellagra.**

    Pellagra is clinically manifested by the 4 *D*s: photosensitive *dermatitis, diarrhea, dementia*, and, if untreated, *death*. Pellagra can be divided into primary and secondary forms.

    Primary pellagra results from inadequate nicotinic acid (i.e., niacin) and/or tryptophan in the diet (long-term parenteral nutrition without appropriate niacin substitution, anorexia nervosa, a self-imposed restriction diet in adult atopics with sensitizations to multiple foodstuffs). Niacin is a pyridine carboxylic acid that is converted into an amide in the body.

    Secondary pellagra occurs when adequate quantities of niacin are present in the diet, but other diseases or conditions interfere with niacin absorption and/or processing. Examples include prolonged diarrhea, chronic alcoholism, chronic dialysis treatment, chronic colitis, cirrhosis of the liver, tuberculosis of the gastrointestinal tract, malignant carcinoid tumor, and Hartnup syndrome. Alcoholism can be considered a risk factor for pellagra. Drugs causing pellagra-like symptoms include isoniazid and 5-fluorouracil. Pellagra has also been reported as an adverse reaction after consumption of Kombucha tea.

    Early cutaneous manifestations: Acute pellagra resembles sunburn. The skin is red, and large blebs or blisters that may develop often exfoliate, leaving large areas of denuded epithelium. The changes subside, leaving a dusky, brown-red coloration. The eruption usually begins as an acute dermatitis with edema and exudative alterations, changing to an erythema on the dorsa of the hands, with pruritus and burning. Vasomotor changes of cyanosis or bleaching may be well defined, with profuse sweating and a sensation of coolness. Initial bright erythema may change to cinnamon brown in color. *Characteristically, the rash is symmetric.* Blisters appear several days after the onset of erythema in some patients. The blisters may coalesce into bullae and then break. In other patients, dry brown scales and blackish crusts, resulting from hemorrhage, form after 2–4 weeks. Redness and superficial scaling appear on areas exposed to sunlight, heat, friction, or pressure.

    Late cutaneous findings: After the early stage, the skin becomes hard, rough, cracked, blackish, and brittle ("goose skin"). When the deficiency state is far advanced, the skin becomes progressively harder, drier, more cracked, and covered with scales and blackish crusts resulting from hemorrhages. Healing usually takes place centrifugally, with the line of demarcation remaining actively inflamed after the center of the lesion has desquamated. Blisters are present when pellagra recurs at the same site (pemphigus pellagrosus).

    Laboratory work-up: The therapeutic response to niacin in a patient with the typical symptoms and signs of pellagra establishes the diagnosis. Low serum niacin, tryptophan, NAD, and NADP levels can reflect niacin deficiency and confirm the diagnosis of pellagra. The combined excretion of *N*-methylnicotinamide and pyridone of less than 1.5 mg in 24 hours indicates severe niacin deficiency. *Histopathology is non-specific and not helpful in making a diagnosis of pellagra.* Early changes include epidermal atrophy with pallor of the superficial epidermis and increased pigmentation of the basal layer, a mild superficial perivascular lymphohistiocytic infiltrate, mild papillary dermal edema and telangiectases. In recurrences in the same site, the blisters (pemphigus pellagrosus) contain lymphocytes, neutrophils, and histiocytes.

20. **E. The best-fit diagnosis for the image shown is acrodermatitis enteropathica (AE).**

    Histopathology of AE is characteristic, although similar, if not identical, findings can be seen in other nutritional disorders such as necrolytic migratory erythema. *Histopathologic changes vary with the age of the lesion.*
    Early lesions: Confluent parakeratosis overlying basket-weave stratum corneum and mild epidermal hyperplasia with hypogranulosis and neutrophil exocytosis. The intracellular edema eventuates into pallor of the upper third of the epidermis. Subsequently, subcorneal and intraepidermal clefts may develop as a result of massive ballooning and reticular degeneration, with necrosis of the keratinocytes.
    Late lesions: Confluent parakeratosis, psoriasiform hyperplasia of the epidermis, minimal epidermal pallor.

    Ultrastructural features include extracellular edema associated with degenerate keratinocytes with multiple cytoplasmic vacuoles and slender, finger-like protrusions. Decreased desmosomes are present, and the basal lamina is typically well preserved.

21. **C. The clinical manifestations of AE are dermatitis, diarrhea and alopecia.**

    Patients with AE have a history of refractory diarrhea, failure to thrive, irritability, dermatitis, and alopecia that gradually appeared shortly after weaning from breast milk. Occasionally, patients have a history of siblings or other family members with similar symptoms in infancy.

22. **C. AE is due to deficiency in the zinc transporter ZIP4.**

    Acrodermatitis enteropathica is an autosomal recessive disorder that is believed to occur as a result of mutations in the *SLC39A4* gene located on 8*q*24.3. This gene encodes a transmembrane protein that is part of the zinc/iron-regulated transporter-like protein (ZIP) family required for zinc uptake. This protein is highly expressed in the enterocytes in the duodenum and jejunum; therefore, affected individuals have a decreased ability to absorb zinc from dietary sources. Absence of a binding ligand needed to transport zinc may further contribute to zinc malabsorption.

23. **B. Necrolytic migratory erythema (NME) is a feature of glucagonoma syndrome.**

Glucagonoma, arising from alpha cells of pancreatic islets of Langerhans, is associated with striking systemic clinical manifestations, referred to as the "glucagonoma syndrome." Systemic manifestations of the syndrome include diabetes mellitus, anemia, venous thrombosis, skin rash (NME), weight loss, glossitis, cheilitis, diarrhea, steatorrhea, and psychiatric disorders.

The cause of skin changes in NME is unclear. Glucagon *per se* has not been found to be the direct cause because there are patients who present with NME without neuroendocrine tumors or hyperglucagonemia. However, normalization of glucagon concentration by surgery or somatostatin analogs almost invariably results in a rapid resolution of the skin lesions. Zinc, essential fatty acid, and amino acid deficiencies are all considered to be possible causes of NME. However, not all patients with skin lesions present with these metabolic changes, and not all patients with these metabolic changes present with resolution of the skin lesions after zinc, essential fatty acid, or amino acid supplementation.

NME is a rare dermatosis that is usually associated with an underlying pancreatic islet cell tumor. The skin eruption may be the first manifestation of the disease. The eruption has a *cyclic nature, with periods of skin lesion resolution*. The lesions consist of erythematous scaling and crusting patches most frequently observed in areas of trauma, such as the groin, intergluteal, and genital areas. Bullous lesions may occur. Cheilitis and glossitis are very common mucosal manifestations. It is commonly observed that these patients present with a history of antibiotic or antifungal treatments without improvements of their skin conditions before the correct diagnosis is made.

The histopathologic features of NME are non-specific and may be seen in pellagra, necrolytic acral erythema, or zinc deficiency. Vacuolated, pale, swollen epidermal cells and necrosis of the superficial epidermis are characteristic. *Biopsy specimens from the edges of active lesions are most likely to show the characteristic upper epidermal necrosis*; however, many biopsy specimens do not have features that are typical, or even suggestive, of NME. Therefore, multiple biopsies are recommended when this diagnosis is suspected.

24. **E. There are no histopathologic features that are specific to secondary syphilis.**

Histopathologic findings in secondary syphilis are diverse and vary with the clinical appearance. The perivascular infiltrate is typically superficial in macular lesions but with clinical progression extends to involve the deep dermis. While plasma cells may be absent or sparse in up to a third of the cases (especially in macular lesions), when present *the presence of perineural plasma cells is a helpful diagnostic clue*. Numerous eosinophils may be seen. Other histopathologic patterns noted include an erythema multiforme-like pattern, a mild non-specific perivascular inflammatory infiltrate, a lichenoid tissue reaction, a pseudolymphomatous appearance, an interstitial granuloma annular-like pattern and even granuloma formation. The mimicry of several other conditions confounds the specificity of the changes and shows that syphilis is a theoretical candidate in considering the etiology of the changes seen. Careful scrutiny of all the histopathologic features may permit a relatively refined differential diagnosis to be established and, either prospectively or retrospectively, alert use of additional investigative techniques.

Immunohistochemically, the lymphocytes are of the cytotoxic (CD8) phenotype and up to 10% of the cells may be CD30 positive.

Treponema pallidum is best identified using immunohistochemistry with an organism-specific antibody. Organisms are typically more commonly found in dermis. The gold standard is the detection of *T. pallidum* using PCR-based techniques.

D2 Spongiotic Reaction Patterns Questions

1. The most likely diagnosis is:

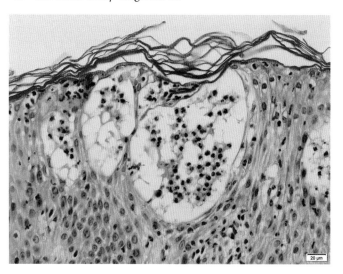

A. IgA pemphigus
B. Allergic contact dermatitis
C. Erythema annulare centrifugum
D. Bullous pemphigoid
E. Incontinentia pigmenti

2. This is a feature of:

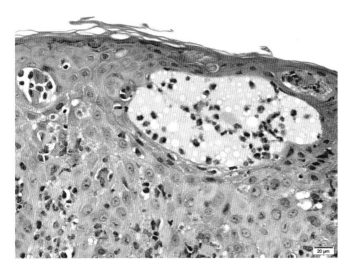

A. Infantile acropustulosis
B. Pityriasis rosea
C. Incontinentia pigmenti
D. Stasis dermatitis
E. IgA pemphigus

3. Precursor lesions of which of the following might demonstrate features similar to that shown above:
A. IgA pemphigus
B. Pemphigus foliaceus
C. Subcorneal pustular dermatosis
D. Erythema annulare centrifugum
E. Epidermolysis bullosa acquisita

4. The diagnosis of acute generalized exanthematous pustulosis (AGEP) is based on:
A. Clinical presentation and histopathology
B. Clinical presentation and serology
C. Clinical presentation and direct immunofluorescence (DIF)
D. Clinical presentation, histopathology and serology
E. Clinical presentation, histopathology and DIF

5. Which of the following best describes acute generalized exanthematous pustular dermatosis (AGEP):
A. Is a chronic, relapsing vesicopustular dermatosis
B. Has a predilection for the intertriginous areas
C. Is specifically associated with paracetamol use
D. Is a variant of pemphigus foliaceus
E. Is a rapidly evolving, pustular dermatosis

6. Which of the following is true regarding IgA pemphigus:
A. Circulating IgA antibodies are present in 50% of cases
B. Is a subepidermal acantholytic, vesicobullous eruption
C. Is typically associated with an IgA monoclonal gammopathy
D. Is clinically homogeneous
E. Direct immunofluorescence shows intercellular IgG deposits

7. All of the following are true regarding pemphigus vegetans EXCEPT:
A. It is a variant of pemphigus foliaceus
B. It is characterized by antibodies to dsg3
C. Two clinical variants have classically been described
D. Histopathologic features include acantholysis and/or eosinophil-rich intraepidermal pustules
E. Direct immunofluorescence and serology are useful diagnostic adjuncts

8. In bullous pemphigoid:
A. Target antigens include BP230, BPAg1 and BP180, BPAg2
B. The major antigenic epitopes of BP230 map within the N-terminal end
C. Serum levels of BP180 do not correlate with disease activity
D. Male patients are more likely to have antibodies to BP230
E. Autoantibodies to BPAg1 and BPAg2 are indicative of underlying bullous pemphigoid

9. Which of the following is true regarding direct immunofluorescence findings in bullous pemphigoid:
A. In early stages of the disease only linear C3 is present
B. In established lesions only linear IgG is noted
C. IgG1 is the predominant subclass of IgG in prodromal lesions
D. IgM and IgA may be seen in up to 80% of cases

10. Which of the following is correct regarding indirect immunofluorescence findings in bullous pemphigoid:
A. Circulating anti-BMZ antibodies are noted in a proportion of patients
B. Antibody titers correlate with disease activity
C. Circulating antibodies may be detected in the presence of circulating immune complexes

11. Which of the following best describes incontinentia pigmenti:
A. Chronic skin disease that occurs in individuals with a personal/family history of atopy
B. Autosomal dominant condition characterized by diagnostic serology and direct immunofluorescence findings
C. X-linked genodermatosis involving multiple organ systems
D. Autoimmune vesicobullous eruption with distinctive direct immunofluorescence findings
E. Chronic relapsing vesiculopustular dermatosis with a predilection for intertriginous areas

12. Which of the following best describes cutaneous manifestations of incontinentia pigmenti:
    A. Dark brown reticulate hyperpigmentation of the trunks with hyperkeratosis of the palms and soles
    B. Evolve through vesicobullous, verrucous and pigmentary stages
    C. Pigmented macules on the buccal mucosa, lips, perioral skin and digits
    D. Ash leaf spots and multiple angiofibromas
    E. Hypopigmented skin and silvery hair

13. The first stage of incontinentia pigmenti is histopathologically characterized by:
    A. Neutrophilic spongiosis
    B. Lymphocytic exocytosis
    C. Hypomelanosis
    D. Pigment incontinence
    E. Eosinophilic exocytosis

14. The most likely diagnosis is:

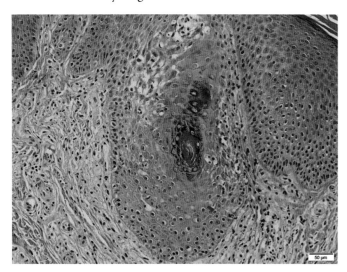

    A. Acute generalized exanthematous pustulosis
    B. Pemphigus (precursor lesion)
    C. Fox-Fordyce disease
    D. Pityriasis rosea
    E. Seborrheic dermatitis

15. Which of the following best describes the clinical correlate of the image shown above:
    A. Chronic papular eruption limited to areas bearing apocrine glands
    B. Chronic papulonodular pustular facial eruption
    C. Acute follicular keratotic papules confined to the extremities
    D. Chronic salmon-pink papulosquamous eruption involving the trunk and extremities
    E. Acute pruritic follicular eruption involving the proximal extremities

16. Which of the following best describes the clinical correlate of the image shown:

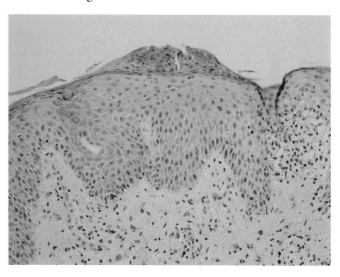

    A. Papular eruption limited to areas bearing apocrine glands
    B. Papulonodular pustular facial eruption
    C. Follicular keratotic papules confined to the extremities
    D. Salmon-pink papulosquamous eruption involving the trunk and extremities
    E. Pruritic follicular eruption involving the proximal extremities

17. Which of the following best describes the horn of pityriasis rosea:
    A. Basket-weave stratum corneum
    B. Scale crust with neutrophils
    C. Mound-like parakeratosis
    D. Absent stratum corneum
    E. Alternating orthokeratosis and parakeratosis

18. Which of the following is correct regarding erythema annulare centrifugum:
    A. Autoimmune etiology
    B. Clinically self-limiting
    C. Diagnostic direct immunofluorescence
    D. Diagnostic histopathology
    E. Diagnostic serology

19. Unifying histopathologic features of irritant contact and allergic contact dermatitis include:
    A. Orthokeratosis and hyperkeratosis
    B. Spongiotic vesiculation
    C. Intraepidermal acantholysis
    D. Pautrier's microabscess
    E. Shoulder parakeratosis

20. Which of the following is correct regarding nummular dermatitis:
    A. Autoimmune etiopathogenesis
    B. Clinical remissions and exacerbations
    C. Diagnostic direct immunofluorescence
    D. Diagnostic histopathology
    E. Diagnostic serology

21. Which of the following best describes the histopathology of nummular dermatitis:
    A. Diagnostic in an early lesion
    B. Diagnostic in an established lesion
    C. Varies with age of the lesion

22. Shoulder parakeratosis is characteristic of:
    A. Nummular dermatitis
    B. Allergic contact dermatitis
    C. Pityriasis rosea
    D. Seborrheic dermatitis
    E. Apocrine miliaria

23. Clinically, lesions of atopic dermatitis are typically seen in:
    A. Sun-exposed areas
    B. Seborrheic areas
    C. Flexural areas
    D. Dorsal hands
    E. Trunk and extremities

24. Histopathologic clues to the diagnosis of seborrheic dermatitis include:
    A. Mound-like parakeratosis
    B. Scale crust with neutrophils
    C. Follicular interface change
    D. Shoulder parakeratosis
    E. Follicular plugging

25. Which of the following histopathologic reaction patterns correctly describes that seen in Giannoti-Crosti syndrome:
    A. Vasculopathic
    B. Psoriasiform
    C. Pityriasiform
    D. Mixed
    E. Vesicobullous

26. The triad of Giannoti-Crosti syndrome includes:
    A. Papular eruption, lymphadenopathy and hepatitis
    B. Vesicobullous eruption, alopecia and a sore throat
    C. Asthma, allergic rhinitis and atopic dermatitis
    D. Cutaneous myxomas, lentigines and endocrine hyperactivity

27. The best-fit diagnosis is:

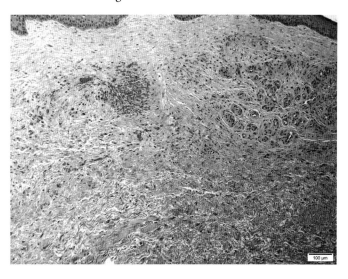

    A. Pigmented purpuric dermatitis
    B. Leukocytoclastic vasculitis
    C. Stasis dermatitis
    D. Senile purpura
    E. Occlusive vasculopathy

28. Histopathologic findings of stasis dermatitis include all of the following EXCEPT:
    A. Neovascularization
    B. Pandermal fibrosis
    C. Thickened vessel walls
    D. Medium vessel vasculitis
    E. Hemosiderin deposits

29. Which of the following best describes the clinical presentation of chronic superficial dermatitis:
    A. Recurrent cyclic urticarial eruption
    B. Well-defined oval patches with a "cigarette-paper" scale
    C. Papular eruption that heals with scarring
    D. Reddish-brown macules with a centrally adherent "mica" scale
    E. Arcuate, polycyclic rash with a trailing "wood grain" scale

30. Which of the following best describes the clinical and histopathologic features of autoimmune progesterone dermatitis:
    A. Urticarial eruption with non-specific histopathology
    B. Maculopapular rash with a pityriasiform reaction pattern
    C. Papular eruption with a pauci-inflammatory subepidermal blister
    D. Reddish-brown macules with a lymphocytic vasculitis
    E. Arcuate, polycyclic rash with a perivascular "coat-sleeve" infiltrate

D2 Spongiotic Reaction Patterns
Answers

Table D2.1 Histopathologic clues based on inflammatory infiltrate

Pattern	Entities	Histopathologic clues	Image
Neutrophilic spongiosis	Pustular psoriasis	Numerous spongiform pustules Psoriasiform epidermal hyperplasia with hypogranulosis and basal keratinocyte atypia Suprapapillary attenuation Papillary dermal telangiectases	
	Prurigo pigmentosa	*Early*: Neutrophilic spongiosis, dyskeratotic keratinocytes at all levels of the epidermis *Established*: acanthosis, variable spongiosis, lymphocyte and neutrophil exocytosis	
	Acute generalized exanthematous pustulosis	Spongiform pustule with an underlying eosinophil-rich inflammatory infiltrate	

Table D2.1 Histopathologic clues based on inflammatory infiltrate (*cont.*)

Pattern	Entities	Histopathologic clues	Image
	IgA pemphigus	Two distinct groups: Subcorneal pustular dermatosis-like group (IgA deposits confined to superficial epidermis) Intraepidermal pustular variant (IgA deposits throughout epidermis)	
Eosinophilic spongiosis	Pemphigus (precursor lesions of vulgaris and foliaceus)	Acantholysis (superficial or suprabasal) with eosinophilic spongiosis	
	Pemphigus vegetans	*Hallopeau type*: Intraepidermal eosinophilic microabscesses, acantholysis	

Table D2.1 Histopathologic clues based on inflammatory infiltrate (*cont.*)

Pattern	Entities	Histopathologic clues	Image
	Bullous pemphigoid	More common in late-stage lesions (in erythematous patches adjacent to bullae)	
	Eosinophilic, polymorphic and pruritic eruption	Variable histopathology, spongiotic vesiculation, superficial and deep dermal infiltrate	
	Allergic contact dermatitis	*Early*: Spongiosis most marked in the lower epidermis *Late*: Spongiotic vesicles at varied horizontal and vertical epidermal levels, superficial dermal infiltrate containing eosinophils *Eosinophil exocytosis characteristic in all stages*	
	Arthropod bite	Eosinophilic spongiosis, superficial and deep perivascular and interstitial eosinophil-rich infiltrate *Focal scale crust with neutrophils and underlying dermal necrosis helpful clues*	

Table D2.1 Histopathologic clues based on inflammatory infiltrate (*cont.*)

Pattern	Entities	Histopathologic clues	Image
	Incontinentia pigmenti	*First stage only*: Eosinophilic spongiosis, superficial dermal infiltrate with eosinophils	
	Vulvar lichen sclerosus	Eosinophilic spongiosis (*portends poor prognostication*), underlying papillary dermal homogenization, lichenoid inflammatory infiltrate	

Table D2.2 Histopathologic clues based on spongiotic pattern/focus and epidermal change

Pattern/ focus	Entity	Histopathologic clues	Image
Miliaria	Miliaria crystallina	Subcorneal vesicle Roof – thin orthokeratotic layer Base – basket-weave keratin	
	Miliaria rubra	Variable spongiosis and spongiotic vesiculation *centered around the acrosyringium*	
	Miliaria profunda	Pronounced papillary dermal edema with subepidermal vesiculation	
Follicular spongiosis	Infundibulofolliculitis	Spongiosis confined to follicular infundibulum with lymphocyte exocytosis, peri-infundibular lymphocytic infiltrate	
	Atopic dermatitis (follicular lesion)	Similar to infundibulofolliculitis	
	Apocrine miliaria	Spongiotic vesiculation of follicular infundibulum (*adjacent to point of entry of apocrine duct*), +/– keratotic plug, perifollicular foam cells	

Table D2.2 Histopathologic clues based on spongiotic pattern/focus and epidermal change (*cont.*)

Pattern/focus	Entity	Histopathologic clues	Image
	Eosinophilic folliculitis	Eosinophilic spongiosis and pustulosis of the infundibular region of the follicle	
Pityriasiform	Pityriasis rosea	*Epidermal*: Patchy parakeratosis in "mounds," diminution of the granular layer, patchy spongiosis (*only* in "herald patch"), Pautrier-like microabscesses (at all layers of the epidermis), individually necrotic, dyskeratotic keratinocytes *Dermal*: Mild papillary dermal edema, mild superficial perivascular lymphocytic infiltrate with occasional eosinophils, red blood cell extravasation	
	Pityriasiform drug reaction	Similar to pityriasis rosea	
	Erythema annulare centrifugum	Well-demarcated, dense perivascular lymphohistiocytic cuffing ("coat-sleeve" distribution) *No epidermal changes*	

Table D2.2 Histopathologic clues based on spongiotic pattern/focus and epidermal change (*cont.*)

Pattern/ focus	Entity	Histopathologic clues	Image
Acute	Irritant contact dermatitis	Superficial ballooning with spongiotic vesiculation, individually necrotic, dyskeratotic keratinocytes	
	Allergic contact dermatitis	Variable spongiosis, spongiotic vesiculation, at different levels of the epidermis, +/− eosinophil exocytosis, a superficial dermal infiltrate with scattered eosinophils	
	Nummular dermatitis	*Vary with age of lesion* "Untidy" appearance (scanning magnification) *Early lesions*: Epidermal hyperplasia with variable spongiosis, spongiotic vesiculation (spongiotic vesicles contain lymphocytes mimicking Pautrier-like microabscesses), lymphocyte and neutrophil exocytosis *Late lesions*: Psoriasiform epidermal hyperplasia, superficial	

Table D2.2 Histopathologic clues based on spongiotic pattern/focus and epidermal change (*cont.*)

Pattern/focus	Entity	Histopathologic clues	Image
	Seborrheic dermatitis	perivascular infiltrate composed of lymphocytes predominantly with admixed neutrophils *Vary with age of lesion* *Acute*: Follicle-centered scale crust, "shoulder" parakeratosis, epidermal hyperplasia with mild spongiosis, a mild superficial perivascular lymphoid infiltrate with occasional neutrophils, papillary dermal edema and telangiectases *Subacute*: Psoriasiform epidermal hyperplasia plus changes seen in an acute lesion *Chronic*: More pronounced psoriasiform epidermal hyperplasia and variable spongiosis	
Subacute	Atopic dermatitis	*Vary with age of lesion* *Acute lesions*: Spongiotic vesiculation, mild superficial perivascular lymphocytic infiltrate, mast cells *Subacute lesions*: Irregular to psoriasiform epidermal hyperplasia, mild to minimal spongiosis *Chronic lesions*: Hyperkeratosis, psoriasiform epidermal hyperplasia, minimal spongiosis, mild superficial perivascular lymphocytic infiltrate with admixed mast cells and eosinophils, increased superficial small blood vessels	

Table D2.2 Histopathologic clues based on spongiotic pattern/focus and epidermal change (*cont.*)

Pattern/ focus	Entity	Histopathologic clues	Image
		with thickened vessel walls, increased Langerhans cells in the epidermis and dermis, vertical "streaking" of collagen in the papillary dermis	
	Papular dermatitis	Patchy parakeratosis, variable spongiosis, superficial and deep, perivascular, eosinophil-rich infiltrate	
	Pompholyx/ dyshidrotic eczema/ acral vesicular dermatitis	Spongiosis of the lower malphigian layer with spongiotic vesiculation, thick stratum corneum (site-related)	
	Hyperkeratotic dermatitis of the palms	Irregular to psoriasiform epidermal hyperplasia, mild spongiosis, mild superficial perivascular lymphocytic infiltrate	
Chronic	Chronic superficial dermatitis/small plaque parapsoriasis	*Entirely non-specific* Subtle, focal spongiosis, focal parakeratosis, mild epidermal hyperplasia with focal lymphocyte exocytosis, mild superficial perivascular lymphohistiocytic infiltrate	

Table D2.3 Skin disorders commonly associated with a monoclonal gammopathy

Association	Entities	Cutaneous clues
Direct correlation	Cutaneous plasmacytoma	Circumscribed, plasma-cell rich dermal infiltrate CD79a, CD117, CD138 positivity in lesional cells
	Hyperviscosity syndrome	None
	Cryoglobulinemia	Type I – Occlusive vasculopathy (fibrin thrombi) Types II/III – Leukocytoclastic vasculitis (fibrinoid necrosis of vessel walls, leukocytoclasia)
	Amyloidosis	Localized cutaneous – Amorphous eosinophilic deposits, HMW keratin positivity in deposits Nodular – Amorphous, eosinophilic interstitial masses, admixed plasma cells
	POEMS syndrome	Glomeruloid hemangioma, M-protein, hypertrichosis, hyperpigmentation, sclerodermoid changes
High association	Scleromyexedema/lichen myxedematosus/papular mucinosis	Variable mucin deposition, interstitial fibroblast proliferation, IgGλ paraproteinemia
	Scleredema	Splaying of thickened collagen bundles by interstitial mucin
	Plane xanthomas	Xanthomatized histiocytes
	Necrobiotic xanthogranuloma	Broad zones of necrobiosis alternating with granulomatous foci, IgG paraproteinemia (IgM may be seen in Waldenström's macroglobulinemia)
	Schnitzler syndrome	Chronic, non-pruritic urticaria, IgM monoclonal gammopathy Approximately 10–15% of patients eventually develop a lymphoproliferative disorder (lymphoplasmacytic lymphoma, Waldenström's macroglobulinemia, or IgM myeloma)
	Erythema elevatum diutinum	Associated with hyper-IgD syndrome, IgA monoclonal gammopathy *Histopathology varies with age* *Early lesion*: Vasculitis, extravasated erythrocytes, reactive endothelial cell atypia *Late lesion*: Fibrosis, "dermatofibroma-like" with admixed foci of neutrophilic vasculitis
	Subcorneal pustular dermatosis	Subcorneal pustule, IgA monoclonal gammopathy

1. **A.** Of entities listed, neutrophilic spongiosis, shown in the image, is seen only in IgA pemphigus.

   Of the other entities, three (allergic contact dermatitis, bullous pemphigoid and incontinentia pigmenti, first stage) are characterized by eosinophilic spongiosis. Erythema annulare centrifugum is primarily a dermal process and epidermal changes are typically pityriasiform and include focal parakeratosis.

   IgA pemphigus is an autoimmune, intraepidermal, vesicobullous eruption with variable acantholysis and intercellular IgA deposits. IgA pemphigus is a clinically heterogeneous condition reflective of the antigenic diversity of the autoantigens. Two distinct groups are recognized: a subcorneal pustular dermatosis-like group in which IgA deposits are confined to the superficial epidermis and an intraepidermal pustular variant in which IgA deposits are distributed throughout the epidermis.

2. **C.** Of entities listed, eosinophilic spongiosis, shown in the image, is seen only in incontinentia pigmenti, first stage.

   Histopathologic findings in incontinentia pigmenti *vary with the stage* of the disease.

First stage: Eosinophilic spongiosis with prominent eosinophil exocytosis, occasional individually necrotic dyskeratotic keratinocytes and a superficial eosinophil-rich inflammatory infiltrate

Verrucous stage: Hyperkeratosis, verrucous epidermal hyperplasia, numerous individually necrotic dyskeratotic keratinocytes and a sparse inflammatory infiltrate

Third stage: Decreased density of basal melanocytes, prominent pigment incontinence in the superficial dermis

3. **B.** Precursor lesions of pemphigus foliaceus demonstrate eosinophilic spongiosis.

   Eosinophilic spongiosis may occur in the preacantholytic stage of pemphigus foliaceus as well as pemphigus vulgaris. Despite the absence of acantholysis, direct immunofluorescence of precursor lesions in both these entities is typically positive.

4. **A.** The diagnosis of acute generalized exanthematous pustulosis (AGEP) is based on clinical presentation and histopathology.

   Diagnosis of AGEP depends on clinical and histologic criteria. An AGEP validation score has been developed by the EuroSCAR (*severe cutaneous adverse reactions*) group. It is a standardized scheme based on morphology, clinical course, and histology that classifies patients with suspected AGEP as having definite, probable, possible, or no AGEP.

Histopathologic features of AGEP include intracorneal, subcorneal, and/or intraepidermal pustules with papillary dermal edema containing neutrophils and eosinophils. The majority of intraepidermal pustules are located in the upper epidermis, often contiguous with the subcorneal pustules. The pustules tend to be large and contain eosinophils. Spongiform changes occur in both the intracorneal and subcorneal pustules. Epidermal changes also include spongiosis with exocytosis of neutrophils and scattered individually necrotic, dyskeratotic keratinocytes.

5. E. Acute generalized exanthematous pustulosis (AGEP) is a rapidly evolving pustular dermatosis in which sterile pustules develop on an erythematous background.

The mucocutaneous features of AGEP include tens to hundreds of small, sterile, non-follicular pustules on an erythematous base with no or minimal mucous membrane involvement (if there is mucous membrane involvement, it is usually confined to a single site, most often the lips or buccal mucosa). The pustules are distributed on the trunk and intertriginous regions. AGEP is typically pruritic. Leukocytosis with an elevated neutrophil count and fever are features of AGEP. Internal organ involvement can be seen in <20% of patients. Hepatic, renal, and pulmonary dysfunction are the most common features in patients with systemic involvement. Elevated absolute neutrophil count and C-reactive protein levels are typically associated with systemic organ involvement. Upon discontinuation of the causative agent, resolution of the cutaneous features typically occurs within a few days. During resolution of AGEP, there is desquamation over the affected area. Mortality is less than 5% in AGEP.

6. A. Circulating IgA antibodies are present in 50% of cases of IgA pemphigus.

IgA pemphigus is an autoimmune, intraepidermal, vesicobullous eruption with variable acantholysis and intercellular IgA deposits. IgA pemphigus is a clinically heterogeneous condition reflective of the antigenic diversity of the autoantigens. Two distinct groups are recognized: a subcorneal pustular dermatosis-like group in which IgA deposits are confined to the superficial epidermis and an intraepidermal pustular variant in which IgA deposits are distributed throughout the epidermis. A monoclonal IgA gammopathy is present in only 20% of cases. Other entities commonly associated with a monoclonal gammopathy are enumerated in Table D2.3.

7. A. Pemphigus vegetans is a variant of pemphigus vulgaris NOT pemphigus foliaceus.

Pemphigus vegetans differs from pemphigus vulgaris by its clinical manifestations of vegetating erosions involving flexural surfaces primarily. Two clinical variants of pemphigus vegetans are recognized: *Neumann type* which presents with vegetating plaques clinically and intraepidermal vesicles with acantholysis but not eosinophilic microabscesses and the *Hallopeau type* which presents with pustular lesions clinically and intraepidermal eosinophilic microabscesses histopathologically. The clinical course of the latter (*Hallopeau type*) is benign in contrast with that of the former (*Neumann type*). Direct IF findings of pemphigus vegetans are similar to those of pemphigus vulgaris with intercellular deposits of IgG and C3, and serology is usually positive for the detection of circulating antibodies. Antibodies to dsg3 have been detected in both types, in keeping with them representing variants of pemphigus vulgaris.

8. A. Target antigens in bullous pemphigoid (BP) include BP230 (BPAg1) and BP180 (BPAg2).

Male patients are more likely to have antibodies to BP180, whereas antibodies to BP230 occur with equal frequency amongst males and females. BP230 is a member of the plakin family of proteins and is restricted to the intracellular hemidesmosomal plaque. BP230 antibodies precipitate and perpetuate disease. Autoantibodies to a complex of BP230 and BP180 are present in up to 80% of patients with BP. Antibodies to BP180 are more often associated with oral lesions, have a poor prognosis with less responsiveness to steroids and serum antibody levels correlate with disease activity. The major antigenic epitopes of the BP230 protein map to the C-terminal end (not the N-terminal end). While autoantibodies to BP230 and BP180 can be seen in normal healthy adults, they do not bind to the NC16A domain (the target antigen in most commercially available ELISA kits).

9. A. In early stages of bullous pemphigoid (BP), only C3 may be seen deposited linearly in direct immunofluorescence.

Direct immunofluorescence (DIF) typically shows a linear deposition of IgG and C3 along the basement membrane zone in established lesions of BP. IgG4 is the predominant subclass of IgG in prodromal lesions. IgM and IgA are present in up to 20% of cases. Some cases with IgA have oral lesions.

10. A. Circulating anti-basement zone antibodies of the IgG subclass are present in 60–80% of patients with bullous pemphigoid.

There is no correlation between antibody titers and disease activity. Antibodies are typically absent in the presence of circulating immune complexes.

11. **C.** Incontinentia pigmenti is an X-linked genodermatosis involving multiple organ systems.

    Incontinentia pigmenti (IP) or Bloch-Sulzberger syndrome is an X-linked dominant genodermatosis characterized by abnormalities of tissues and organs derived from the ectoderm and neuroectoderm. It essentially represents a type of ectodermal dysplasia. Involvement of the skin, hair, teeth, and nails is seen in conjunction with neurologic and ophthalmologic anomalies. In female IP patients, lyonization results in functional mosaicism of X-linked genes, which is manifested by the blaschkoid distribution of cutaneous lesions. Late-onset incontinentia pigmenti is occasionally reported in older infants. Neurologic and ophthalmologic sequelae often manifest during early infancy.

12. **B.** Cutaneous manifestations in incontinentia pigmenti evolve through vesiculobullous, verrucous and pigmentary stages.

    Characteristic skin lesions compatible with the early, vesicular and/or verrucous stages of incontinentia pigmenti are present at birth or develop in the first few weeks of life in approximately 90% of patients. The cutaneous manifestations of the hyperpigmented stage develop during infancy and persist during childhood. The hyperpigmented lesions usually fade during adolescence. The cutaneous manifestations of the atrophic/hypopigmented stage develop during adolescence and early adulthood and persist indefinitely. Hair, nail, and dental anomalies often first manifest during infancy and are permanent.

13. **E.** The first stage of incontinentia pigmenti is histopathologically characterized by eosinophilic exocytosis.

    Other findings seen in the early/first stage include eosinophilic spongiosis with prominent eosinophil exocytosis, occasional individually necrotic dyskeratotic keratinocytes and a superficial eosinophil-rich inflammatory infiltrate.

14. **C.** The most likely diagnosis for the image shown is that of Fox-Fordyce disease.

    Fox-Fordyce disease is an infrequently occurring chronic pruritic papular eruption that localizes to areas where apocrine glands are found. The etiology of Fox-Fordyce disease currently is unknown. Fox-Fordyce disease is a disease of the skin alone, with some proposing apocrine miliaria as the cause. Clinically, it presents as dome-shaped discrete follicular papules in the axilla, anogenital and periareolar areas. A paucity of hair in the affected areas is typically observed and intense pruritus is common. The observed pathophysiology is a keratin plug in the hair follicle infundibulum obstructing the apocrine

acrosyringium and producing apocrine anhidrosis. Rupture of the apocrine excretory duct results in spongiotic inflammation. Extravasation of sweat and inflammation is postulated to cause the intense itching.

15. **A.** The clinical correlate of Fox-Fordyce disease is a chronic papular eruption limited to areas bearing apocrine glands.

    Clinically, it presents as dome-shaped discrete follicular papules in the axilla, anogenital and periareolar areas. A paucity of hair in the affected areas is typically observed and intense pruritus is common.

16. **D.** Image shown is that of pityriasis rosea (PR), which clinically presents as a salmon-pink papulosquamous eruption involving the trunk and the extremities.

    PR manifests as an acute, self-limiting, papulosquamous eruption with duration of 6–8 weeks. It evolves rapidly, usually beginning with a patch that heralds the eruption, the so-called "herald patch." PR-like eruptions can also occur in association with many drugs (e.g., acetylsalicylic acid, barbiturates, bismuth, captopril, clonidine, gold, imatinib, isotretinoin, ketotifen, levamisole, metronidazole, omeprazole, D-penicillamine, and terbinafine), as well as certain vaccines (e.g., bacille Calmette-Guérin (BCG), human papilloma virus, and diphtheria). Anti-tumor necrosis factor (TNF)-α agents such as adalimumab and etanercept have also been implicated. PR-like drug eruptions have been reported to be related to use of rituximab, nortriptyline, and clozapine. While PR-like drug eruptions may be difficult to distinguish from non-drug-induced cases on a histopathologic basis alone, clinically, drug-induced PR often lasts longer than non-drug-induced PR. Lesions are also thought to be increased in individuals with high stress levels. PR is very common in the general population, and most cases occur in the spring and winter in temperate climates.

17. **C.** The horn of pityriasis rosea is characterized by "mound-like" parakeratosis.

    Although not pathognomonic, the histopathology of PR is sufficiently characteristic to allow for a diagnosis to be rendered even in the absence of a clinical history. Briefly, these include:

    Epidermal changes: Vaguely undulating epidermis with patchy parakeratosis in "mounds," diminution of the granular layer, patchy spongiosis (especially in the "herald patch"), Pautrier-like microabscesses (at all layers of the epidermis) and individually necrotic, dyskeratotic keratinocytes

    Dermal changes: Mild papillary dermal edema, mild superficial perivascular lymphocytic infiltrate with occasional eosinophils and red blood cell extravasation

18. **B.** Erythema annulare centrifugum is clinically self-limiting.

    Erythema annulare centrifugum (EAC) is classified as one of the figurate or gyrate erythemas and is characterized by a scaling or non-scaling, non-pruritic, annular or arcuate, erythematous eruption that tends to spread peripherally while clearing centrally. The prognosis for EAC is excellent, except when associated with an underlying malignancy and other systemic disease. The mean duration of erythema annulare centrifugum is 11 months. Most cases require no treatment and resolve spontaneously. Others have been reported in association with malignancy, with the eruptions responding to treatment of the underlying neoplasm. The etiology is uncertain, but it may be due to a hypersensitivity to malignancy, infection, drugs, or chemicals, or it may be idiopathic.

    Histopathologically, a dense, well-demarcated lymphohistiocytic cuffing occurs about the superficial and deep dermal vessels ("coat-sleeve" distribution) without epidermal involvement.

    Controversy exists in the classification of the gyrate erythemas, and the literature is wrought with ambiguity and contradictions. Since its initial description, the term erythema annulare centrifugum has grown to include several histologic and clinical variants. Ackerman, and later Bressler and Jones, suggested a classification in which only 2 types of gyrate erythema are considered: superficial (pruritic, scaling) and deep (non-pruritic, non-scaling). The original description of EAC was of the latter type. However, the superficial type is more commonly seen with its characteristic trailing scale behind an advancing, erythematous border. The pathogenesis of EAC is unknown, but it is probably due to a hypersensitivity reaction to a variety of agents, including drugs, arthropod bites, infections (bacterial, mycobacterial, viral, fungal, filarial), ingestion (blue cheese *Penicillium*), and malignancy.

19. **B.** Spongiotic vesiculation is common to both irritant contact and allergic contact dermatitis.

    Both entities fall under the acute spongiotic dermatitis reaction pattern (Table D2.2). Helpful differentiating features include the presence of individually necrotic dyskeratotic keratinocytes in irritant contact dermatitis and an eosinophil-rich superficial dermal infiltrate with occasional eosinophilic exocytosis in allergic contact dermatitis.

20. **B.** Nummular dermatitis is characterized clinically by remissions and exacerbations.

    Nummular dermatitis is a chronic, pruritic inflammatory dermatitis that clinically presents as coin-shaped plaques composed of grouped small papules and vesicles on an erythematous base. It is particularly common on the lower extremities of older males in the winter months. There is a predisposition in individuals with a history of atopy. The etiopathogenesis is unknown. Histopathology is non-diagnostic and serology and direct immunofluorescence non-contributory.

21. **C.** Histopathologic features of nummular dermatitis vary with age of the lesion.

    At scanning magnification, nummular dermatitis has an "untidy" appearance (see Table D2.2).
    Early lesion: Epidermal hyperplasia with variable spongiosis, spongiotic vesiculation (spongiotic vesicles contain lymphocytes mimicking Pautrier-like microabscesses) and lymphocyte and neutrophil exocytosis
    Established/late lesion: Psoriasiform epidermal hyperplasia, superficial perivascular infiltrate composed of lymphocytes predominantly with admixed neutrophils

22. **D.** Shoulder parakeratosis is characteristic of seborrheic dermatitis.

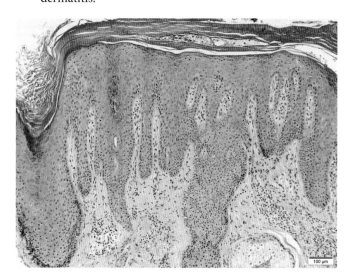

Other patterns of parakeratosis useful as a clue to the underlying disease include the following:
"Mound-like" parakeratosis – Pityriasis rosea, pityriasiform drug reaction
Parakeratosis with neutrophils but no serum – Psoriasis, psoriasiform drug reaction
Parakeratosis with neutrophils and serum – Fungal infection
Parakeratosis in tiers – Porokeratosis, palmoplantar psoriasis
"Capped" parakeratosis – Verruca vulgaris
Horizontally oriented alternating parakeratosis and orthokeratosis – Actinic keratosis, ILVEN
Horizontally and vertically oriented alternating parakeratosis and orthokeratosis – Pityriasis rubra pilaris

Parakeratosis with overlying orthokeratosis – Resolving dermatosis, NOS

"Thick" parakeratosis – Glucagonoma, deficiency states, granular parakeratosis, pityriasis lichenoides

23. **C. Lesions of atopic dermatitis are typically seen in flexural areas.**

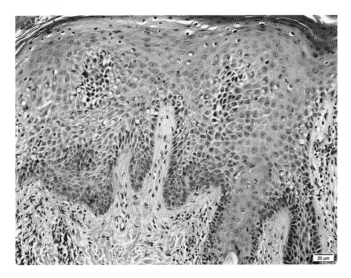

Atopic dermatitis (AD) is a chronic, pruritic inflammatory skin disease of unknown origin that usually starts in early infancy, but also affects a substantial number of adults. AD is commonly associated with elevated levels of immunoglobulin E (IgE). That it is the first disease to present in a series of allergic diseases – including food allergy, asthma, and allergic rhinitis, in order – has given rise to the "atopic march" theory, which suggests that AD is part of a progression that may lead to subsequent allergic disease at other epithelial barrier surfaces.

Incessant pruritus is the central and most debilitating symptom of atopic dermatitis; children often scratch themselves uncontrollably. The disease typically has an intermittent course with flares and remissions occurring, often for unexplained reasons. AD patients often present with a personal or family history of type I hypersensitivity, allergic rhinitis, and asthma. Essential historical features (must be present) are pruritus and a chronic or relapsing history of disease. Important historical features (supports the diagnosis) are early age of onset and atopy, i.e. a personal and/or family history.

Histopathologic features of AD vary with stage of the disease and include:

Acute lesion: Spongiotic vesiculation, mild superficial perivascular lymphocytic infiltrate, mast cells

Subacute lesion: Irregular to psoriasiform epidermal hyperplasia

Chronic lesion: Hyperkeratosis, psoriasiform epidermal hyperplasia with mild to minimal spongiosis and Langerhans cell microabscesses, mild superficial perivascular lymphocytic infiltrate with admixed mast cells and eosinophils, increased number of superficial small blood vessels with thickened vessel walls and vertical streaking of collagen in the papillary dermis

24. **D. Shoulder parakeratosis is a histopathologic clue to a diagnosis of seborrheic dermatitis.**

Histopathologic features of seborrheic dermatitis vary with age of the lesion and to varying degrees involve both the epidermis and dermis.

Epidermal: Shoulder parakeratosis, mild epidermal hyperplasia with spongiosis

Dermal: A mild superficial perivascular infiltrate with occasional neutrophils

Acute lesion: Scale crust centered around the follicle, papillary dermal edema and telangiectases and a mild superficial perivascular lymphoid infiltrate with occasional neutrophils

Subacute lesion: Psoriasiform epidermal hyperplasia plus changes seen in an acute lesion

Chronic lesion: More pronounced psoriasiform epidermal hyperplasia, minimal spongiosis

AIDS-related seborrheic dermatitis: Individually necrotic, dyskeratotic keratinocytes plus changes observed in an acute lesion

25. **D. A mixed histopathologic reaction is typical of Giannoti-Crosti syndrome (GCS).**

Although not diagnostically specific, histopathologic features of GCS are sufficiently characteristic to allow for a diagnosis.

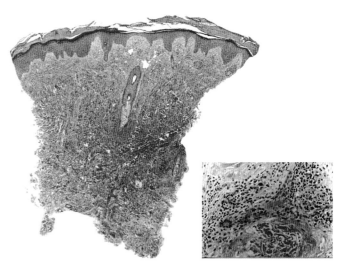

At scanning magnification, three distinct patterns – lichenoid, spongiotic and vasculitic – *are present at the same time*. Other features include prominent exocytosis of mononuclear cells, interface change and a perivascular inflammatory infiltrate that extends up to the mid dermis. The absence of fibrinoid necrosis of vessel walls has led some to conclude that the vasculitis is a lymphocytic vasculitis.

26. **A.** The triad of Giannoti-Crosti syndrome includes a papular eruption, lymphadenopathy and hepatitis.

    Gianotti-Crosti syndrome (GCS) is a distinct infectious exanthem with associated lymphadenopathy and acute anicteric hepatitis. Gianotti and Crosti described GCS as associated with a hepatitis B virus exanthem, which they initially termed papular acrodermatitis of childhood. A similar constellation of characteristics was later found to be associated with several infectious agents and immunizations that were called papulovesicular acrolocated syndromes. Subsequent retrospective studies have shown that these 2 entities are indistinguishable from one another, and they are now consolidated under the unifying title of GCS. The rash is usually present for 2–4 weeks but can last as long as 4 months.

27. **C.** The best-fit diagnosis for the image shown is stasis dermatitis.

    Histopathologic features of stasis dermatitis are essentially confined to the dermis and include *from top to bottom*:
    - Superficial neovascularization
    - Variable pandermal fibrosis (which increases with chronicity of the disease)
    - Interstitial pandermal deposits of hemosiderin
    - Thick-walled vessels in the deep dermis and subcutis

28. **D.** Medium vessel vasculitis is NOT a histopathologic feature of stasis dermatitis.

    Entities characterized under the umbrella medium vessel vasculitis include:
    - Polyarteritis nodosa
    - Kawasaki disease

    Features typically seen in stasis dermatitis are listed above in answer to question 27.

29. **B.** Chronic superficial dermatitis typically presents clinically as well-defined oval patches with a cigarette-paper scale.

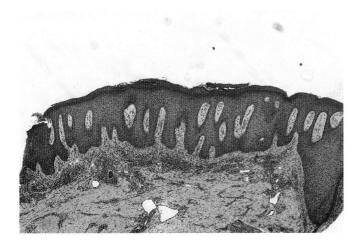

Other names for chronic superficial dermatitis include small plaque parapsoriasis or digitate dermatosis. Current terminology of parapsoriasis refers to 2 disease processes that are caused by T-cell-predominant infiltrates in the skin. These disease processes are large plaque parapsoriasis and small plaque parapsoriasis. As the nomenclature and description of the disease spectrum under the descriptive term parapsoriasis evolved, the primary focus has been on the distinction of whether the disorder progresses to mycosis fungoides (MF) or cutaneous T-cell lymphoma (CTCL).

Small plaque parapsoriasis is a benign disorder that rarely if ever progresses.

Large plaque parapsoriasis is more ominous in that approximately 10% of patients progress to MF/CTCL. Controversy exists currently in the classification of large plaque parapsoriasis because some believe it is equivalent to the earliest stage CTCL, the patch stage. The duration of parapsoriasis can be variable. Small plaque disease lasts several months to years and can spontaneously resolve.

Histopathologic features of small plaque parapsoriasis, shown above, *are entirely non-specific* and include:
- Subtle, focal spongiosis
- Focal parakeratosis
- Mild epidermal hyperplasia with focal lymphocyte exocytosis
- Mild superficial perivascular lymphohistiocytic infiltrate

30. **A.** Autoimmune progesterone dermatitis clinically presents as a cyclical urticarial eruption with non-specific histopathology.

    The condition presents with a variety of skin eruptions characterized by recurrent cyclical premenstrual exacerbation secondary to progesterone fluctuations during a woman's menstrual cycle. Skin eruptions include urticaria, erythema multiforme, eczema, and papulovesicular eruptions. These eruptions typically occur 5 to 8 days prior to menses and subside at the start of menarche.

    Histopathologic features vary from a non-specific picture to one that mimics specific dermatosis such as erythema multiforme or urticaria.

D3 Vesicobullous Diseases
Questions

1. Which of the following is NOT an adhesion molecule:
   A. Cadherin
   B. Plakoglobulin
   C. Integrin
   D. Desmoglein
   E. Selectin

2. Impetigo:
   A. Is caused by *Staphylococcus aureus*
   B. Results from production of an epidermolytic toxin by *Staphylococcus aureus*
   C. Occurs predominantly in immunocompromised adults
   D. Histopathologic features of an early lesion include a subepidermal blister

3. Staphylococcal scaled skin syndrome:
   A. Affects immunocompromised children
   B. Affects healthy infants
   C. Has an adverse prognosis
   D. Histopathologic features include a subepidermal pustule

4. Pemphigus foliaceus:
   A. Is associated with vancomycin use
   B. Is associated with autoantibodies of the IgG4 subclass
   C. Is associated with antibodies to dsg3
   D. Is characterized by a subepidermal blister containing neutrophils
   E. Is associated with linear IgG and C3 in DIF

5. Which of the following is correct regarding the image shown:

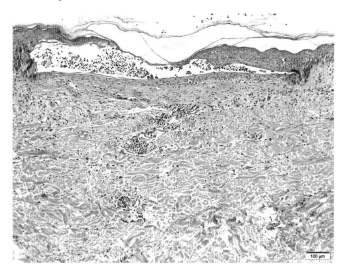

   A. Is a congenital relapsing vesicopustular genodermatosis
   B. Exhibits a predilection for the intertriginous areas
   C. Is an autoimmune-mediated dermatosis
   D. Is associated with diagnostic DIF
   E. Is associated with antibodies to dsg1

6. IgA pemphigus:
   A. Is clinically homogeneous
   B. Is a subepidermal acantholytic, vesicobullous eruption
   C. Is associated with circulating IgA antibodies

   D. Is typically associated with an IgA monoclonal gammopathy
   E. Direct immunofluorescence demonstrates linear, granular IgA

7. Which of the following best describes acute generalized exanthematous pustular dermatosis (AGEP):
   A. Is a chronic, relapsing vesicopustular dermatosis
   B. Is associated specifically with paracetamol use
   C. Is a rapidly evolving, pustular dermatosis
   D. Is a variant of pemphigus foliaceus

8. Which of the following is correct regarding the image shown:

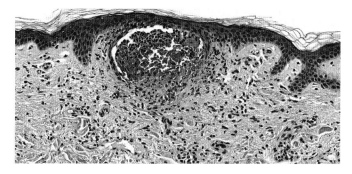

   A. Results from superficial obstruction in the stratum corneum
   B. Is caused by infection with *Staphylococcus epidermidis*
   C. Occurs in the setting of immunocompromise
   D. Is commonly associated with atopic dermatitis
   E. Is associated with diagnostic direct immunofluorescence

9. Regarding the image shown:

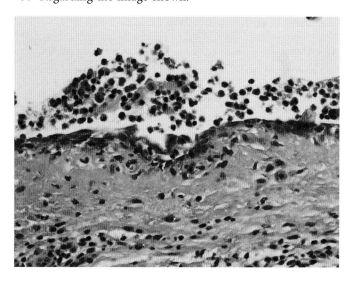

   A. Is associated with a monoclonal gammopathy
   B. Is associated with antibodies to dsg3

C. Serology is non-diagnostic
D. Direct immunofluorescence is non-diagnostic
E. Is associated with IgA antibodies in active disease

10. Pemphigus vegetans:
   A. Is a variant of pemphigus vulgaris
   B. Is characterized by antibodies to dsg1
   C. Is clinically homogeneous
   D. Is associated with superficial acantholysis
   E. Is associated with non-diagnostic serology

11. Paraneoplastic pemphigus:
   A. Has a monomorphous clinical presentation
   B. Is associated with antibodies to plectin
   C. Is associated with non-diagnostic histopathology
   D. Is associated with non-diagnostic direct immunofluorescence

12. Hailey-Hailey disease:
   A. Clinically presents with tense bullae on sun-exposed areas
   B. Is autosomal dominant
   C. Is associated with *PTEN* mutations
   D. Exhibits non-diagnostic histopathology
   E. Is associated with diagnostic direct immunofluorescence

13. Darier's disease:
   A. Is autosomal recessive
   B. Has a "seborrheic" distribution
   C. Has a predilection for intertriginous areas
   D. Is associated with non-diagnostic histopathology
   E. Is associated with diagnostic direct immunofluorescence

14. Grover's disease:
   A. Has a predilection for intertriginous areas
   B. Is not associated with *ATP2A2* mutations
   C. Is associated with superficial acantholysis
   D. Is associated with a plasma cell-rich dermal infiltrate

15. Epidermolysis bullosa (EB):
   A. Is typically acquired
   B. Is clinically homogeneous
   C. Is not associated with trauma-induced blisters
   D. Is associated with non-diagnostic serology
   E. Is associated with non-diagnostic ultrastructural findings

16. Epidermolysis bullosa acquisita:
   A. Is not associated with trauma-induced blisters
   B. Is typically acquired
   C. Is not associated with mucous membrane involvement
   D. Is associated with non-diagnostic serology
   E. Is associated with diagnostic histopathology

17. Which of the following would NOT be expected to demonstrate the histopathologic reaction pattern shown:

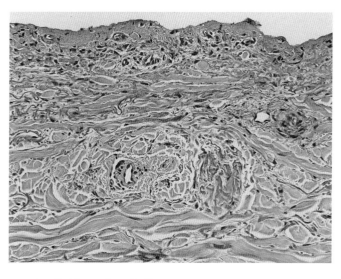

   A. Epidermolysis bullosa
   B. Paraneoplastic pemphigus
   C. Porphyria cutanea tarda
   D. Kindler's syndrome
   E. Bullous solar elastosis

18. Porphyria cutanea tarda is due to:
   A. Reduced activity of aminolevulinic acid (ALA)-synthase
   B. Reduced activity of ALA-dehydratase
   C. Reduced activity of porphobilinogen deaminase
   D. Reduced activity of uroporphyrinogen III cosynthase
   E. Reduced activity of uroporphyrinogen decarboxylase

19. The entity shown in this image:

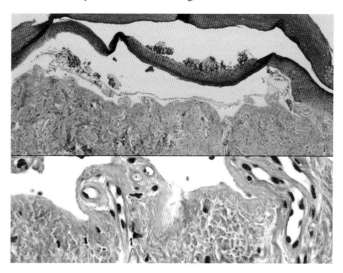

   A. Is associated with hepatic porphyrin underproduction
   B. Is associated with HIV infection
   C. Clinically presents predominantly in sun-protected areas

D. Is associated with PAS+ "caterpillar bodies"

E. Is associated with diagnostic serology

20. Ultrastructural features of porphyria cutanea tarda include:
    A. Oval/round juxtanuclear inclusions
    B. Intracytoplasmic Farber bodies
    C. Reduplication of the basal laminae
    D. Vacuolation of fibroblasts
    E. Intranuclear Zebra bodies

21. In bullous pemphigoid:
    A. Target antigens map within the N-terminal end
    B. Target antigens include BP230 (BPAg1) and BP180 (BPAg2)
    C. Serologic antibodies are clinically irrelevant
    D. Anti-BP180 antibodies are more common in female patients

22. Which of the following would NOT demonstrate the histopathologic reaction pattern shown:

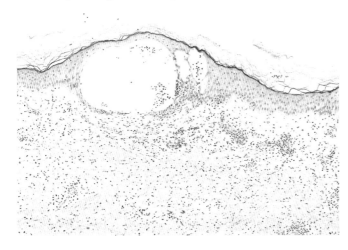

    A. Arthropod bite reaction
    B. Bullous pemphigoid
    C. Bullous lupus erythematosus
    D. Incontinentia pigmenti
    E. Ofuji's disease

23. Regarding direct immunofluorescence findings in bullous pemphigoid:
    A. In early stages of the disease only linear C3 is present
    B. In established lesions only linear IgG is noted
    C. IgG1 is the predominant subclass of IgG detected
    D. IgM and IgA may be seen in up to 80% of cases

24. Regarding indirect immunofluorescence findings in bullous pemphigoid:
    A. Circulating anti-BMZ antibodies are noted in a proportion of patients
    B. Antibody titers correlate with disease activity

C. Circulating antibodies may be detected in the presence of circulating immune complexes

25. Pemphigoid gestationis:
    A. Typically occurs in the first trimester of pregnancy
    B. Does not recur in subsequent pregnancies
    C. Autoantibodies target the BP180 antigen
    D. Is associated with specific histopathology
    E. Is associated with non-specific serology

26. Which of the following circulating antibodies is diagnostic of dermatitis herpetiformis:
    A. Anti-reticulin
    B. Anti-gliadin
    C. Anti-endomysial
    D. Anti-thyroid
    E. Anti-nuclear

27. Dermatitis herpetiformis:
    A. Exhibits a predilection for sun-exposed areas
    B. Is associated with a gluten-sensitive enteropathy in 10% of cases
    C. Typically occurs in adults
    D. Is associated with an IgA monoclonal gammopathy in 50% of cases
    E. Is associated with non-diagnostic serology

28. Early lesions of dermatitis herpetiformis may be characterized by all of the following EXCEPT:
    A. Acantholysis
    B. Eosinophils
    C. Vasculitis
    D. Fibrin deposits
    E. Neutrophils

29. Anti-endomysial antibodies in dermatitis herpetiformis are typically of which class of immunoglobulins:
    A. IgA
    B. IgE
    C. IgG1
    D. IgG2
    E. IgG4

30. Linear IgA bullous dermatosis:
    A. Is sulfone resistant
    B. Is clinically homogeneous
    C. Is associated with antibodies targeting a 97 kDa antigen
    D. Is an intraepidermal blistering process
    E. Is characterized by an eosinophil-rich inflammatory infiltrate

31. Target antigen/s in linear IgA bullous dermatosis:
    A. Are not selectively restricted to the basement membrane zone

B. Include plectin
C. Include BP230, in vancomycin-induced disease
D. Are degradation products of desmocollin

32. Distinguishing histopathologic findings between linear IgA bullous dermatosis (LABD) and dermatitis herpetiformis (DH) include:
    A. Plane of cleavage
    B. Predominance of neutrophils in the inflammatory infiltrate in LABD
    C. Localization of neutrophils in the dermal papillae in DH
    D. Fibrin deposits in dermal papillae in DH
    E. None of the above

33. Regarding direct immunofluorescence findings in linear IgA bullous dermatosis (LABD):
    A. IgA is the only immunoreactant
    B. Linear deposition of IgA is a non-specific finding
    C. IgA deposits are exclusively IgA1

34. Mucous membrane pemphigoid:
    A. Occurs predominantly in children
    B. Is clinically a homogeneous entity
    C. Cutaneous involvement typically precedes mucosal involvement

35. Which of the following is NOT a target antigen in mucous membrane pemphigoid:
    A. BP180
    B. BP230
    C. Type VII collagen
    D. Dsg1
    E. Laminin 5

36. Histopathologic features of mucous membrane pemphigoid include:
    A. Subepidermal blister
    B. Pautrier microabscesses (early lesions)
    C. Neutrophil-rich infiltrate (older lesions)
    D. Scarring (older lesions alone)
    E. Naked hair shafts within the blister

37. In localized cicatricial pemphigoid:
    A. Scarring of intertriginous areas is typical
    B. Mucous membrane involvement is uncommon
    C. Plane of clefting is intraepidermal
    D. Histopathology does not vary with age of the lesion
    E. Basal lamina and anchoring fibrils are fragmented ultrastructurally

38. Deep lamina lucida pemphigoid:
    A. Is a non-scarring subepidermal bullous dermatosis
    B. Is a scarring subepidermal bullous dermatosis
    C. Has the same target antigen as bullous pemphigoid
    D. Is characterized by an intraepidermal blister

E. Is characterized by immunoreactants within the epidermis (intercellular pattern) in direct immunofluorescence

39. The histopathologic reaction pattern shown may be seen in all of the following EXCEPT:

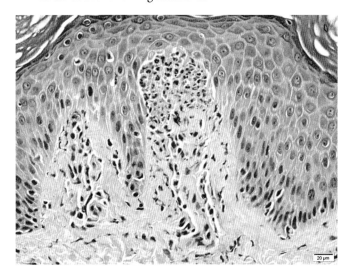

    A. Deep lamina lucida pemphigoid
    B. Localized cicatricial pemphigoid (early lesions)
    C. Dermatitis herpetiformis
    D. Pemphigus vegetans
    E. Erysipelas

40. Distinguishing features between bullous lupus and inflammatory epidermolysis bullosa acquisita include:
    A. Plane of clefting
    B. Composition of the inflammatory infiltrate
    C. Target antigen
    D. Predilection for sun-exposed surfaces
    E. Direct immunofluorescence findings

41. The best-fit diagnosis is:

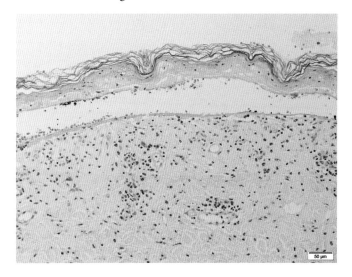

A. Bullous lupus erythematosus
B. Bullous pemphigoid
C. Pemphigus vulgaris
D. Cicatricial pemphigoid
E. Dermatitis herpetiformis

42. The best site to biopsy for direct immunofluorescence of vasculitis is:
    A. Edge of the lesion
    B. Perilesional of normal skin
    C. Lesional skin
    D. Exposed normal skin

43. The best site to biopsy for direct immunofluorescence of systemic lupus erythematosus is:
    A. Edge of the lesion
    B. Perilesional of normal skin
    C. Lesional skin
    D. Exposed normal skin

D3 Vesicobullous Diseases Answers

Table D3.1 Classification of vesicobullous reaction pattern (plane of cleavage/composition of inflammatory infiltrate based)

Plane of cleavage	Inflammatory infiltrate	Disease/s
Intracorneal/subcorneal blister	Minimal inflammation Neutrophils	Staphylococcal scalded skin syndrome Impetigo Pemphigus foliaceus Subcorneal pustular dermatosis
	Neutrophils and eosinophils	Acute generalized exanthematous pustulosis
Intraepidermal blister	Minimal inflammation Neutrophils	Friction blister Palmoplantar pustulosis Erosive pustular dermatosis of the leg EBS (localized type)
Suprabasilar blister	Minimal inflammation	Hailey-Hailey disease Darier's disease
	Eosinophils	Pemphigus vulgaris Pemphigus vegetans
	Lymphocytes and eosinophils	Grover's disease
Suprabasilar and subbasilar	Lymphocytes	Paraneoplastic pemphigus
Subepidermal	Minimal inflammation	EB PCT BP (cell-poor variant) Burns TEN Suction blister Bullous elastosis Bullous amyloidosis Waldenström's macroglobulinemia Kindler's syndrome
	Lymphocytes	Erythema multiforme Lichen planus Lichen planus pemphigoides Lichen sclerosus Bullous mycosis fungoides Polymorphic light eruption
	Eosinophils	Bullous pemphigoid Pemphigoid gestationis Epidermolysis bullosa Bullous urticaria

Table D3.1 Classification of vesicobullous reaction pattern (plane of cleavage/composition of inflammatory infiltrate based) (*cont.*)

Plane of cleavage	Inflammatory infiltrate	Disease/s
	Neutrophils	Dermatitis herpetiformis
		Linear IgA bullous dermatosis
		Mucous membrane pemphigoid
		Ocular cicatricial pemphigoid
		Localized cicatricial pemphigoid
		Deep lamina lucida pemphigoid
		EBA
		Sweet's syndrome
		Bullous lupus erythematosus
		Bullous vasculitis
	Mast cells	Bullous mastocytosis

EB = Epidermolysis bullosa; EBS = EB simplex; PCT = Porphyria cutanea tarda; BP = Bullous pemphigoid; TEN = Toxic epidermal necrolysis; EBA = EB acquisita

Table D3.2 Target antigens in autoimmune bullous disease

Disease	Antigenic target	Antigen location	Other antigens implicated
Pemphigus foliaceus	Dsg1	Desmosomes, upper epidermis	Dsc
IgA pemphigus (subcorneal pustular dermatosis type)	Dsc	Desmosomes, transmembrane	
IgA pemphigus (intraepidermal neutrophilic type)	Dsg1 or dsg3	Desmosomes, transmembrane	Dsc
Pemphigus vulgaris	Dsg3	Desmosomes, lower epidermis	Dsc
Epidermolysis bullosa acquisita	Type VII collagen	Anchoring fibrils	IgA antibody to plectin
Paraneoplastic pemphigus	Dsg1, dsg3, Dpk1, Dpk2	Cytoplasmic plaque	BP230, plectin, desmocollin
Bullous pemphigoid	BPAg1 (BP230, 80%), BPAg2 (BP180, 30%)	Hemidesmosome, transmembrane protein	20% have antibodies to BP180 alone, plectin, dsg3
Pemphigoid gestationis	BPAg2 (BP180)	Transmembrane protein	BP230
Dermatitis herpetiformis	Tissue transglutaminase	GIT, ?skin	Papillary dermal deposits of IgA
Linear IgA bullous dermatosis	LABD97, LAD-1 LABD285 (10–25%)	Lamina lucida Sublamina densa	Degradation products of BP180, NC-1 domain of type VII collagen
Ocular cicatricial pemphigoid	Plectin	Conjunctiva	Heterogeneous IgA antibody
Cicatricial pemphigoid	BPAg2 (BP180) Epiligrin (laminin 332, in 10%)	C-terminal domain A3 subunit of laminin5	
Deep lamina lucida pemphigoid	105 kDa	Lower lamina lucida	Resembles TEN, PV clinically

Dsg = Desmoglein; Dsc = Desmocollin; Dpk = Desmoplakin; BPAg = Bullous pemphigoid antigen; GIT = Gastrointestinal tract; LABD = Linear IgA bullous dermatosis; PV = Pemphigus vulgaris; TEN = Toxic epidermal necrolysis

Table D3.3 Genetic classification of inherited epidermolysis bullosa

Type		Gene involved	Target protein/s
EBS	Suprabasal	*DSP*	Desmoplakin
	Basal	*PKP*	Plakophilin
Junctional	Herlitz	*LAMA3, LAMB3, LAMC2*	Laminin 5
	Others	*LAMA3, LAMB3, LAMC2, COL17A1, ITG176, ITGB4*	Laminin 5, type XVII collagen, α6β4 integrin, laminin 332
Dystrophic EB	Dominant	*COL7A1*	Type VII collagen
	Recessive	*COL7A1*	Type VII collagen
	Kindler's syndrome	*KIND1*	Kindlin 1

EB = Epidermolysis bullosa; EBS = EB simplex

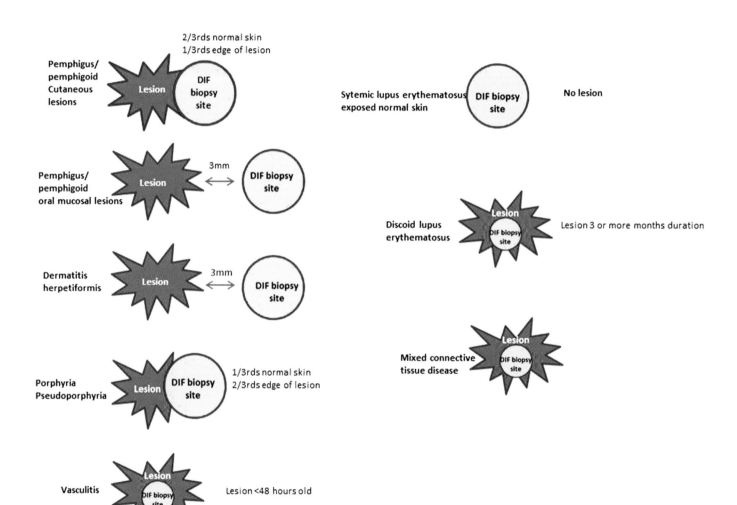

Figure D3.1 Biopsy sites for direct immunofluorescence

1. **B.** Plakoglobulin is NOT an adhesion molecule.

    Plakoglobulin is part of the cytoplasmic plaque. Adhesion molecules include those that mediate cell–cell adhesion (cadherin and immunoglobulin superfamily members), those mediating cellular adhesion to matrix molecules (selectins) and those that mediate both (integrins).

2. **A.** Impetigo is caused by *Staphylococcus aureus*.

    Impetigo is acute superficial pyoderma that occurs more frequently in childhood and is caused most commonly by *Staphylococcus aureus*. It is *the most common* bacterial cutaneous infection in childhood and does not have a predilection for immunocompromised adults. Of the two clinical forms of impetigo, the vesicopustular type is more common than the bullous variant. Common impetigo is rarely biopsied as a diagnosis can be easily made on clinical grounds alone. Histopathologic features of an early lesion reveal a subcorneal pustule.

    Staphylococcal scalded skin syndrome is caused by an epidermolytic toxin produced by select strains of *Staphylococcus aureus* (most notable type 71 of phage group II).

3. **B.** Staphylococcal scalded skin syndrome (SSSS) affects healthy infants and children <6 years of age.

    SSSS does not have a predilection for immunocompromised children.

    It results from production of an epidermolytic toxin produced by select strains of *Staphylococcus aureus* (notably type 71 of phage group II). Clinically, it is characterized by sudden onset skin tenderness, a scarletiniform eruption followed by the development of flaccid blisters and a positive Nikolsky sign. The disease has a good prognosis in children with spontaneous resolution after several days due to formation of neutralizing antibodies to the toxin. Histopathologic features include a subcorneal split and acantholysis.

4. **B.** Pemphigus foliaceus (PF) results from autoantibodies mainly of the IgG4 subclass.

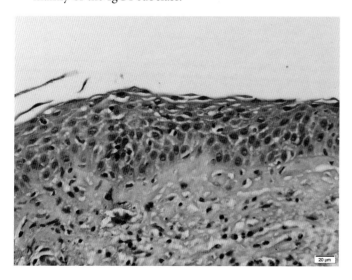

These autoantibodies react with several different antigenic epitopes on the amino-terminal region of dsg1. Dsg1 is expressed primarily in the upper regions of the epidermis, at a much lower level than dsg3 in the mucosa and is highest in the upper torso and scalp. Pemphigus foliaceus accounts for <10% of all cases of pemphigus and is one of the less severe forms of the disease. It is clinically characterized by recurrent crops of flaccid bullae that rupture easily. It is the most common form of pemphigus complicating the use of penicillamine not vancomycin.

Histopathologic features of PF, shown above, include a superficial bulla with a split high in the granular layer. With direct immunofluorescence, there is intercellular staining for IgG and C3 *in both the affected as well as normal skin*.

5. **B.** Image shown is that of a subcorneal pustule, the histopathologic *sine qua non* of subcorneal pustular dermatosis (SPD), a chronic, relapsing, vesicopustular dermatosis with a predilection for the intertriginous areas.

    SPD also affects the flexor aspect of limbs. While the etiology and pathogenesis of SPD are unknown, a small proportion of cases have an associated IgA monoclonal gammopathy. The distinctive histopathologic feature is the presence of a subcorneal pustule filled predominantly with neutrophils and occasional eosinophils and not acantholysis. Direct immunofluorescence and serology are typically non-diagnostic.

6. **C.** Circulating IgA antibodies are present in 50% of cases of IgA pemphigus.

    IgA pemphigus is an autoimmune, intraepidermal, vesicobullous eruption with variable acantholysis and intercellular IgA deposits. It is a clinically heterogeneous condition reflective of the antigenic diversity of the autoantigens. Two distinct groups are recognized: a subcorneal pustular dermatosis-like group in which IgA deposits are confined to the superficial epidermis and an intraepidermal pustular variant in which IgA deposits are distributed throughout the epidermis. A monoclonal IgA gammopathy is present in only 20% of cases of IgA pemphigus.

7. **C.** Acute generalized exanthematous pustulosis (AGEP) is a rapidly evolving pustular eruption.

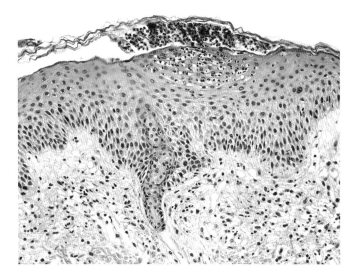

AGEP is clinically characterized by the development of sterile pustules on an erythematous background. The spectrum of drugs implicated is broad and includes antibiotics (particularly β-lactams and cephalosporins) in addition to several others.

Histopathologic features of AGEP, shown above, include a subcorneal or superficial epidermal pustule containing eosinophils in addition to neutrophils.

8. **A.** Image shown is that of *miliaria crystallina* which results from superficial obstruction in the stratum corneum.

Miliaria is clinically heterogeneous with 3 distinct variants:

- *Miliaria crystallina* which results from superficial obstruction in the stratum corneum and is clinically characterized by asymptomatic small vesicles that rupture easily
- *Miliaria rubra* characterized by spongiotic vesiculation adjacent to the acrosyringium and presenting as an erythematous papulovesicular eruption
- *Miliaria profunda* characterized by profound subepidermal vesiculation

9. **B.** Pemphigus vulgaris is characterized by production of autoantibodies to dsg3.

Cutaneous lesions of pemphigus vulgaris (PV) present as flaccid blisters with application of pressure leading to extension of the blister (positive Nikolsky's sign or the Asboe-Hansen sign). Serology is useful in confirming the diagnosis and the critical antigen is believed to reside in amino terminal residues 1–161. Circulating antibodies are found in 80–90% of patients with active disease, *although they may be absent in early cases*. Established lesions are characterized by suprabasal bullae, acantholysis and an infiltrate with admixed eosinophils. Direct immunofluorescence demonstrates IgG in the intercellular regions of the epidermis. Antibodies of the IgG1 and IgG4 subclasses, not IgA, are most commonly found in patients with active lesions.

10. **A.** Pemphigus vegetans is a rare variant of pemphigus vulgaris.

Pemphigus vegetans differs from pemphigus vulgaris by its clinical manifestations of vegetating erosions involving flexural surfaces primarily. Two distinct clinical variants of pemphigus vegetans are recognized:
- *Neumann type* which presents with vegetating plaques clinically and intraepidermal vesicles with acantholysis but not eosinophilic microabscesses
- *Hallopeau type* which presents with pustular lesions clinically and intraepidermal eosinophilic microabscesses histopathologically.

The clinical course of the latter (*Hallopeau type*) is benign in contrast with that of the former (*Neumann type*). Direct immunofluorescence findings of pemphigus vegetans are similar to those of pemphigus vulgaris with intercellular deposits of IgG and C3, and serology is usually positive for the detection of circulating antibodies to dsg3.

11. **C.** Histopathologic features of paraneoplastic pemphigus (PNP) are non-diagnostic in keeping with the clinical heterogeneity of this entity.

Histopathologic features of PNP are variable and include a lichenoid and interface dermatitis in conjunction with suprabasal acantholysis. Paraneoplastic pemphigus (PNP) is an autoimmune blistering disorder characterized by antibodies to multiple antigens including members of the plakin and desmoglein family. Antibodies to dsg1 and/or dsg3 are usually present. Of note, and in contrast to pemphigus vulgaris (in which the dominant subclass is IgG4), the antibody response to dsg3 includes IgG1 and IgG2 subclasses. Direct immunofluorescence shows intercellular and basement membrane zone staining.

12. **B.** Hailey-Hailey disease is inherited as an autosomal dominant condition.

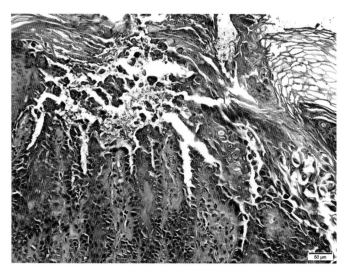

Hailey-Hailey disease (familial benign chronic pemphigus) is clinically characterized by a chronic course with spontaneous remission and subsequent exacerbation. Vesicular plaques progress to flaccid bullae with a predilection for the neck and intertriginous areas. The responsible gene is *ATP2C1* mapped to *3q21–q24*.

Histopathologic features of Hailey-Hailey disease, shown above, are distinctive and include acanthosis and acantholytic dyskeratosis ("dilapidated brick wall").

13. **B.** Darier's disease characteristically involves the head, neck and trunk ("seborrheic distribution").

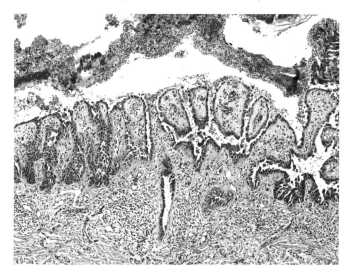

Darier's disease is an uncommon autosomal dominant genodermatosis that is clinically characterized by greasy, yellow/brown crusted lesions involving the head, neck and trunk ("seborrheic distribution"). Areas devoid of follicles such as palms, soles and oral mucosa may also be involved in Darier's disease. The mechanisms underlying the acantholysis are still a subject of debate although most believe that it is due to a defect in the synthesis or maturation of the tonofilament-desmosome complex.

Histopathologic features of Darier's disease, shown above, include suprabasal acantholysis with lacunae formation and corps ronds (solitary or groups of dyskeratotic cells in the stratum malphigian and corneum layers) and corps grains (small cells with elongate nuclei in the superficial epidermal layers).

14. **B.** Grover's disease does not share an abnormality in the *ATP2A2* gene (despite the histopathologic similarity to Darier's disease).

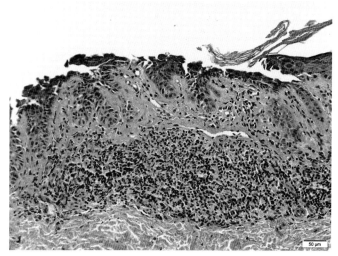

Grover's disease, clinically characterized by a pruritic papulovesicular rash, typically develops in the trunks of older men.

Histopathologic features of Grover's disease *vary with the age of the lesion* but typically include acantholysis, dyskeratotic keratinocytes and a dermal infiltrate containing eosinophils not plasma cells, shown in the above image. Older lesions may have pronounced acanthosis and only subtle acantholysis.

15. **D.** Electron microscopy and NOT serology is the gold standard for the diagnosis of epidermolysis bullosa.

Epidermolysis bullosa (EB) encompasses a heterogeneous group of disorders inherited in an autosomal dominant or recessive form and characterized by the development of blisters following minor trauma. The 3 types include:
- EB simplex (intraepidermal)
- Junctional EB (intralamina lucida)
- Dystrophic EB (sublamina densa)

In EB simplex, the plane of cleavage is so low that in routine H&E stained sections, it appears as a cell-poor subepidermal blister.

16. **B.** Epidermolysis bullosa acquisita (EBA) is typically acquired.

EBA is a non-hereditary subepidermal bullous disorder in which blisters typically develop at the site of trauma. Involvement of the mucous membranes occurs in 30–50% of cases. The target antigen in EBA is type VII collagen ("EBA antigen") with a molecular weight of 290 kDa. Serology using ELISA is diagnostic. Histopathologic features are that of a pauci-inflammatory subepidermal blister. With PAS stain, the basement membrane is split with most of the PAS+ material on the roof. Laminin and type IV collagen can be identified using immunohistochemical techniques.

17. **B. Image shown is that of a pauci-inflammatory subepidermal blister, which would not be seen in paraneoplastic pemphigus.**

    Suprabasilar and *not subepidermal* blisters are a feature of paraneoplastic pemphigus. Entities characterized by a pauci-inflammatory subepidermal blister include epidermolysis bullosa, porphyria cutanea tarda, bullous pemphigoid (cell-poor variant), Kindler's syndrome (a variant of epidermolysis bullosa) and bullous solar elastosis. Other entities include bullous amyloidosis, and Waldenström's macroglobulinemia (Table D3.1).

18. **E. Reduced activity of UPG decarboxylase leads to porphyria cutanea tarda and hepatoerythropoietic porphyria.**

    Biosynthesis of heme consists of the following steps:

    Glycine + succinyly COA catalyzed by aminolevulinic acid (ALA) synthetase is converted to ALA

    ALA to porphobilinogen catalyzed by ALA-dehydratase

    Porphobilinogen (PBG) to hydroxymethylbilane catalyzed by PBG deaminase (*reduced activity leads to acute intermittent porphyria*)

    Hydroxymethylbilane to uroporphyrinogen (UPG) III catalyzed by UPG III cosynthase (*reduced activity leads to congenital erythropoietic porphyria*)

    UPG III to coproporphyrinogen (CPG) III catalyzed by UPG decarboxylase (*reduced activity leads to porphyria cutanea tarda and hepatoerythropoietic porphyria*)

    CPG III to protoporphyrinogen (PPG) IX catalyzed by CPG oxidase (*reduced activity leads to hereditary coproporphyria*)

    PPG IX to protoporphyrin IX catalyzed by PPG oxidase (*reduced activity leads to variegate porphyria*)

    Protoporphyrin IX to heme catalyzed by ferrochelatase (*reduced activity leads to erythropoietic protoporphyria*)

19. **D. Image shown is that of a pauci-inflammatory subepidermal blister with festooning, a feature of** porphyria cutanea tarda, also associated with PAS+ caterpillar bodies.

    "Caterpillar bodies" in porphyria cutanea tarda (PCT) represent basement membrane material and colloid bodies, have a high specificity for PCT and are PAS positive and contain collagen IV. The segmented, elongated shape of the bodies is reminiscent of the larvae of butterflies, hence the name "caterpillar bodies" was coined to describe them. These bodies are similar in their composition to the Kamino bodies of Spitz's nevi, cylindrical bodies in adenoid cystic carcinoma, Civatte bodies of lichen planus, and the collagenous spherules seen in a number of conditions, and provide a unique clue to the diagnosis of the porphyric bullous eruptions. Porphyria cutanea tarda comprises three major forms: *familial, sporadic* and *toxic*. The unifying feature of all types is the reduction in activity of uroporphyrinogen decarboxylase leading to *overproduction of hepatic porphyrins*. The *familial form* is inherited in an autosomal dominant manner and tends to present earlier than the others. The *sporadic form* typically has its onset in mid-life and has a very strong association with hepatitis C. The *toxic form* results from exposure to polychlorinated aromatic hydrocarbons. Cutaneous changes occur predominantly on sun-exposed sites such as the face, arms and dorsal aspect of arms. Histopathologic features include a pauci-inflammatory subepidermal blister with festooning and the presence of "caterpillar bodies."

20. **C. Ultrastructural features of porphyria cutanea tarda (PCT) include prominent reduplication of the basal laminae with concentric encasement of vessels.**

    Of other inclusions mentioned:

    - Oval/round juxtanuclear inclusions are seen in Lafora disease
    - Farber bodies are seen in Farber's disease
    - Vacuolation of fibroblasts and endothelial cells is seen in gangliosidosis
    - Zebra bodies are seen in Fabry's disease

21. **B. Target antigens in bullous pemphigoid (BP) include BP230 (BPAg1) and BP180 (BPAg2).**

    Male patients are more likely to have antibodies to BP180, whereas antibodies to BP230 occur with equal frequency. BP230 is a member of the plakin family of proteins and is restricted to the intracellular hemidesmosomal plaque. BP230 antibodies precipitate and perpetuate disease. Autoantibodies to a complex of BP230 and BP180 are present in up to 80% of patients with BP. The major antigenic epitopes of the BP230 protein map to the C-terminal end (not the N-terminal end). Antibodies to BP180 are more often associated with oral lesions, have a poor prognosis with less responsiveness to steroids and serum antibody levels correlate with disease activity. While autoantibodies to BP230 and BP180 can be seen in normal healthy adults, they do not bind to the NC16A domain (the target antigen in most commercially available ELISA kits).

22. **C.** Eosinophilic spongiosis would not be an expected histopathologic feature of bullous lupus erythematosus (LE).

    Bullous LE histopathologically resembles dermatitis herpetiformis and is characterized by a subepidermal blister *with neutrophils not eosinophils.* Eosinophilic spongiosis is a histopathologic reaction pattern seen in a heterogeneous group of dermatoses. These include:
    - Arthropod bite reaction
    - Bullous pemphigoid
    - Incontinentia pigmenti
    - Ofuji's disease (eosinophilic folliculitis)
    - Pemphigus (precursor lesions and vegetans)
    - Eosinophilic, polymorphous and pruritic eruption
    - "Id" reaction

23. **A.** In early stages of bullous pemphigoid (BP), only linear C3 is seen in direct immunofluorescence.

    In established lesions of BP, direct immunofluorescence typically shows a linear deposition of IgG and C3 along the basement membrane zone. IgG4 is the predominant subclass of IgG in prodromal lesions. IgM and IgA are present in only a small proportion (up to 20%) of cases. Some cases with IgA have oral lesions.

24. **A.** In indirect IF, circulating anti-basement zone antibodies of the IgG subclass are present in 60–80% of patients with BP.

    The precise proportion depends upon the substrate used. There is no correlation between antibody titers and disease activity. Antibodies are *typically absent in the presence* of circulating immune complexes.

25. **C.** All patients with pemphigoid gestationis possess a circulating antibody that targets the same antigen as the BP antigen (BP180).

Pemphigoid gestationis is an uncommon vesicobullous dermatosis of pregnancy that typically manifests in the second or third trimester with urticarial plaques and papules in a periumbilical distribution. It usually recurs in subsequent pregnancies and manifests earlier in subsequent pregnancies.

Histopathologic features of pemphigoid gestationis, shown above, are non-specific and include papillary dermal edema (that can be so marked as to produce "teardrop-shaped" papillae), and a mixed inflammatory infiltrate composed of lymphocytes, histiocytes and eosinophils. Direct immunofluorescence reveals C3 and sometimes IgG in a linear pattern along the basement membrane zone. Serology using the commercially available BP180 NC16A ELISA is helpful in clinching the diagnosis.

26. **C.** The presence of anti-endomysial antibodies (of the IgA class) is diagnostic of dermatitis herpetiformis (DH).

    Anti-endomysial antibodies have been noted in up to 70% of DH patients on a normal diet and in 100% of patients with villous atrophy.

    Circulating antibodies to reticulin, gliadin, nuclear components and thyroid antigens may be seen in variable percentages in DH but are not diagnostic.

27. **C.** Dermatitis herpetiformis (DH) typically occurs in adults.

    Onset of DH is most common in adult life although select studies have indicated that a pediatric population can be affected. Dermatitis herpetiformis is a relatively uncommon autoimmune bullous disorder characterized by an intensely pruritic papulovesicular symmetric rash that is "grouped" and has a predilection for extensor surfaces. A gluten-sensitive enteropathy has been noted in approximately 90% of cases and circulating anti-endomysial antibodies of the IgA subclass are diagnostic. Direct immunofluorescence findings reveal granular deposits of IgA in the dermal papillae.

28. **B.** Vasculitis is NOT a feature of an early lesion of dermatitis herpetiformis (DH).

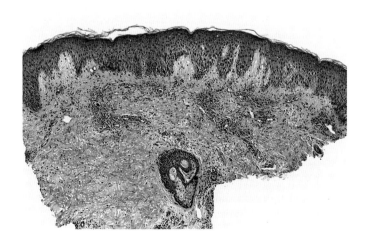

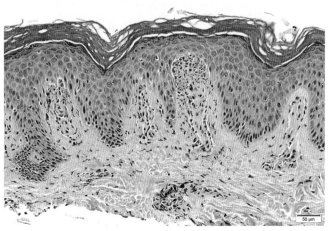

Histopathologic features of early lesions of DH include aggregates of neutrophils and eosinophils in the dermal papillae (forming microabscesses), fibrin deposits in the dermal papillae and occasional acantholytic cells.

29. **A.** Circulating anti-endomysial antibodies are typically IgA.

These are diagnostic of dermatitis herpetiformis and present in 70% of patients on a normal diet and in 100% of patients with villous atrophy. The target autoantigen is tissue transglutaminase (TG).

30. **C.** Linear IgA bullous dermatosis is associated with antibodies targeting a 97 kDa antigen.

The other target antigen is a 285 kDa antigen. Both antigenic targets are located in the lamina lucida. There are 2 clinical variants of linear IgA bullous dermatosis: chronic bullous dermatosis of childhood and adult linear IgA bullous dermatosis. Both variants share the same target antigen and are thus regarded as different expressions of the same disease. Linear IgA bullous dermatosis is a sulfone-responsive bullous dermatosis that is histopathologically characterized by a subepidermal blister with neutrophils as the predominant cell in the inflammatory infiltrate.

31. **A.** Target antigens in linear IgA bullous dermatosis are not restricted to a single component or specific area of the basement membrane zone.

Linear IgA bullous dermatosis (LABD) is a heterogeneous disease as far as localization of the target antigen and deposition of the antibody is concerned. The target antigen of LABD in the major (lamina lucida) type is a 97 kDa protein (ladinin) or a 120 kDa protein (LAD-1). Both of these are degeneration products of the bullous pemphigoid antigen (BP180) which has a key role to play in the pathogenesis of this disease. The target antigen in the drug-induced form of the disease is also heterogeneous with autoantibodies targeting BP180 as well as LAD285. Circulating IgA antibodies are found in 70% of childhood cases and 20% of adult cases. Ultrastructural studies have revealed diverse findings (a split within the lamina lucida as well below the basal lamina), echoing the heterogeneous nature of the disease.

32. **E.** No single histopathologic finding is of utility in distinguishing linear IgA bullous dermatosis (LABD) from dermatitis herpetiformis (DH).

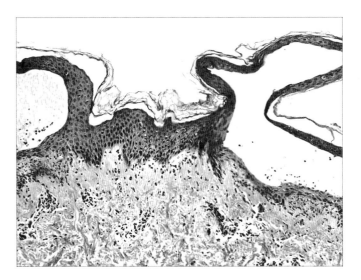

Both entities share unifying features of having the same plane of cleavage (subepidermal) and a predominance of neutrophils in the inflammatory infiltrate.

While the spread of neutrophils in LABD, shown in the image above, is more widespread than in DH, where it is concentrated in the dermal papillae, in most cases distinguishing both entities based on this feature alone is impossible. Furthermore, while fibrin deposits in dermal papillae have been noted in nearly all cases of DH, they have also been reported in up to 75% of cases LABD.

33. **B.** The linear deposition of IgA is NOT specific for linear IgA bullous dermatosis (LABD) as it may be seen in other autoimmune bullous diseases.

Direct immunofluorescence reveals IgA deposition in a linear homogeneous pattern in LABD. While IgA is the sole immunoreactant in only 80% of cases, IgG/M and/or C3 have been detected in the rest. IgA deposits may be of the IgA1 or IgA2 subclass.

34. **C.** In mucous membrane pemphigoid cutaneous lesions precede mucosal involvement.

In only 10% of cases of mucous membrane pemphigoid do cutaneous lesions precede mucosal involvement. Mucous membrane pemphigoid is a relatively uncommon chronic autoimmune vesicobullous disease that is characterized by a predilection for oral and ocular mucous membranes. Lesions have a tendency to scar (hence the old name of cicatricial pemphigoid). It tends to occur more commonly in the elderly although scattered reports of children and adolescents being affected do exist. There is considerable heterogeneity in clinical presentation.

35. **D.** Target antigens in mucous membrane pemphigoid do NOT include dsg1.

Target antigens in mucous membrane pemphigoid are diverse and include BP180, BP230, laminin 5, type VII collagen, uncein and β_4 integrin. Dsg1 is the target antigen in pemphigus foliaceus.

36. **A.** In mucous membrane pemphigoid, the plane of cleavage is subepidermal.

    In lesions of mucous membrane pemphigoid that are <48 hours old, neutrophilic microabscesses in the dermal papillae (similar to those seen in dermatitis herpetiformis) may be seen. As the lesion ages, the proportions of eosinophils as well as lymphocytes in the inflammatory infiltrate increase. Scarring may be a feature of an early lesion. *The presence of a sebaceous gland within the blister is a clue to the diagnosis of this entity.*

37. **B.** Mucous membranes are typically NOT involved in localized cicatricial pemphigoid.

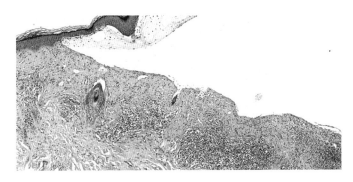

    Localized cicatricial pemphigoid (Brunsting-Perry type) is clinically characterized by the development of plaques in the head and neck area.

    Histopathologic features of cicatricial pemphigoid, shown in the image above, include a subepidermal blister with an inflammatory infiltrate that varies with age of the lesion with neutrophils predominating in lesions <48 hours old (forming DH-like papillary dermal microabscesses). Ultrastructurally, the basal lamina and anchoring fibrils are well preserved and attached to the "roof" (intact epidermis).

38. **A.** Deep lamina lucida pemphigoid is a unique non-scarring, subepidermal bullous dermatosis with involvement of skin and mucous membranes.

    The target antigen is a 105 kDa antigen and NOT the bullous pemphigoid antigens (BP180 and/or BP230). Histopathologic features include a subepidermal blister with neutrophils (forming DH-like papillary dermal microabscesses) and direct immunofluorescence findings reveal immunoreactants ONLY at the basement membrane zone.

39. **D.** Neutrophilic microabscesses shown in the image would not be an expected histopathologic finding of pemphigus vegetans.

    Pemphigus vegetans, an uncommon variant of pemphigus vulgaris, has two clinical variants: *Neumann type* which presents with intraepidermal vesicles with acantholysis but not eosinophilic microabscesses and

Hallopeau type which presents with intraepidermal eosinophilic (NOT neutrophilic) microabscesses histopathologically.

Neutrophilic microabscesses within the papillary dermis are seen in:
- Dermatitis herpetiformis and linear IgA bullous dermatosis (typically)
- Mucous membrane pemphigoid
- Localized cicatricial pemphigoid (Brunsting-Perry type), early lesions (<48 hours old)
- Deep lamina lucida pemphigoid
- Bullous urticaria
- Bullous lupus, erysipelas
- Sweet's syndrome
- Epidermolysis bullosa acquisita

40. **D.** While clinical lesions of bullous lupus have a predilection for sun-exposed surfaces, lesions of epidermolysis bullosa acquisita (EBA) are clinically heterogeneous and rarely precipitated by sun exposure.

    Features shared by bullous lupus and inflammatory EBA include histopathologic features of a subepidermal blister with neutrophils, presence of autoantibodies to type VII collagen and direct immunofluorescence findings of deposition of immunoreactants along the basement membrane zone.

41. **B.** Image shown is that of bullous pemphigoid.

    Bullous pemphigoid (BP) falls into the category of subepidermal blisters with eosinophils. It occurs primarily in the elderly and clinically presents as tense bullae on normal or erythematous skin. Oral lesions have been noted in up to 40% of cases but involvement of other mucosal surfaces is uncommon. Histopathologic features are that of a subepidermal blister with eosinophils in the lumen. In older lesions, the plane of cleavage may appear intraepidermal because of partial re-epithelialization.

42. **C.** Lesional skin is the most informative in terms of direct immunofluorescence (DIF) for cases of vasculitis.

    Typically, the biopsy should be of a lesion that is <48 hours old. DIF of lesions >72 hours are low yield. If no fresh lesions are available or if the age of the lesion is unknown, biopsy should be of normal skin at the edge of the biopsy (also see Figure D3.1).

43. **D.** Exposed normal skin is most informative for direct immunofluorescence (DIF) in systemic lupus erythematosus (SLE).

    Positive DIF in a biopsy of lesional skin in SLE is a non-diagnostic finding. In contrast, if discoid lupus erythematosus is suspected, the DIF biopsy site should be a lesion in an exposed area of 3 or months duration (also see Figure D3.1).

D4 Connective Tissue Disease and Other Interface Dermatitis
Questions

1. Entities with a similar histopathologic reaction pattern include all of the following EXCEPT:

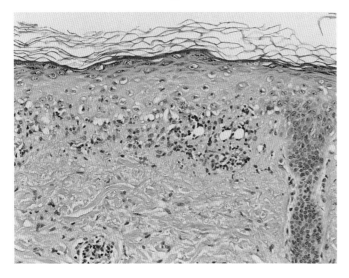

   A. Vitiligo
   B. Subacute lupus erythematosus
   C. Kindler's syndrome
   D. Atrophie blanche
   E. Eruption of lymphocyte recovery

2. Rowell's syndrome is BEST regarded as:
   A. A variant of lupus with antibodies to histone
   B. A variant of lupus with antibodies to Ro/La
   C. A variant of lupus with antibodies to Jo-1
   D. A variant of lupus with anti-mitochondrial antibodies
   E. A variant of lupus with antibodies to Scl-70

3. Which of the following antibody specificity associations is INCORRECT:
   A. Sm and systemic lupus erythematosus
   B. Scl-70 and systemic sclerosis
   C. Anti-Ro and subacute cutaneous lupus erythematosus
   D. Anti-myeloperoxidase and Wegener's granulomatosis
   E. Anti-histone and drug-induced lupus

4. The antibody with the *lowest* specificity for autoimmune disease, NOS, is:
   A. ANA
   B. dsDNA
   C. Ro/SSA
   D. Smith
   E. Centromere

5. All of the following are correct regarding clinical manifestations of subacute cutaneous lupus erythematosus (SCLE) EXCEPT:
   A. Lesions are annular or psoriasiform
   B. Follicular plugging is prominent
   C. Scarring is minimal
   D. Rash is photosensitive
   E. Arthralgia may be present

6. Which of the following is INCORRECT regarding the lupus anticoagulant:
   A. Is a circulating, IgG/IgM or both
   B. Interferes with one or more phospholipid-dependent coagulation tests
   C. Is diagnostic for systemic lupus erythematosus
   D. Is associated with an increased risk for thrombosis

7. Cutaneous manifestations of lupus anticoagulant include all of the following EXCEPT:
   A. Thrombophlebitis
   B. Stasis dermatitis
   C. Raynaud's phenomenon
   D. Subungual splinter hemorrhages
   E. Sneddon's syndrome

8. Laboratory findings in the work-up of lupus anticoagulant include all of the following EXCEPT:
   A. Abnormal prothrombin time
   B. Abnormal screening test
   C. Identification of an inhibitor
   D. Demonstration of a phospholipid-dependent inhibitor
   E. Factor VIII deficiency

9. The *most commonly found circulating antibody specific* for the diagnosis of systemic lupus erythematosus is:
   A. ssDNA
   B. dsDNA
   C. ENA
   D. Sm
   E. Histone

10. The target autoantigen in bullous systemic lupus erythematosus is:
    A. Fibrillin 1
    B. Collagen II
    C. Collagen IV
    D. Collagen VII
    E. Collagen IX

11. The target autoantigen in neonatal lupus erythematosus is:
    A. dsDNA
    B. SSA

C. SSB

D. ssDNA

E. Histone

12. Extracutaneous manifestations of neonatal lupus erythematosus include all of the following EXCEPT:

    A. Cardiomyopathy

    B. Heart block

    C. Hepatitis

    D. Thrombocytopenia

    E. Pneumonia

13. All of the following are correct regarding the entity shown EXCEPT:

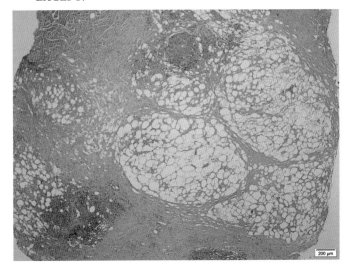

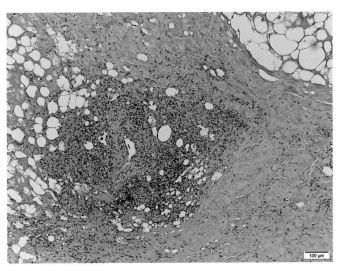

    A. Onset typically precedes other manifestations of disease

    B. Clinically presents as tender subcutaneous nodules

    C. Direct immunofluorescence is diagnostic

    D. Involves dermis and epidermis in >50% cases

    E. Presence of reactive lymphoid follicles common

14. Histopathologic findings in early lesions of graft-versus-host disease (GVHD) include all of the following EXCEPT:

    A. Normal skin

    B. Squamatization of the basal layer

    C. Individually necrotic, dyskeratotic keratinocytes

    D. Satellite cell necrosis

    E. Leukocytoclastic vasculitis

15. Which of the following is characterized by this histopathologic reaction pattern:

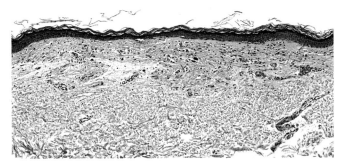

    A. Kindler's syndrome

    B. Muir-Torre syndrome

    C. Birt-Hogg-Dubé syndrome

    D. Basal cell nevus syndrome

    E. Chediak-Higashi syndrome

16. Clinical correlates of this might include:

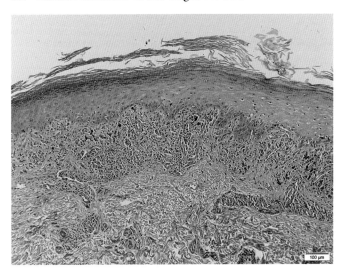

    A. Linear plaques

    B. Ulcerated papules

    C. Erythematous scales

    D. Polygonal papules

    E. Tense bullae

17. The best-fit diagnosis is:

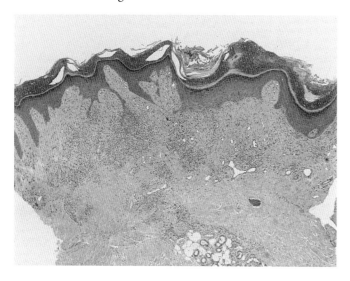

    A. Hypertrophic actinic keratosis
    B. Hypertrophic lichen planus
    C. Hypertrophic lupus erythematosus
    D. Lichenoid contact dermatitis
    E. Lichenoid drug eruption

18. Which of the following best describes the direct immunofluorescence findings typical of lichen planus:
    A. Intercellular IgG
    B. Shaggy fibrin band
    C. Linear IgG and C3
    D. Granular IgM and C3

19. Identities synonymous with ashy dermatosis include all of the following EXCEPT:
    A. Erythema dyschromicum perstans
    B. Lichen planus pigmentosus
    C. Lichen planopilaris
    D. Lichen planus pigmentosus

20. Which of the following is NOT a typical histopathologic feature of lichen planus:
    A. Interface change
    B. Lichenoid infiltrate
    C. Irregular acanthosis
    D. Eosinophil-rich infiltrate
    E. Caspary-Joseph space

21. Graham Little-Picccardi-Lasseur syndrome is characterized by:
    A. Violaceous papular and nodular lesions on the extremities
    B. Cicatricial alopecia and follicular keratotic lesions
    C. Violaceous itchy papular and nodular lesions on flexor surfaces
    D. Asymptomatic flesh-colored papules in the genital areas
    E. Scaly plaques in "seborrheic areas"

22. Scalp biopsy from a 53-year-old female presenting with keratotic follicular lesions and alopecia. The most likely diagnosis is:

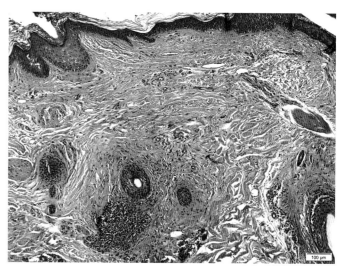

    A. Folliculitis decalvans
    B. Alopecia areata
    C. Androgenetic alopecia
    D. Lichen planopilaris
    E. Trichotillomania

23. Biopsy from a papule of a 23-year-old male presenting with an asymptomatic papular eruption. The most likely diagnosis is:

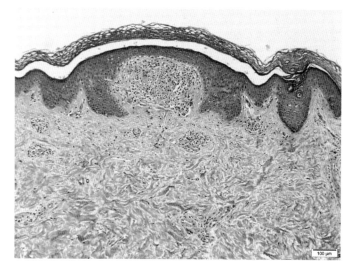

    A. Lichen amyloidosus
    B. Lichen planus
    C. Lichen nitidus
    D. Lichen aureus
    E. Lichen planus-like keratosis

24. A 14-year-old male presenting with an asymptomatic linear papular eruption in a "blaschkoid" distribution. The most likely diagnosis is:

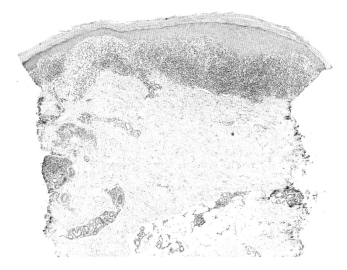

   A. Lichen striatus
   B. Inflammatory linear verrucous epidermal nevus (ILVEN)
   C. Linear lichen planus
   D. Linear lichen aureus
   E. Lichen planus-like keratosis

25. Histopathologic distinguishing features of a lichenoid drug eruption of utility in differentiating it from lichen planus include the presence of:
   A. Satellite cell necrosis and histiocytes
   B. Parakeratosis and eosinophils
   C. Interface change and density of infiltrate
   D. Interface change and Caspary-Joseph spaces
   E. Civatte bodies and density of infiltrate

26. A 38-year-old male with no prior significant medical history presents with erythematous iris-shaped papules and plaques involving the palms and soles. The best-fit diagnosis is:

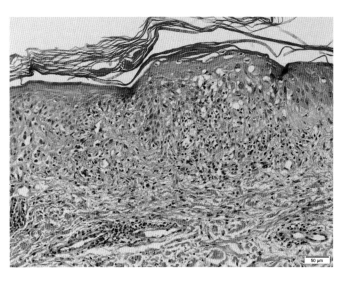

   A. Secondary syphilis
   B. Lichen planus
   C. Erythema multiforme
   D. Toxic epidermal necrolysis
   E. Graft-versus-host disease

27. Biopsy from a sudden-onset blistering rash involving mucocutaneous surfaces. The most likely diagnosis is:

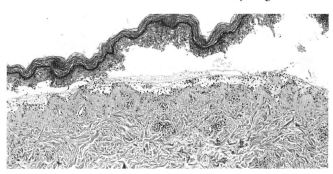

   A. Toxic epidermal necrolysis
   B. Erythema multiforme
   C. Bullous pemphigoid
   D. Lichen planus
   E. Primary syphilis

28. Pityriasis lichenoides et varioliformis acuta (PLEVA/ Mucha-Habermann disease) is best classified as:
   A. An occlusive vasculopathy
   B. A leukocytoclastic vasculitis
   C. A non-inflammatory purpura
   D. A lymphocytic vasculitis
   E. A septic vasculitis

29. Which of the following is INCORRECT regarding pityriasis lichenoides chronica (PLC):
   A. Clinical exacerbations and remissions common
   B. Lymphomatoid papulosis is part of the same spectrum

C. Unknown etiopathogenesis

D. Histopathologic features include lymphocytic vasculitis

E. Histopathologic features include interface dermatitis

30. Histopathologic distinguishing features found in primary perniosis but not in lupus-related perniosis include:
    A. Interface change
    B. Lymphocytic vasculitis
    C. Papillary dermal edema
    D. "Fluffy edema" of endothelial cells
    E. None of the above

31. Which of the following is INCORRECT regarding the entity shown:

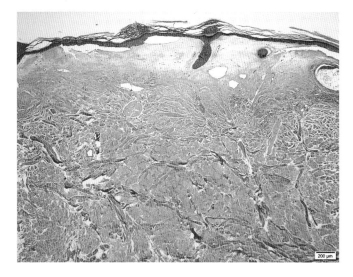

A. Affects children primarily
B. Present for years prior to detection
C. Predilection for genital areas
D. Typically associated with morphea

32. Which of the following is NOT a histopathologic feature of lichen sclerosus?
    A. Lymphocytic vasculitis
    B. Interface change
    C. Leukocytoclastic vasculitis
    D. Follicular plugging
    E. Pautrier microabscess

33. Which of the following BEST characterizes the histopathology of small plaque parapsoriasis:
    A. Satellite cell necrosis and interface dermatitis
    B. Deep dermal lymphocytic infiltrate
    C. Hyperchromatic enlarged dermal lymphocytes
    D. Hyperchromatic lymphocytes tagging the dermoepidermal junction
    E. Parakeratosis and acanthosis with mild spongiosis

34. Which of the following is INCORRECT regarding paraneoplastic pemphigus:
    A. Polymorphous clinical presentation
    B. Target antigens include plakins and/or desmogleins
    C. Diagnostic histopathology
    D. Diagnostic direct immunofluorescence findings

35. Clinical variants of pigmented purpuric dermatosis include all of the following EXCEPT:
    A. Schamberg's disease
    B. Lichen aureus
    C. Gougerot-Blum disease
    D. Majocchi's granuloma
    E. Purpuric contact dermatitis

36. An early lesion of pigmented purpuric dermatosis will demonstrate all of the following EXCEPT:
    A. Band-like lichenoid infiltrate
    B. Lymphocytic vasculitis
    C. Hemosiderin deposits
    D. Predominance of CD4+ T lymphocytes
    E. Extravasated erythrocytes

37. Entities characterized by infiltrates "filling" the papillary dermis include all of the following EXCEPT:
    A. Pigmented purpuric dermatoses
    B. Mycosis fungoides
    C. Lichenoid dermatitis
    D. Urticaria pigmentosa
    E. Perniosis

38. The most likely diagnosis is:

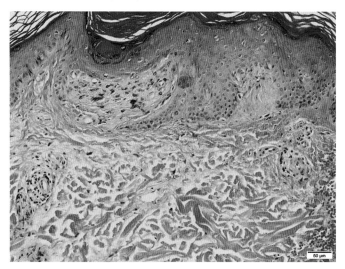

A. Prurigo pigmentosa
B. Lichen sclerosus
C. Post-inflammatory hyperpigmentation
D. Lichen amyloidosus
E. Lichen nitidus

39. The most useful stain in confirming the diagnosis of the above is:
    A. CK5/6
    B. CK7
    C. EVG
    D. CK20
    E. Giemsa

40. The best-fit diagnosis is:

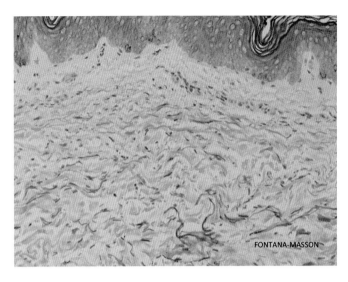

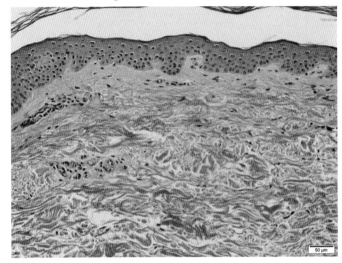

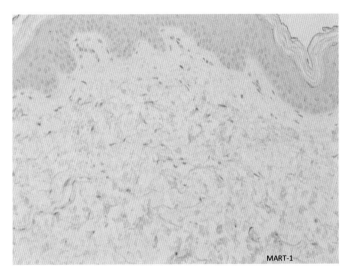

A. Nevus depigmentosus
B. Oculocutaneous albinism
C. Chediak-Higashi syndrome
D. Vitiligo
E. Pityriasis alba

41. This is believed to be due to:

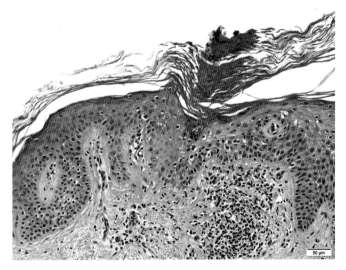

A. Retention hyperkeratosis
B. Faulty keratinization
C. Profilaggrin deficiency
D. Transglutaminase mutations

D4 Connective Tissue Disease and Other Interface Dermatitis
Answers

Table D4.1 Distinguishing histopathologic findings of entities with a lichenoid reaction pattern

Entity		Histopathology	Image
Lichen planus	Regular	Irregular epidermal hyperplasia with wedge-shaped hypergranulosis Interface change with prominent Civatte bodies Positive DIF (colloid bodies IgM+ C3, BMZ with fibrin)	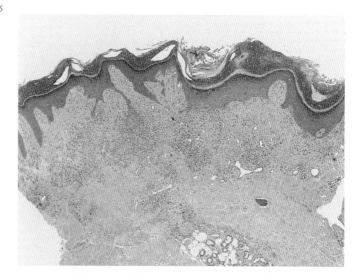
	Hypertrophic variant	Interface change *confined to the tips of the rete ridges*	
	Atrophic variant	Effaced epidermis with loss of rete ridges Infiltrate less dense than in regular LP	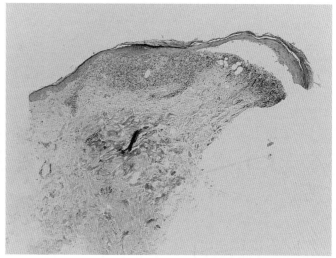

Table D4.1 Distinguishing histopathologic findings of entities with a lichenoid reaction pattern (*cont.*)

Entity	Histopathology	Image
Erosive	Ulceration with more typical LP-like changes at the periphery Plasma-cell rich infiltrate (*mucosal lesions alone*)	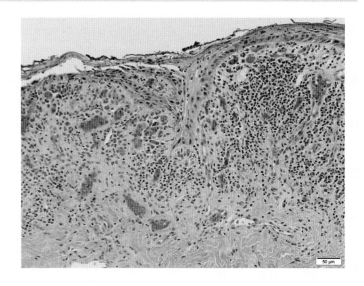
Oral	Mimics regular LP Heavy infiltrate with plasma cells and neutrophils Dyskeratotic keratinocytes higher up in epidermis Positive DIF positive ("shaggy" BMZ fibrin)	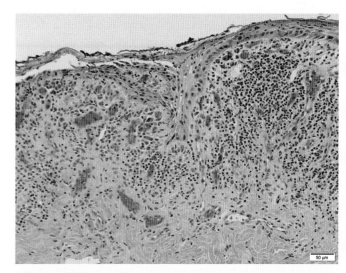
Erythema dyschromicum perstans (LP pigmentosus)	Interface change plus dyskeratotic keratinocytes Prominent pigment incontinence (may be the *only* feature in older lesions) DIF similar to regular LP	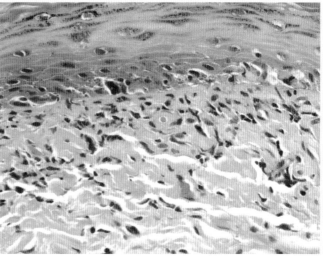

Table D4.1 Distinguishing histopathologic findings of entities with a lichenoid reaction pattern (*cont.*)

Entity	Histopathology	Image
Lichen planopilaris	Interface change involving follicular epithelia plus perifollicular inflammation (peri-infundibular and peri-isthmic) Positive DIF (adjacent to involved follicle)	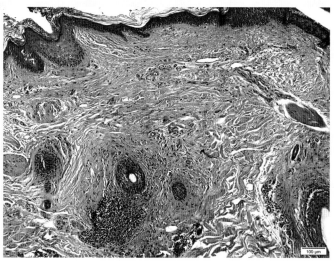
Lichen planus pemphigoides	Cell-poor subepidermal blister Mild mixed perivascular infiltrate Positive linear DIF (IgG + C3)	
Lichen nitidus	Interface change confined to a single papilla ("ball and claw") Lichenoid mixed inflammatory cell infiltrate (lymphocytes + histiocytes + MNGCs) with pigment incontinence	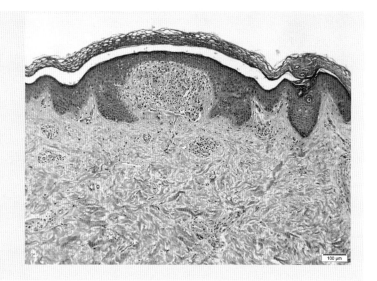
Lichen striatus	Interface change Lichenoid and periadnexal mixed inflammatory cell infiltrate (lymphocytes + histiocytes) with pigment incontinence	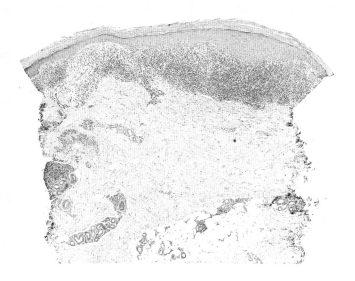

Table D4.1 Distinguishing histopathologic findings of entities with a lichenoid reaction pattern (*cont.*)

Entity	Histopathology	Image
Lichen planus-like keratosis	Confluent interface change plus scattered individually necrotic, dyskeratotic keratinocytes Lichenoid lymphoid cell infiltrate	
Lichenoid drug eruption	Features of regular lichen planus Parakeratosis and presence of eosinophils in the inflammatory infiltrate (*distinguishing features from LP*)	

BMZ = Basement membrane zone; DIF = Direct immunofluorescence; LP = Lichen planus; MNGCs = Multinucleate giant cells

Table D4.2 Distinguishing histopathologic findings of connective tissue diseases

Entity	Key histopathologic findings	Image
Subacute lupus erythematosus	Epidermal atrophy, interface change, scattered individually necrotic dyskeratotic keratinocytes, minimal dermal mucin	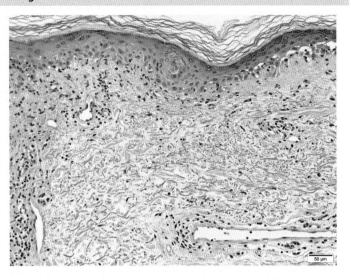
Systemic lupus erythematosus	Interface change (with extension along follicular epithelia), perivascular and periadnexal lymphocytic inflammatory infiltrate, increased dermal mucin	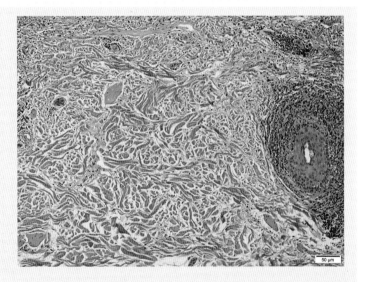
Discoid lupus erythematosus	Epidermal atrophy, follicular plugging, interface change (with extension along follicular epithelia), scattered individually necrotic dyskeratotic keratinocytes, minimal dermal mucin	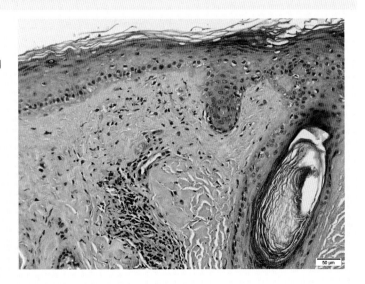

Table D4.2 Distinguishing histopathologic findings of connective tissue diseases (*cont.*)

Entity	Key histopathologic findings	Image
Tumid lupus erythematosus	Perivascular and periadnexal lymphocytic inflammatory infiltrate, increased dermal mucin *No epidermal change*	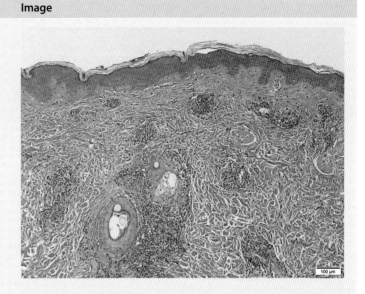
Dermatomyositis	Interface change, scattered individually necrotic dyskeratotic keratinocytes, minimal dermal mucin	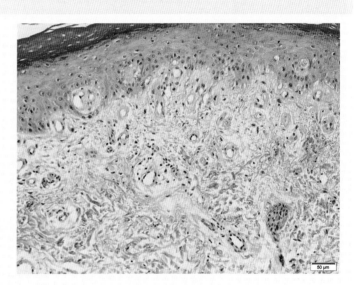

Table D4.3 Antigenic targets in non-blistering cutaneous disorders

Antigenic target	Disease association/s	Comments
ANA	SLE (95%) Subacute LE (80%) DLE (25%)	Non-specific, low levels of positivity found normally in older people, more commonly in females
B$_2$-glycoprotein 1	Lupus anticoagulant, thromboembolic events	
CCP	Rheumatoid arthritis, several autoimmune diseases	More specific than RF for rheumatoid arthritis
Centromere	Systemic sclerosis, scleroderma (57–82% in limited, 8% in diffuse)	Specific for CREST, associated with a high incidence of pulmonary hypertension
dsDNA	SLE (40–60% of cases), MCTD (low titers) DLE (low titers) Rheumatoid arthritis (low titers)	Relatively specific for SLE, high titers associated with an increased risk of lupus nephritis, titers correlate with disease activity

Table D4.3 Antigenic targets in non-blistering cutaneous disorders (*cont.*)

Antigenic target	Disease association/s	Comments
	Progressive systemic sclerosis (low titers) Sjogren's syndrome (low titers) Dermatomyositis (low titers)	
Histone	Drug-induced lupus (95% cases), SLE	Drugs commonly implicated include procainamide, hydralazine
Jo-1	Polymyositis	Often associated with pulmonary fibrosis, not seen in dermatomyositis
MPO	Microscopic polyangiitis	
NMDAR	SLE	Presence correlates with neuropsychiatric manifestations
Nuclear RNP (U1RNP)	Mixed connective tissue disease (MCTD), SLE, associated with Raynaud's phenomenon	
Phospholipid	Thromboembolic events	
Pm-Scl	Polymyositis/scleroderma overlap	
RAP (SS-C)	Primary Sjogren's syndrome (5%)	
RF	Rheumatoid arthritis (higher the titer, the higher the specificity), several autoimmune diseases	Non-specific
SS-A (Ro)	Sjogren's syndrome, subacute cutaneous lupus, neonatal lupus with heart block, SLE with interstitial pneumonia	Constitutes a diagnostic marker for Sjogren's syndrome, helpful in ANA-negative lupus
SS-B (La)	Sjogren's syndrome, SLE	Constitutes a diagnostic marker for Sjogren's syndrome
ssDNA	Found in most systemic autoimmune diseases	No clinical utility
Scl-70	Scleroderma (70% in diffuse, 13% in limited)	Associated with a high incidence of pulmonary fibrosis
Serine protease	Wegener's granulomatosis (found in >80% of patients)	Specific for Wegener's, correlates with disease activity
Sm	SLE (20–30%)	Helpful in RNP negative subset of LE Highly specific for SLE, serves as a disease marker for SLE
Thyroglobulin	Autoimmune thyroiditis	
TSH receptor	Graves's disease	

ANA = Antinuclear antibody; CCP = Cyclic citrullinated peptide; DLE = Discoid lupus erythematosus; dsDNA = Double stranded deoxyribonucleic acid; Jo 1 = histidyl tRNA synthetase; NMDAR = *N*-methyl-D-aspartate receptor; RNP = Ribonucleoprotein; Pm-Scl = Polymyositis-scleroderma overlap syndrome-associated autoantigen; RF = Rheumatoid factor; Scl-70 = Topoisomerase 1; SLE = Systemic lupus erythematosus; Sm = Smith antigen

1. **D.** Atrophie blanche is a thrombogenic vasculopathy and NOT an interface dermatitis, shown in the image.

   While the histopathology varies with age of the lesion in atrophie blanche, the initial event is the formation of occlusive fibrin thrombi in small dermal vessels of the superficial and mid dermis.

   The primary histopathologic reaction pattern seen in vitiligo, subacute cutaneous lupus erythematosus (SCLE), eruption of lymphocyte recovery and Kindler's syndrome (autosomal recessive dermatosis characterized by acral trauma-induced blistering that improves with age and progressive poikiloderma in later life) is that of an interface dermatitis.

   Differentiating features of each include:

   Vitiligo – Interface dermatitis plus loss of pigment in basal keratinocytes plus loss of melanocytes

   SCLE – Pronounced interface dermatitis plus numerous dyskeratotic keratinocytes plus inflammation confined to the superficial dermis, direct immunofluorescence positive for "lupus band" (in only 60%)

   Kindler's syndrome – Interface dermatitis plus epidermal atrophy plus sparse inflammatory infiltrate

   Eruption of lymphocyte recovery – Interface dermatitis plus satellite cell necrosis plus perivascular infiltrate composed of small lymphocytes

2. **B.** Rowell's syndrome is best regarded as a variant of lupus with antibodies to Ro/La.

   First described in 1963 by Rowell *et al.*, Rowell's syndrome (RS) is clinically characterized by lupus erythematosus (LE)-like and erythema multiforme (EM)-like lesions, positive tests for rheumatoid factor (RF), speckled antinuclear antibody (ANA), and precipitating antibodies to Ro/La. Major and minor diagnostic criteria have been proposed for the diagnosis of this syndrome.

Major criteria include coexistence of LE- and EM-like lesions, and positive ANA with a speckled pattern.

Minor criteria include chilblains, positive anti-La (SS-B) or anti-Ro (SS-A) antibodies, and reactive RF.

All the major criteria and at least one of the minor criteria are required to confirm the diagnosis of RS.

3. **D.** Wegener's granulomatosis (WG) is characterized by antibodies to serine protease NOT myeloperoxidase.

Circulating antibodies to serine protease 3 are found in >80% of patients with WG *and are specific for WG.* While antibodies to myeloperoxidase are also seen occasionally in WG, they are not specific to Wegener's but are more commonly associated with microscopic polyangiitis.

All other antibody associations listed are specific (also see Table D4.2).

4. **A.** Antinuclear antibody (ANA) is not specific for any autoimmune disease entity.

Low levels of positivity may be found normally in older people and more commonly in females.

dsDNA – Specific for systemic lupus erythematosus (SLE)

Smith – Specific for SLE

Ro/SS-A – Found in subacute cutaneous LE (70%), primary Sjogren's syndrome (60–70%), SLE (30%), Rowell's syndrome, systemic sclerosis (<5%) and neonatal lupus (congenital heart block); it is particularly useful in ANA-negative lupus

La/SS-B – Found in primary Sjogren's syndrome (40–50%), SLE

SS-C (RAP) – Found in rheumatoid arthritis (67%) and SLE (7%)

Centromere – Found in CREST syndrome (70–95%) and progressive systemic sclerosis (10%); it is specific for CREST

Also see Table D4.2.

5. **B.** Follicular plugging is NOT a feature of subcutaneous lupus erythematosus (SCLE).

Cutaneous lesions of SCLE may be annular or psoriasiform. Follicular plugging, and scarring are typically absent. Criteria of SLE as defined by the American Rheumatism Association (ARA) include photosensitivity, arthralgias, serositis, renal disease and serologic abnormalities in the form of antibodies to Ro/SS-A and La/SS-B. Follicular plugging is a feature of discoid lupus erythematosus.

6. **C.** The lupus anticoagulant is NOT diagnostic for systemic lupus erythematosus (SLE).

The name lupus anticoagulant itself is a misnomer because the vast majority of patients actually do not have SLE. The lupus anticoagulant (LA) is a circulating IgG/IgM or both that interferes with one or more of the *in vitro* phospholipid dependent tests of coagulation. Clinical conditions associated with LA are several and include autoimmune disease (such as SLE and rheumatoid arthritis), drugs (chlorpromazine, procainamide, hydralazine, quinidine, phenytoin and antibiotics), infections (bacterial, viral and protozoa), and hematopoietic malignancies (such as lymphoma and hairy cell leukemia). While most inhibitors of coagulation are associated with clinical bleeding, LA is paradoxically associated with an increased risk of thrombosis.

7. **B.** Cutaneous manifestations of lupus anticoagulant (LA) do NOT include stasis dermatitis.

Cutaneous manifestations of LA include thrombophlebitis, Raynaud's phenomenon, subungual splinter hemorrhages, Sneddon's syndrome and livedo reticularis.

Stasis dermatitis, commonly seen in middle-aged or older individuals, is a consequence of impaired venous drainage of the legs and is not an autoimmune disease.

8. **E.** Factor VIII deficiency is not an observation associated with work-up of the lupus anticoagulant.

Factor VIII deficiency is observed in hemophilia A and is not an observation associated with work-up of the lupus anticoagulant.

The laboratory diagnosis of the lupus anticoagulant requires 3 distinct steps:

Step 1: Identification of an abnormal screening test (including prothrombin time, activated partial thromboplastin time)

Step 2: Proof that the abnormality is the result of an inhibitor

Step 3: Demonstration that the inhibitor is phospholipid dependent

9. **B.** dsDNA is the most commonly found circulating antibody specific for the diagnosis of systemic lupus erythematosus (SLE).

Autoantibodies to dsDNA, found in approximately 70% of patients with SLE, have both diagnostic and prognostic utility. High titers of anti-dsDNA are also associated with an increased risk of lupus nephritis. The other antibody specific for SLE is anti-smith (Sm). However, it is found in only 30% of patients with SLE.

10. **D.** The target antigen in bullous lupus erythematosus is collagen VII.

Type VII collagen, a component of anchoring fibrils, *is also targeted in epidermolysis bullosa acquisita (EBA).*

The diagnosis of bullous systemic lupus erythematosus requires the following elements:

- Fulfillment of the American College of Rheumatology criteria for systemic lupus erythematosus
- An acquired vesiculobullous eruption
- Histopathologic evidence of a subepidermal blister and a predominantly neutrophilic dermal infiltrate
- Direct immunofluorescence demonstrating immunoglobulin G (IgG, with or without immunoglobulin A (IgA) and immunoglobulin M (IgM)) deposits at the basement membrane zone (BMZ))
- Evidence of antibodies to type VII collagen *via* direct or indirect immunofluorescence on salt-split skin, immunoblotting, immunoprecipitation, enzyme-linked immunosorbent assay (ELISA), or immunoelectron microscopy

All 5 criteria listed above are needed for a diagnosis of type 1 bullous systemic lupus erythematosus, whereas only the first 4 criteria are needed to diagnose type 2 (undetermined location of antigen or dermal antigen other than type VII collagen) and type 3 (epidermal antigen) bullous systemic lupus erythematosus.

11. **B.** The target antigen in neonatal lupus erythematosus (NLE) is SSA/Ro.

Serum containing anti-SSA/Ro antibodies recognizes either the 52 kDa or 60 kDa protein from the Ro-RNP complex. The 52 kDa SSA/Ro (Ro52) ribonucleoprotein is an antigenic target strongly linked with the autoimmune response in mothers whose children have NLE and cardiac conduction disturbances, mainly congenital heart block. Anti-SSA/Ro52 autoantibodies recognize the Ro52 protein cardiac 5-HT4 serotoninergic receptor and inhibit serotonin-activated L-type calcium currents. This effect could explain the pathogenesis of the cardiac rhythm disturbances, which lead to an increased risk of diminished cardiac output and the subsequent development of congestive heart failure in these infants. The incidence of congenital heart block in infants with NLE is 15–30%. The mother produces immunoglobulin G (IgG) autoantibodies against Ro (SSA), La (SSB), and/or U1-ribonucleoprotein (U1-RNP), and they are passively transported across the placenta. The presence of maternal anti-SSA/Ro and anti-SSB/La antibodies increases the risk of bearing infants with NLE; rarely, NLE is due to maternal passage of U1-RNP antibodies. These autoantibodies can be found alone or in combination; *however, anti-Ro is present in almost 95% of patients.*

12. **E.** Pneumonia is NOT an extracutaneous manifestation of neonatal lupus erythematosus.

Neonatal lupus erythematosus (NLE) is thought to be caused by the transplacental passage of maternal autoantibodies; however, only 1–2% of infants with positive maternal autoantibodies develop neonatal lupus erythematosus. The most common clinical manifestations are dermatologic, cardiac, and hepatic. Some infants may also have hematologic, central nervous system, or splenic abnormalities. Although cutaneous, hematologic, and hepatic manifestations of NLE are transient, NLE has substantial associated morbidity and mortality, particularly when the heart is affected, which may occur in up to 65% of patients.

Cardiac NLE may manifest as complete or incomplete congenital heart block. Heart block may be evident in utero, detected during the second or third trimester, but is often undiagnosed until birth. The neonatal mortality rate of those with cardiac NLE is 20–30%. Most patients with NLE of the skin, liver, or blood have transient disease that spontaneously resolves within 4–6 months. Skin and hematologic manifestations usually improve with the disappearance of maternal autoantibodies. In some cases, severe liver failure may occur and is associated with a poor prognosis; death due to hepatitis may occur. Although cytopenias are self-limited, when severe thrombocytopenia is present, bleeding can affect the prognosis.

13. **C.** Image shown is that of a lymphocytic lobular panniculitis consistent with lupus profundus for which direct immunofluorescence is NOT diagnostic.

Lupus panniculitis, or lupus profundus, is a variant of lupus erythematosus that primarily affects subcutaneous fat. In nearly all cases there are deep, erythematous plaques and nodules, and some ulcers, which usually involve the proximal extremities, trunk, breasts, buttocks, and face. Lesions may be tender and painful and frequently heal with atrophy and scars. In 70% of patients with lupus panniculitis there will be preceding, subsequent, or concomitant lesions of discoid lupus erythematosus. Conversely, between 10 and 50% of patients with lupus panniculitis will have or eventually develop systemic lupus erythematosus. Most patients are adults between 20 and 60 years old, with a female:male ratio of approximately 2:1. Lupus panniculitis is a chronic condition that often involves persistent lesions that subsequently heal with disfigurement.

Diagnosis is confirmed primarily by both clinical and histologic findings. Diagnostic histopathologic features, as shown in the image, are that of a lymphocytic lobular panniculitis with hyalinized fat necrosis. A characteristic feature is the presence of reactive lymphoid follicles noted in 20–50% of cases. Mucinous changes and foci of calcification can be seen. Involvement of the overlying epidermis in the form of epidermal atrophy, interface change and a perivascular and periappendageal lymphocytic inflammation can be seen and is typically more common in cases in which lupus profundus develops as a complication of discoid lupus erythematosus. *Direct immunofluorescence is typically negative.*

Although often normal, serological analysis may show a positive antinuclear antibody titer. Less frequently, anti-double stranded DNA antibodies will be present. Syphilis serology may be falsely positive. Other possible laboratory findings are lymphopenia, anemia, reduction of C4 levels, and rheumatoid factor.

14. E. Leukocytoclastic vasculitis is not a histopathologic finding observed in early lesions of graft-versus-host disease (GVHD).

Based upon the time of onset of disease, GVHD has been divided into acute and chronic forms:

Acute GVHD – Manifestations of GVHD occurring within 100 days after hematopoietic cell transplant (HCT)
Chronic GVHD – Manifestations of GVHD occurring more than 100 days after HCT

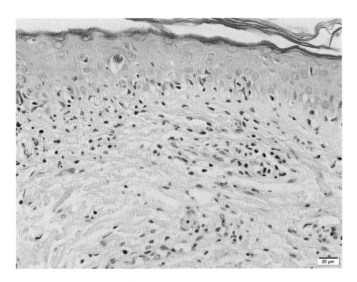

Key histopathologic findings in acute cutaneous GVHD, shown in the image above, include epidermal apoptotic keratinocytes, interface dermatitis and a mild lymphocytic infiltrate in the superficial dermis. Apoptotic keratinocytes may also be present in the follicular epithelium. The lymphocytic infiltrate can be sparse and perivascular or more extensive. Migration of lymphocytes into the superficial layers of the epidermis (lymphocyte exocytosis) is common. The presence of satellite cell necrosis (two or more lymphocytes surrounding an apoptotic keratinocyte) also supports a diagnosis of acute GVHD. Fulminant lesions demonstrate subepidermal clefting and full-thickness necrosis of the epidermis.

The criteria often used for categorizing the histopathologic findings in acute GVHD are as follows:

Grade 0 – Normal skin or changes not referable to GVHD
Grade 1 – Vacuolization of the basal layer at the dermal-epidermal junction

Grade 2 – Basal layer vacuolization, necrotic epidermal cells, lymphocytic infiltrate
Grade 3 – Grade 2 changes plus cleft formation at the dermal-epidermal junction
Grade 4 – Grade 2 changes plus separation of the epidermis from the dermis

The sensitivity and specificity of skin biopsy for acute GVHD has not been definitively established. In general, a diagnosis of acute cutaneous GVHD is supported by the appearance of a consistent cutaneous eruption occurring in a time period that correlates with the return of lymphocytes to the peripheral circulation (lymphocyte recovery) and at least grade 2 changes on histopathologic examination. Biopsies taken early in the course of GVHD may reveal non-diagnostic findings and essentially normal skin.

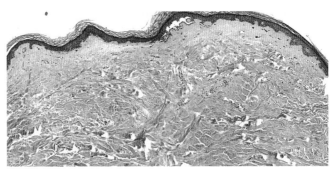

The histopathologic changes in chronic GVHD, shown in the image above, vary according to the type of skin involvement. The classic findings in lichen planus-like and sclerotic lesions include:

Lichen planus-like lesions – Lichen planus-like papules and plaques reveal findings that resemble lichen planus, with hyperkeratosis, hypergranulosis, acanthosis, saw-tooth rete, interface dermatitis, and dyskeratotic keratinocytes. Periadnexal inflammation, particularly around eccrine glands, is evident in some cases.
Sclerotic lesions – Sclerotic skin involvement may or may not demonstrate overlying epidermal changes of lichen planus-like disease. Lichen sclerosus-like lesions characteristically show epidermal atrophy with edema and homogenization of collagen in the superficial dermis. Morpheaform lesions demonstrate thickened collagen bundles in the dermis with loss of adnexal structures, and in the absence of epidermal changes, may be indistinguishable from specimens from true morphea or systemic sclerosis. As in these other disorders, specimens from lesions of sclerotic chronic GVHD often have a square or "box car" shape to the biopsy. Sclerotic GVHD involving the subcutaneous tissue demonstrates a lymphocytic infiltrate near the interface of dermis and fat with thickening of the septae.

15. **A.** Kindler's syndrome is characterized histopathologically by poikiloderma shown in the image.

    Kindler's syndrome is a rare autosomal recessive genodermatosis characterized by acral trauma-induced blistering that improves with age and by progressive poikiloderma later in life.

    Cutaneous manifestations of other entities listed include:

    Muir-Torre syndrome – Sebaceous neoplasms (outside of the head and neck area in individuals <40 years of age) and keratoacanthomas
    Birt-Hogg-Dubé syndrome – Fibrofolliculomas
    Basal cell nevus syndrome – Multiple basal cell carcinomas, palmoplantar pits, skeletal malformations
    Chediak-Higashi syndrome – Oculocutaneous albinism

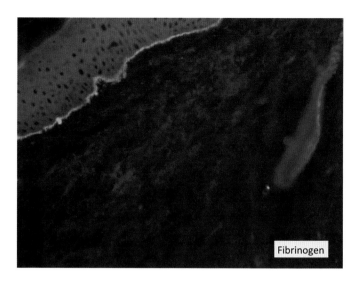

Fibrinogen

16. **D.** Clinical correlates of lichen planus (LP) shown in the image include the presence of polygonal papules.

    Histopathologic features of LP include hyperkeratosis, irregular epidermal hyperplasia ("saw-toothed") with hypergranulosis and scattered individually necrotic dyskeratotic keratinocytes, interface change and a mild to moderate lichenoid lymphoid cell infiltrate with pigment incontinence. Clinically, lesions of LP initially develop on flexural surfaces of the limbs, with a generalized eruption developing after a week or more and maximal spreading within 2–16 weeks. Pruritus of varying severity, depending on the type of lesion and the extent of involvement, is typical. In addition to the widespread cutaneous eruption, lichen planus can involve the mucous membranes, genitalia, nails and scalp. Oral lesions may occur and may be asymptomatic, burning, or even painful. In cutaneous disease, lesions typically resolve within 6 months (>50%) to 18 months (85%); chronic disease is more likely with oral lichen planus or with large, annular, hypertrophic lesions and mucous membrane involvement.

17. **B.** The best-fit diagnosis for the image shown is hypertrophic lichen planus (LP).

    Key histopathologic features of hypertrophic LP include irregular epidermal hyperplasia with hypergranulosis and interface change with an underlying lichenoid inflammatory infiltrate that is *confined to the tips of the rete ridges*. Clinically, hypertrophic LP lesions are typically confined to the shins. They appear as single or multiple pruritic plaques which can have a verrucous appearance. Squamous cell carcinoma may develop in long-standing lesions.

18. **B.** A shaggy fibrin band is the single best indicator of the diagnosis of lichen planus.

This finding is however only observed in approximately 50% of cases of lichen planus. The presence of Civatte bodies, which is a poorer indicator than the shaggy deposition of fibrin along the dermoepidermal junction, is found in even fewer cases (approximately 20%).

19. **C.** Lichen planopilaris is NOT synonymous with ashy dermatosis.

    Ashy dermatosis or erythema dyschromicum perstans or lichen planus pigmentosus is a slowly progressive, asymptomatic, ash-colored macular area of hyperpigmentation. Its prevalence is highest in Latin America. Lesions are often widespread. This entity is regarded by some as a macular variant of lichen planus.

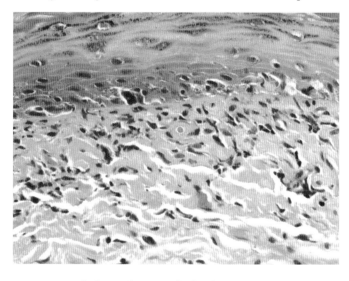

Histopathologic changes of ashy dermatosis, shown in the image, include an interface dermatitis and a lichenoid lymphoid inflammatory infiltrate with pigment incontinence. In active lesions, the interface change is prominent, while in older lesions pigment incontinence may be the only feature. The inflammatory infiltrate, although milder than in lichen planus, extends deeper. Lichen planopilaris is a clinically heterogeneous variant of lichen planus in which keratotic follicular lesions are present, often in association with other manifestations of lichen planus.

20. **D.** An eosinophil-rich inflammatory infiltrate is NOT a typical histopathologic feature of lichen planus (LP).

The presence of eosinophils with/without parakeratosis argues away from LP and is more indicative of a lichenoid drug reaction. Histopathologic features of LP include irregular/saw-toothed or wedge-shaped acanthosis with hypergranulosis, interface change with Civatte bodies and a lichenoid inflammatory infiltrate with pigment incontinence.

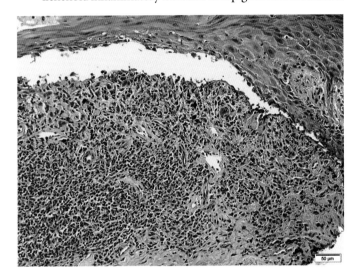

Small clefts known as Caspary-Joseph spaces, shown in the image above, may be seen at the dermoepidermal junction secondary to damage to the basal layer. Involvement of the eccrine ducts adjacent to the acrosyringium has been noted in select cases.

21. **B.** Graham Little-Picccardi-Lasseur (GLPL) syndrome is characterized by cicatricial alopecia and follicular keratotic lesions.

GLPL syndrome is essentially a variant of lichen planopilaris. The syndrome consists of a triad of spinous/ acuminated follicular lesions, typical cutaneous/mucosal lichen planus and alopecia of the scalp with/without atrophy. These features *need not be present simultaneously.*

22. **D.** Based on the clinical presentation and histopathologic features shown in the image, the most likely diagnosis is lichen planopilaris (LPP).

Key histopathologic features of LPP include an interface dermatitis with involvement of the follicular epithelium (infundibulum and isthmus mainly) and a lichenoid and perifollicular lymphoid inflammatory infiltrate. LPP is *the*

prototypic lymphocyte scarring alopecia. Differentiating features from discoid lupus erythematosus (DLE), also a lymphocyte scarring alopecia, include the presence of a predominantly peri-infundibular and peri-isthmic inflammatory infiltrate in LPP and perifollicular mucin ("perifollicular mucinous fibrosis"). In DLE, the mucin is in the interstitium and typically confined to the interfollicular dermis, and interface change is not confined merely to follicular epithelia but is also noted between follicles at the dermoepidermal junction. Key histopathologic features of central centrifugal cicatricial alopecia (CCCA), also a lymphocyte scarring alopecia, include follicular miniaturization and asymmetry, premature desquamation of the inner root sheath and compound follicles with perifollicular fibrosis ("goggle" sign).

23. **C.** The most likely diagnosis for the image shown is lichen nitidus.

Key histopathologic features of lichen nitidus consist of a lymphohistiocytic inflammatory cell infiltrate that lies in close proximity to the epidermis with overlying interface change. The overlying epidermis is flattened and may be parakeratotic. At the lateral margins of the papule, the rete ridges extend downward and seem to hug ("ball and claw") the inflammatory infiltrate, which may be granulomatous. Lichen nitidus is a relatively rare, chronic skin eruption that is characterized clinically by asymptomatic, flat-topped, skin-colored "micropapules." Lichen nitidus mainly affects children and young adults. The primary lesions consist of multiple 1–3 mm, sharply demarcated, round or polygonal, flat-topped, skin-colored shiny papules that often appear in groups. The Köbner phenomenon (or an isomorphic response) may be observed. This phenomenon causes the occasional linear pattern of the lesions associated with lichen nitidus. The most common sites of involvement are the trunk, flexor aspects of upper extremities, dorsal aspects of hands, and genitalia.

24. **A.** Based on the clinical presentation and histopathologic features shown in the image, the most likely diagnosis is lichen striatus.

Histopathologic findings in lichen striatus vary depending on the stage of evolution, but typically consist of a patchy interface and lichenoid dermatitis. Of note, and a diagnostic finding, is that the inflammatory infiltrate extends deep into the dermis and surrounds the hair follicles and eccrine sweat glands and ducts. Clinically, lichen striatus is a rare, benign, self-limited linear dermatosis of unknown origin that predominantly affects children. It is clinically diagnosed on the basis of its appearance and characteristic developmental pattern following the lines of Blaschko. Lichen striatus often appears as a sudden eruption of small papules on an extremity. The papules are usually asymptomatic, reaching maximum involvement within several days to weeks. When lichen striatus patients are symptomatic, the most common complaint is pruritus. It is self-limited, but may resolve with post-inflammatory hyperpigmentation or hypopigmentation.

25. **B.** The presence of parakeratosis and eosinophils in the infiltrate is typical of a lichenoid drug eruption.

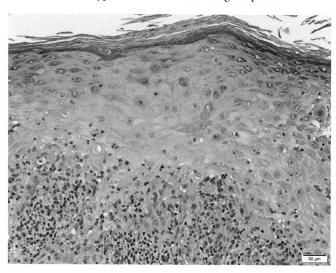

Histopathologic findings that are more typical of lichenoid drug eruption, also called drug-induced lichen planus, include focal parakeratosis, cytoid bodies in the cornified and granular layers, presence of eosinophils, a higher number of necrotic keratinocytes as well as plasma cells and eosinophils, exocytosis of lymphoid cells into the upper epidermis and a deeper perivascular infiltrate. *These features are seen more often in non-photodistributed lesions. Photodistributed lesions are usually indistinguishable from idiopathic lichen planus.* Direct immunofluorescence shows findings indistinguishable from classic lichen planus.

Clinically, a lichenoid drug eruption is characterized by a symmetric eruption of flat-topped, erythematous or violaceous papules resembling lichen planus on the trunk and extremities. The time interval between the initiation of the offending drug and the appearance of the cutaneous lesions varies from months to a year or more and depends upon the class of drug, dose, host reaction, and concurrent medications.

Drugs commonly associated with a cutaneous lichenoid eruption include:
- ACE inhibitors
- Thiazide diuretics
- Antimalarials
- Beta blockers
- Gold salts
- Penicillamine

Cases induced by tumor necrosis factor-alpha antagonists (e.g., infliximab, adalimumab, etanercept, and lenercept) and tyrosine kinase inhibitors (e.g., imatinib) have also been reported.

Drugs commonly associated with lichenoid eruptions primarily involving the oral mucosa include:
- Allopurinol
- ACE inhibitors
- Gold salts
- Ketoconazole
- NSAIDs
- Anticonvulsants
- Antiretrovirals

26. **C.** Based on the clinical presentation and histopathologic features shown in the image, the most likely diagnosis is erythema multiforme.

In established lesions of erythema multiforme (EM), the histopathologic reaction pattern is that of an interface dermatitis with scattered individually necrotic dyskeratotic keratinocytes within or just above the basal layer of the epidermis and an accompanying dermal infiltrate of varied densities composed predominantly of lymphocytes (although occasional eosinophils have been noted in scattered reports). Typically *there are no changes in the horn* which is usually basket-weave.

Erythema multiforme is an acute, self-limited, and sometimes recurring skin condition that is considered to be a type IV hypersensitivity reaction associated with certain infections, medications, and other various triggers. Erythema multiforme can present with a wide spectrum of severity. Cutaneous papules evolve into pathognomonic target or iris lesions that appear within a 72-hour period and typically begin on the extremities. Lesions remain in a fixed location for at least 7 days and then begin to heal. Precipitating factors include herpes simplex virus, Epstein-Barr virus, and histoplasmosis. Because this condition may be related to a persistent antigenic stimulus, *recurrence is the rule* rather than the exception, with most affected individuals experiencing 1–2 recurrences per year.

27. **A.** Based on the clinical presentation and histopathologic features shown in the image, the most likely diagnosis is toxic epidermal necrolysis (TEN).

TEN is a clinical diagnosis, confirmed by histopathologic analysis of lesional skin. Skin biopsy, harvested at the earliest possible stage, *is important in establishing an accurate diagnosis* and directing specific therapeutic modalities. Necrotic keratinocytes with full-thickness epithelial necrosis and detachment and a minimal inflammatory infiltrate is consistent with the diagnosis of TEN. Clinically, TEN is a potentially life-threatening dermatologic disorder characterized by widespread erythema, necrosis, and bullous detachment of the epidermis and mucous membranes, resulting in exfoliation and possible sepsis and/or death. Mucous membrane involvement can result in gastrointestinal hemorrhage, respiratory failure, ocular abnormalities, and genitourinary complications. Mucous membrane erosions (seen in 90% of cases) generally *precede the skin lesions* by 1–3 days. The most frequently affected mucosal membrane is the oropharynx, followed by the eyes and genitalia. Most cases of TEN are drug induced, typically occurring within 1–3 weeks of therapy initiation and rarely occurring after more than 8 weeks. The most commonly implicated agents include:

- Sulfonamide antibiotics
- Antiepileptic drugs
- Non-steroidal anti-inflammatory drugs
- Allopurinol

28. **D.** Pityriasis lichenoides et varioliformis acuta (PLEVA/ Mucha-Habermann disease) is best classified as a lymphocytic vasculitis.

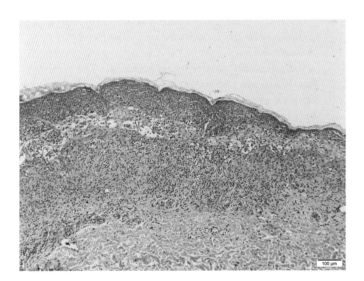

Histopathologic findings of PLEVA, shown in the image, typically encompass three distinct reaction patterns: a lymphocytic vasculitis, interface dermatitis with numerous individually necrotic, dyskeratotic keratinocytes at all levels of the epidermis, and a lichenoid dermatitis with an infiltrate that is composed predominantly of lymphocytes.

29. **B.** Lymphomatoid papulosis is not part of the same spectrum as pityriasis lichenoides chronica.

Pityriasis lichenoides chronica (PLC) represents one end of a self-limiting dermatosis with pityriasis lichenoides et varioliformis acuta (PLEVA) and *not* lymphomatoid papulosis at the other. Despite the unifying features of lymphomatoid papulosis and PLEVA in terms of clinical presentation (hemorrhagic and ulcerating papulonodular lesions) and presence of CD30+ atypical lymphocytes, they are *pathogenetically distinct entities*. Pityriasis lichenoides is a self-limiting dermatosis of unknown etiopathogenesis with a spectrum of clinical and histopathologic changes. At one end is PLEVA, clinically characterized by hemorrhagic papules and nodules and histopathologically by a lymphocytic vasculitis and an interface and lichenoid dermatitis (see above). At the other end is PLC, clinically characterized by a scaly, red/brown maculopapular rash.

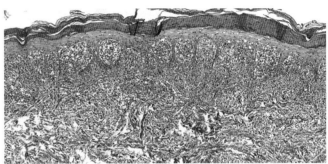

Unifying histopathologic features of PLEVA and PLC, shown in the image above, are a lymphocytic vasculitis and interface dermatitis. Overall, the density of the infiltrate in PLC is less than that observed in PLEVA.

30. **E.** No single histopathologic feature is of utility in differentiating primary perniosis from lupus-related perniosis.

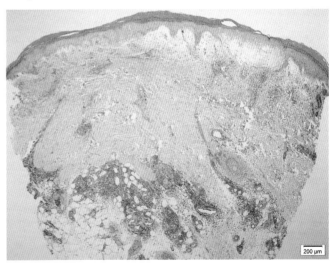

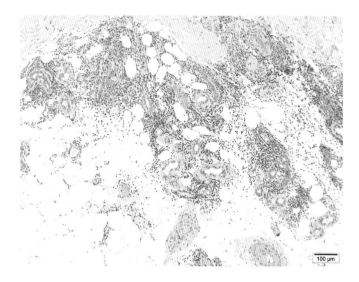

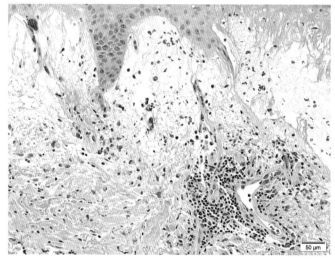

Both primary perniosis and lupus-related perniosis exhibit similar histopathologic findings. These include (from top to bottom):

- Papillary dermal edema
- Interface change (more widespread in lupus-related perniosis)
- Lymphocytic vasculitis involving superficial and deep vessels
- Perivascular and periadnexal lymphocytic infiltrate
- Extravasated erythrocytes

31. **D.** Image shown is that of lichen sclerosus which is NOT always associated with morphea.

    Histopathologic findings of an established lesion of lichen sclerosus (LS) demonstrate hyperkeratosis, follicular plugging, epidermal atrophy, basal vacuolar change, subepidermal edema with homogenization of papillary dermal collagen and a lichenoid lymphoid cell infiltrate. While the inflammatory infiltrate abuts the epidermis in very early lesions, as the lesion ages, it gets pushed further below the epidermis.

Elastophagocytosis may be noted in extragenital lesions. A spectrum of vascular changes may be associated. Briefly, these include leukocytoclastic vasculitis, lymphocytic vasculitis and, albeit rarely, granulomatous phlebitis. While the coexistence of morphea and LS has been noted in more than one case report, lichen sclerosus is not always associated with morphea. Guttate lesions of morphea are more superficial and can resemble LS.

Clinically, LS is a chronic inflammatory dermatosis that results in white plaques ("porcelain-white" plaques) with epidermal atrophy and scarring. Lichen sclerosus has both genital and extragenital presentations and also goes by the names lichen sclerosus et atrophicus (dermatological literature), balanitis xerotica obliterans (glans penis presentation), and kraurosis vulvae (older description of vulvar presentation). An increased risk of squamous cell carcinoma may exist in genital disease, but the precise increase in risk and what cofactors (human papillomavirus infection or prior radiotherapy) may be involved are not yet completely defined. In terms of incidence, vulvar and penile LS outnumber extragenital LS by >5:1. Male genital lichen sclerosus is seen almost exclusively in uncircumcised or incompletely circumcised men and boys. A genetic predisposition, based on family clustering, is apparent. The male-to-female ratio is 1:6, with female genital cases making up the bulk of reports. Up to 15% of cases are in children with the majority being vulvar presentations. A study of foreskins submitted after therapeutic circumcision for phimosis revealed many cases of unrecognized lichen sclerosus. Extragenital lichen sclerosus is rare in children. The isomorphic (Koebner) phenomenon has been described in LS, with the resultant lesions in old surgical scars, burn scars, sunburned areas, and areas subject to repeated trauma.

32. **E.** Pautrier microabscesses are NOT a histopathologic feature of lichen sclerosus.

    Histopathologic findings have been described in the previous answer. Pautrier microabscesses are a feature of mycosis fungoides not lichen sclerosus.

33. **E.** Parakeratosis and acanthosis with mild spongiosis are the histopathologic findings observed in small plaque parapsoriasis.

    Histopathology of small plaque parapsoriasis is entirely non-specific and includes epidermal changes in the form of parakeratosis and acanthosis with mild/minimal spongiosis and dermal changes in the form of a mild superficial perivascular lymphocytic infiltrate composed of both CD4+ and CD8+ T-cells (although CD4+ T-cells are predominant). In terms of cytomorphology, lesional lymphocytes are small and do not show atypical features. Clinically, small plaque parapsoriasis (persistent superficial dermatitis, digitate dermatosis, chronic superficial dermatitis) presents as well-defined, round to oval patches with a fine "cigarette-paper" scale that have a predilection for the trunk and proximal portion of extremities. Onset typically occurs in middle life with a male predominance.

34. **C.** Histopathologic features of paraneoplastic pemphigus (PNP) are NOT diagnostic.

    Paraneoplastic pemphigus (PNP) is an autoimmune blistering disorder characterized by antibodies to multiple antigens including members of the plakin and desmoglein family. Antibodies to dsg1 and/or dsg3 are usually present. Of note, and in contrast to pemphigus vulgaris (in which the dominant subclass is IgG4), the antibody response to dsg3 includes IgG1 and IgG2 subclasses. In keeping with the clinical heterogeneity, histopathologic features of paraneoplastic pemphigus are variable and include a lichenoid and interface dermatitis in conjunction with suprabasal acantholysis. Direct immunofluorescence is diagnostic and shows intercellular as well as basement membrane zone staining.

35. **D.** Majoccchi's granuloma is not a variant of pigmented purpuric dermatosis.

    Clinical variants of pigmented purpuric dermatosis (PPD) include the following:

    Schamberg's disease (progressive pigmentary dermatosis) – The most common type, clinically presents as pin-head sized macules with a reddish-brown ("cayenne pepper") color with a predilection for the pretibial region and ankles
    Majocchi's disease – Is essentially an annular form of Schamberg's disease with a perifollicular distribution
    Gougerot-Blum disease – Clinically presents as lichenoid papules and macules, usually in association with Schamberg's disease
    Lichen aureus – Clinically presents as grouped macules or lichenoid papules with a predilection for the head and neck area
    Purpuric contact dermatitis – The least well known and a form of allergic contact dermatitis clinically presents as purpuric and hemorrhagic areas distributed in clothed areas

    Majocccchi's granuloma is the clinical term used for a nodular lesion of the lower leg with a predilection for females and showing a histopathologic picture consistent with a granulomatous perifolliculitis. Fungi that have been implicated are several and include *Trichophyton rubrum, Microsporum canis, T. violaceum, T. tonsurans, T. mentographytes* and *Aspergillus fumigatus.*

36. **C.** Hemosiderin deposits would not be present in an early lesion of pigmented purpuric dermatosis (PPD).

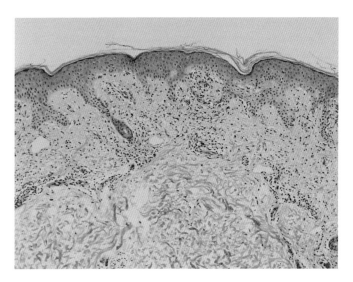

Histopathologic features of an early lesion of PPD, shown in the image above, include a band-like infiltrate composed of lymphocytes of the T helper phenotype (CD4+), a lymphocytic vasculitis and extravasated erythrocytes.

While epidermotropism is typically not a feature of an early lesion of PPD, there are several reports indicating an overlap between the histopathologic picture of early PPD and that of an early lesion of mycosis fungoides. Overlapping histopathologic features include lymphocyte epidermotropism and a lichenoid infiltrate composed predominantly of CD4+ T lymphocytes.

37. **E.** The inflammatory infiltrate in perniosis involves the papillary as well as the reticular dermis.

    Infiltrates filling the papillary dermis are best characterized by the mnemonic LUMP – which stands for *l*ichenoid dermatitis, *u*rticarial pigmentosa, *m*ycosis fungoides and *p*igmented purpuric dermatosis. Histopathologic features of perniosis include a superficial and deep perivascular and periadnexal lymphocytic infiltrate, lymphocytic vasculitis, papillary dermal edema, +/− interface change and extravasated erythrocytes.

38. **D.** The most likely diagnosis for the image shown is lichen amyloidosus.

    Lichen amyloidosus and macular amyloidosis are clinical variants of primary localized cutaneous amyloidosis (LCA) and represent the same process. Histopathologic features of lichen amyloidosus and macular amyloidosis are essentially the same and consist of amorphous, eosinophilic deposits in the papillary dermis with pigment incontinence. *The presence of pigmented cells is an important clue to the diagnosis of LCA.*

    Patients with features of both or transformation from one to another (biphasic form) are well documented in the literature. Clinically, lichen amyloidosus typically presents as an intensely itchy eruption. It presents as intensely pruritic, red-brown hyperkeratotic papules most commonly seen on the pretibial surfaces, but it can also occur on the feet and the thighs.

Lichen amyloidosus has been reported in association with few syndromes. The most intriguing is the association with multiple endocrine neoplasia type 2A (MEN 2A), also known as Sipple syndrome. The cardinal triad of this autosomal dominant syndrome is medullary thyroid carcinoma, pheochromocytoma, and hyperparathyroidism. The lichen amyloidosus in this syndrome is usually localized to the interscapular region and consists of lichenoid papules, with hyperpigmentation and fine scaling.

39. **A.** The most useful stain in confirming the presence of localized cutaneous amyloidosis (LCA) is CK5/6.

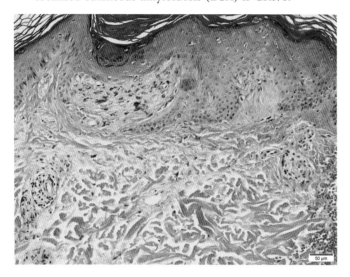

Amongst special stains, crystal violet has been shown to be superior to the Congo red stain in identifying deposits in LCA. LCA deposits typically do not exhibit the apple-green birefringence noted in systemic amyloidosis. Positive staining of the deposits with the high molecular weight cytokeratins (5/6 and 903) is the gold standard for the identification of localized cutaneous amyloidosis as it is keratinocyte-derived amyloid.

40. **D.** Given the complete absence of melanin in the basal layer and loss of basal melanocytes, the most likely diagnosis for the image shown is vitiligo.

Of other entities listed:

- Oculocutaneous albinism and Chediak-Higashi syndrome are characterized histopathologically by complete loss of melanin in the basal layer as well as the hair bulbs but by a normal density and morphology of basal melanocytes
- Nevus depigmentosus and pityriasis alba are characterized by decreased melanin but a normal density of basal melanocytes

41. **B.** Image shown is that of cornoid lamellae which represents an area of faulty keratinization.

The cornoid lamella is a column of parakeratotic cells with an underlying absent granular cell layer and

occasional, individually necrotic, dyskeratotic keratinocytes. As the lesion ages, the parakeratotic column tends to become more horizontal and less protuberant. Although the key histopathologic feature of porokeratosis, it can be seen as an incidental finding as a reaction pattern in almost any entity. Historically, porokeratosis is a misnomer in that it was erroneously coined on the assumptions that cornoid lamellae emerged from pores of the sweat glands. Clinically recognized variants of porokeratosis include:

- Classic porokeratosis of Mibelli
- Disseminated superficial actinic porokeratosis and its non-actinic variant disseminated superficial porokeratosis
- Linear porokeratosis
- Porokeratosis palmaris et plantaris disseminata
- Punctate porokeratosis

A patient may develop more than one type of porokeratosis simultaneously or consecutively.

D5 Vasculopathic Reaction Patterns Questions

1. The image shown is best characterized as:

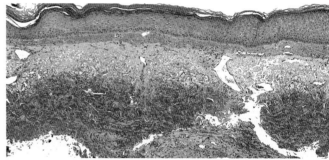

   A. An occlusive vasculopathy
   B. Non-inflammatory purpura
   C. A drug reaction
   D. Autoimmune purpura

2. Livedo reticularis:
   A. Is a clinical manifestation of vascular occlusive disease
   B. Is a clinical feature of chronic lymphocytic vasculitis
   C. Exhibits distinct serology
   D. Is typically associated with Henoch-Schönlein purpura

3. Protein C:
   A. Is usually autosomal recessive
   B. Deficiency protects against warfarin-induced necrosis
   C. The inactivated form has an anticoagulant function
   D. Is a vitamin K dependent glycoprotein
   E. Is independent of protein S for anticoagulant function

4. Protein S:
   A. Is not a serine protease

B. Deficiency protects against warfarin-induced necrosis

C. Is only produced by plasma cells

D. Is a vitamin K independent glycoprotein

E. Serves as a cofactor for prothrombin

5. Warfarin-induced necrosis:
   A. Manifests as non-tender plaques on the extremities
   B. Typically occurs within the first week of warfarin therapy
   C. Is related to low levels of factor IX
   D. Occurs independent of factor V Leiden deficiency
   E. Is characterized histopathologically by leukocytoclastic vasculitis

6. The primary event in atrophie blanche is a/n:
   A. Non-inflammatory purpura
   B. Leukocytoclastic vasculitis
   C. Lymphocytic vasculitis
   D. Occlusive vasculopathy
   E. Urticarial vasculitis

7. Atrophie blanche:
   A. Is secondary to increased fibrinolytic activity
   B. Is secondary to warfarin-induced necrosis
   C. Is synonymous with livedoid vasculopathy
   D. Is never seen in association with livedo reticularis
   E. Is characterized by a non-inflammatory purpura histopathologically

8. Which of the following is correct regarding disseminated intravascular coagulation (DIC):
   A. Typically acquired
   B. Cutaneous involvement is typical
   C. Early lesions characterized by leukocytoclastic vasculitis
   D. Typically associated with increased protein C

9. Laboratory abnormalities in acute disseminated intravascular coagulation (DIC) include:
   A. Shortened activated partial thromboplastin time (APTT)
   B. Shortened prothrombin time (PT) and thrombin time (TT)
   C. Increased protein C
   D. Decreased fibrinogen
   E. Decreased D-dimer

10. Regarding cryoglobulins:
    A. Type I is a cold-insoluble monoclonal protein
    B. Type I is associated with hepatitis C
    C. Type II is a cold-insoluble monoclonal protein
    D. Type I may have rheumatoid factor activity
    E. Type III is a cold-insoluble monoclonal protein

11. Regarding histopathologic reaction pattern/s of cryoglobulinemia:
    A. Type I is characterized by lymphocytic vasculitis
    B. Type III is characterized by leukocytoclastic vasculitis
    C. Type II is characterized by senile purpura

D. Type III is characterized by a mixed pattern (occlusive vasculopathy and vasculitis)

12. Which of the following does NOT exhibit the histopathologic reaction pattern shown:

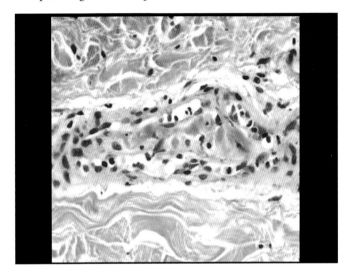

   A. Senile purpura
   B. Protein C/S deficiency
   C. Factor V Leiden deficiency
   D. Atrophie blanche
   E. Warfarin necrosis

13. The lupus anticoagulant:
    A. Is a circulating IgA
    B. Does not interfere with phospholipid-dependent coagulation tests
    C. Is not diagnostic for systemic lupus erythematosus
    D. Is associated with an increased risk of bleeding

14. Which of the following is NOT a cutaneous manifestation of the lupus anticoagulant:
    A. Thrombophlebitis
    B. Stasis dermatitis
    C. Raynaud's phenomenon
    D. Subungual hemorrhages
    E. Sneddon's syndrome

15. Laboratory findings in the work-up of lupus anticoagulant include:
    A. Normal prothrombin time
    B. Normal screening test
    C. Absence of an inhibitor
    D. Demonstration of a phospholipid-independent inhibitor
    E. Normal factor VIII levels

16. Regarding skin biopsies in Sneddon's syndrome:
    A. A superficial biopsy is diagnostic
    B. Deep dermal vessels are typically affected
    C. Biopsy of a "red" area increases the sensitivity
    D. Papillary dermal edema is an early change
    E. Leukocytoclastic vasculitis is a late change

17. Regarding histopathology of leukocytoclastic vasculitis:
    A. Diagnostic features are best seen in lesions that are <1 day old
    B. Changes characteristically involve deep dermal vessels
    C. Fibrin thrombi within vessels is typical
    D. Eosinophils are present in early lesions

18. Regarding direct immunofluorescence in leukocytoclastic vasculitis :
    A. In fully developed lesions only IgM deposits are evident
    B. In late lesions, only IgG deposits are evident
    C. Biopsy of non-lesional skin is most informative
    D. Biopsy of lesional skin is most informative
    E. Serology is helpful in confirming the diagnosis

19. In the 2012 Chapel Hill Consensus Conference criteria, Henoch-Schönlein purpura is best described as:
    A. An ANCA-associated small vessel vasculitis
    B. A medium vessel vasculitis
    C. A large vessel vasculitis
    D. An immune-complex small vessel vasculitis
    E. An anti-endothelial cell antibody vasculitis

20. Which of the following does NOT typically involve small vessels:
    A. Henoch-Schönlein purpura
    B. Cryoglobulinemia
    C. Kawasaki disease
    D. Microscopic polyangiitis
    E. Leukocytoclastic vasculitis

21. Which of the following is NOT a feature of urticarial vasculitis:
    A. Papillary dermal edema
    B. Leukocytoclasia and fibrinoid necrosis
    C. Eosinophilic infiltration of vessel walls
    D. Involvement of the superficial plexus
    E. Involvement of deep dermal vessels

22. A mixed (occlusive vasculopathic and leukocytoclastic vasculitis) pattern is typically seen in:
    A. Protein C deficiency
    B. Warfarin-induced necrosis
    C. Cryoglobulinemia I
    D. Factor V Leiden mutation
    E. Levamisole-induced vasculopathy, ecchymosis and necrosis (LIVEN)

23. Regarding histopathologic features of erythema elevatum diutinum:
    A. Changes are static throughout the disease
    B. Acute and chronic lesions involve medium-sized vessels
    C. Early lesions are characterized by vasculitis
    D. Early lesions resemble dermatofibroma
    E. Established lesions demonstrate a pandermal eosinophilic infiltrate

24. Regarding the entity shown:

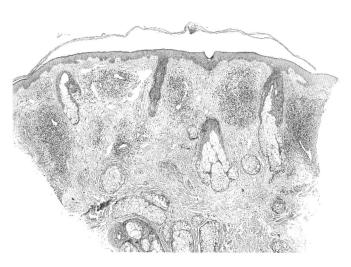

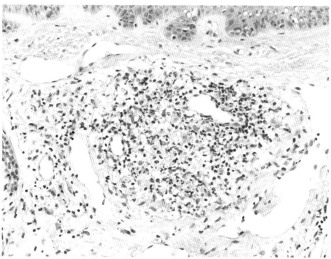

    A. Extrafacial involvement is uncommon
    B. Solitary lesions are uncommon
    C. Grenz zone is uncommon
    D. Monomorphous infiltrate is common
    E. Occlusive vasculopathy is common

25. The 2012 Chapel Hill Consensus Conference definitions of anti-neutrophil cytoplasmic antibody-associated vasculitis (AAV) include all of the following EXCEPT:
    A. Granulomatosis with polyangiitis
    B. Microscopic polyangiitis
    C. Leukocytoclastic vasculitis
    D. Eosinophilic granulomatosis with polyangiitis

26. Proteinase 3 (PR3)-specific anti-neutrophil cytoplasmic antibodies are most often associated with:
    A. Granulomatosis with polyangiitis
    B. Microscopic polyangiitis
    C. Leukocytoclastic vasculitis

D. Eosinophilic granulomatosis with polyangiitis

E. Henoch-Schönlein purpura

27. Myeloperoxidase (MPO) anti-neutrophil cytoplasmic antibodies are most often associated with:

A. Granulomatosis with polyangiitis

B. Microscopic polyangiitis

C. Leukocytoclastic vasculitis

D. Eosinophilic granulomatosis with polyangiitis

E. Henoch-Schönlein purpura

28. The lesion shown is best regarded as a latent form of:

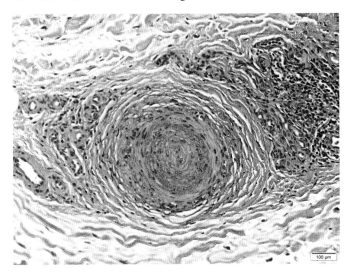

A. Granuloma faciale

B. Erythema elevatum diutinum

C. Urticarial vasculitis

D. Polyarteritis nodosa

E. Kawasaki syndrome

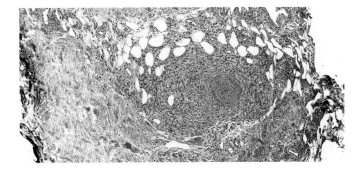

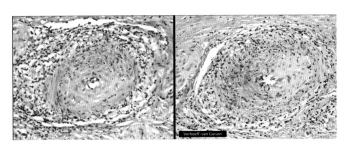

29. The cutaneous variant of the entity shown:

A. Is typically ANCA positive

B. Has an acute clinical course

C. Involves superficial dermal vessels

D. Is diagnostic in a superficial biopsy

E. Serology is non-diagnostic

30. Pruritic urticarial papules and plaques of pregnancy (PUPPP):

A. Is synonymous with polymorphous eruption of pregnancy

B. Usually begins in the first trimester

C. Is more common in multigravidas

D. Adversely effects on fetal outcome

31. Pruritic urticarial papules and plaques of pregnancy (PUPPP):

A. Is best classified as an occlusive vasculopathy

B. Typically involves the deep dermis and subcutis

C. Is characterized by a neutrophil-rich infiltrate

D. Can be diagnosed by serology alone

E. Has negative direct immunofluorescence findings

32. Unifying features of herpes gestationis and pruritic urticarial papules and plaques of pregnancy (PUPPP) include:

A. Onset in the last trimester

B. Absence of recurrence in subsequent pregnancies

C. Lack of association with other autoimmune disease

D. Similar histopathologic reaction pattern

E. Direct immunofluorescence findings

33. A 27-year-old primigravida presents with an erythematous papular abdominal rash in an annular distribution in the third trimester. Direct immunofluorescence findings of C3 are shown in the image. The most likely diagnosis is:

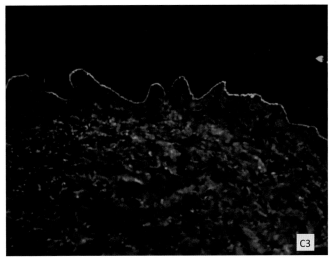

A. Lupus erythematosus

B. Pruritic urticarial papules and plaques of pregnancy (PUPPP)

C. Herpes gestationis
D. Erythema annular centrifugum
E. Erythema gyratum repens

34. Erythema annulare centrifugum:
    A. Is primarily drug related
    B. Is clinically self-limiting
    C. Does not exhibit epidermal changes
    D. Serology is diagnostic
    E. Direct immunofluorescence is diagnostic

35. Pityriasis lichenoides et varioliformis acuta (PLEVA/Mucha-Habermann disease) is best classified as:
    A. An occlusive vasculopathy
    B. A leukocytoclastic vasculitis
    C. A non-inflammatory purpura
    D. A lymphocytic vasculitis
    E. A septic vasculitis

36. Pityriasis lichenoides chronica (PLC):
    A. Is part of the lymphomatoid papulosis spectrum
    B. Is part of the PLEVA spectrum
    C. Is vancomycin triggered
    D. Is an occlusive vasculopathy
    E. Is associated with "shoulder" parakeratosis

37. Which of the following is NOT a clinical variant of pigmented purpuric dermatosis:
    A. Schamberg's disease
    B. Lichen aureus
    C. Gougerot-Blum disease
    D. Majocchi's granuloma
    E. Purpuric contact dermatitis

38. An early lesion of pigmented purpuric dermatosis will not be expected to demonstrate:
    A. Band-like lichenoid infiltrate
    B. Lymphocytic vasculitis
    C. Hemosiderin deposits
    D. Epidermotropism
    E. Extravasated erythrocytes

39. Entities characterized by infiltrates "filling" the papillary dermis include all of the following EXCEPT:
    A. Pigmented purpuric dermatoses
    B. Mycosis fungoides
    C. Lichenoid dermatitis
    D. Urticaria pigmentosa
    E. Perniosis

40. Histopathologic features of Degos disease (malignant atrophic papulosis) include:
    A. Periadnexal infiltrate
    B. Subepidermal blister

C. Lymphocytic vasculitis
D. Fibrinoid necrosis of vessels
E. Lobular panniculitis

41. Histopathologic features found in primary perniosis but not in lupus-related perniosis include:
    A. Interface change
    B. Lymphocytic vasculitis
    C. Papillary dermal edema
    D. "Fluffy edema" of endothelial cells
    E. None of the above

42. Histopathologic changes in pyoderma gangrenosum:
    A. Vary with age of the lesion
    B. Typically do not involve the follicle
    C. Include an occlusive vasculopathy
    D. Include lobular panniculitis
    E. Typically involve medium-sized vessels

43. Which of the following is NOT a lymphocytic vasculitis:
    A. Pruritic urticarial papules and plaques of pregnancy
    B. Pyoderma gangrenosum
    C. Erythema annulare centrifugum
    D. Cryoglobulinemia
    E. Perniosis

44. Approximately 80% of patients with Wegener's granulomatosis have antibodies to:
    A. Anti-neutrophil elastase
    B. Myeloperoxidase
    C. Serine proteinase 3
    D. Histone
    E. Smith

45. Histopathologic changes in Wegener's granulomatosis include:
    A. Confluent subepidermal clefting
    B. Primary septal panniculitis
    C. Intravascular granulomas
    D. Neovascularization
    E. Necrotizing angiitis

46. Regarding serology from patients with Wegener's granulomatosis:
    A. Antibodies to serine proteinase 3 are typically not found
    B. Antibodies to myeloperoxidase are typically not found
    C. Antibody titers to serine proteinase 3 correlate with disease activity
    D. Antibody titers to myeloperoxidase correlate with disease activity

47. Which of the following is not included in the American College of Rheumatology (ACR) diagnostic criteria for Wegener's granulomatosis:
    A. Nasal/oral inflammation
    B. Abnormal chest X-ray
    C. Urinary sediment
    D. Granulomatous inflammation on biopsy
    E. Antibodies to serine proteinase 3

48. Diagnostic histopathologic findings in Churg-Strauss syndrome (CSS) include:
    A. Necrotizing panniculitis
    B. Occlusive vasculopathy of small/medium-sized vessels
    C. Extravascular granulomas
    D. Interstitial neutrophils
    E. Superficial neovascularization

49. Which of the following is not included in the American College of Rheumatology (ACR) diagnostic criteria for Churg-Strauss syndrome CSS:
    A. Bronchial asthma
    B. Peripheral eosinophilia
    C. Mono/poly neuropathy
    D. Extravascular eosinophils
    E. Hepatic infiltrate

50. The best-fit diagnosis for the image shown is:

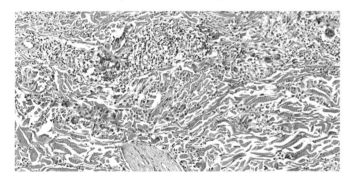

    A. Wells's syndrome
    B. Black spider bite reaction
    C. Polyarteritis nodosa
    D. Churg-Strauss syndrome
    E. Wegener's granulomatosis

51. Regarding the clinical presentation of the entity characterized by the histopathologic reaction pattern shown in the image:

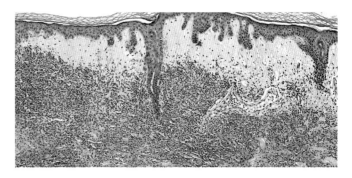

    A. Confined to intertriginous areas
    B. Typically painful
    C. More common in children
    D. Associated with hepatitis C
    E. Associated with leukopenia

52. Leukocytoclastic vasculitis is a feature of all of the following EXCEPT:
    A. Mixed cryoglobulinemia
    B. Sweet's syndrome
    C. Erythema elevatum diutinum
    D. Henoch-Schönlein purpura
    E. Microscopic polyangiitis

53. Neutrophilic dermatoses include:
    A. Warfarin necrosis
    B. Atrophie blanche
    C. Sneddon's syndrome
    D. Pityriasis lichenoides
    E. Behcet's disease

54. This entity is a form of:

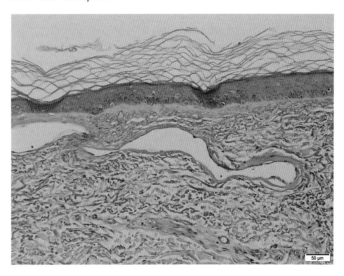

    A. Hypersensitivity vasculitis
    B. Septic vasculitis
    C. Non-inflammatory purpura
    D. Microangiopathy
    E. Generalized essential telangiectasia

D5 Vasculopathic Reaction Patterns Answers

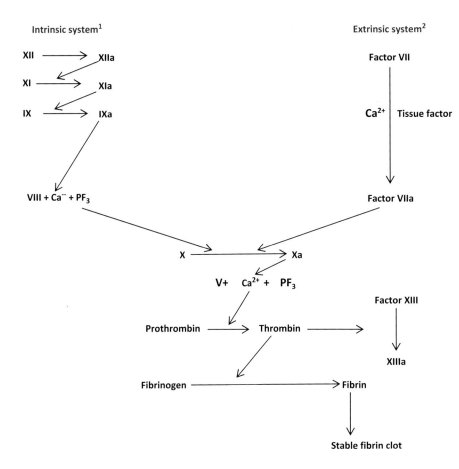

Intrinsic system[1]

$XII \longrightarrow XIIa$

$XI \longrightarrow XIa$

$IX \longrightarrow IXa$

$VIII + Ca^{..} + PF_3$

Extrinsic system[2]

Factor VII

Ca^{2+} | Tissue factor

Factor VIIa

$X \longrightarrow Xa$

$V+ \quad Ca^{2+} + \quad PF_3$

Prothrombin $\longrightarrow$ Thrombin $\longrightarrow$

Factor XIII

XIIIa

Fibrinogen $\longrightarrow$ Fibrin

Stable fibrin clot

Figure D5.1 Overview of the coagulation cascade
[1]Intrinsic system measured by the activated partial thromboplastin time (**APTT**)
[2]Extrinsic system measured by the prothrombin time (**PT**)

Clues provided by patterns of bleeding:

Mucocutaneous bleeding (epistaxis and ecchymosis), genitourinary bleeding = platelet disorder

Soft tissue bleed (hematoma, hemarthrosis), retroperitoneal bleeding = coagulation disorder

Delayed bleeding = fibrinolytic-type bleeding

Table D5.1 Clinical states associated with disseminated intravascular coagulation (DIC)

Obstetric complications		Abruption placentae, placenta previa, amniotic fluid infusion, dead fetus, placenta accrete, cesarean section, abortion, hydatid mole, extrauterine pregnancy, forceps delivery, normal delivery
Tissue trauma		Major surgery, trauma, burns, fat embolism, transplant rejection, heatstroke
Hemolytic processes		Mismatched blood transfusion, drowning, acute hemolysis secondary to infection, acid ingestion
Neoplastic disease		Solid tumors, leukemias (particularly AML3, AML5)
Snakebites		
Infections	**Bacterial**	Gram-negative, pneumococcal, meningococcal, septicemia
	Rickettsial	Rocky mountain spotted fever
	Viral	Smallpox and hemorrhagic fever
	Mycotic	Acute histoplasmosis
	Parasitic	Malaria (blackwater fever)
Miscellaneous		Cirrhosis, glomerulonephritis, acute pancreatitis, purpura fulminans, thrombotic thrombocytopenic purpura, hemolytic uremic syndrome, shock, acute heart failure, Kasabach-Meritt syndrome, large aortic aneurysm

Table D5.2 Vascular reaction patterns

Pattern		Entities	Specifics
Non-inflammatory purpura		Senile purpura	
Occlusive vasculopathy		Protein C/S deficiency	
		Warfarin necrosis	Vessels in deep dermis and subcutis
		Atrophie blanche	Early lesions (pre-ulcerative stage)
		Disseminated intravascular coagulation (DIC)	
		Purpura fulminans	
		Cryoglobulinemia	Monoclonal (type I)
		Cholesterol emboli	
		Antiphospholipid syndrome	
		Factor V Leiden mutation	
		Sneddon's syndrome	Late stage
Vasculitis	Acute	Leukocytoclastic vasculitis	
		Drug	
		Henoch-Schönlein purpura	
		Infectious disease	
		Microscopic polyarteritis	
		Mixed cryoglobulinemia	Types II and III
		Hypergammaglobulinemic purpura	
	Chronic	Erythema elevatum diutinum	
		Granuloma faciale	
Chronic lymphocytic vasculitis		Collagen vascular disease	
		Pruritic urticarial papules and plaques of pregnancy	
		Erythema annulare centrifugum	
		Erythema chronicum migrans	
		Pityriasis lichenoides	
		Pigmented purpuric dermatosis	
		Malignant atrophic papulosis	
		Perniosis	
		Infection	Rickettsial, viral
		Polymorphic light eruption (PMLE)	
Granulomatous vasculitis		Wegener's granulomatosis	
		Lymphomatoid granulomatosis	
		Churg-Strauss syndrome	
		Lethal midline granuloma	
		Giant cell (temporal) arteritis	
		Takayasu's arteritis	
Leukocytoclasia without vasculitis		Familial Mediterranean fever	
		Sweet's syndrome	
		Behcet's disease	
		Rheumatoid neutrophilic dermatosis	
		Bowel-associated dermatosis-arthritis syndrome	
		Abscess-forming neutrophilic dermatosis	
		Amicrobial pustulosis of the folds	

Table D5.3 Vasculitis, etiopathogenesis – based on the 2012 International Chapel Hill Consensus Conference

Large vessel vasculitis	Giant cell temporal arteritis	
	Takayasu's arteritis	
Medium vessel vasculitis	Polyarteritis nodosa	
	Kawasaki's disease	
Small vessel vasculitis	ANCA-associated vasculitis	Granulomatosis with polyangiitis
		Microscopic polyangiitis
		Eosinophilic granulomatosis with polyangiitis

Table D5.3 Vasculitis, etiopathogenesis – based on the 2012 International Chapel Hill Consensus Conference (*cont.*)

	Immune complex vasculitis	Anti-glomerular basement membrane disease Cryoglobulinemic vasculitis IgA vasculitis (including Henoch-Schönlein purpura) Hypocomplementemic urticarial vasculitis
Variable vessel vasculitis	Behcet's disease Cogan's syndrome	
Single organ vasculitis	Cutaneous leukocytoclastic angiitis Cutaneous arteritis Primary CNS vasculitis Isolated aortitis	
Vasculitis associated with systemic disease	Lupus vasculitis Rheumatoid vasculitis Sarcoid vasculitis	
Vasculitis associated with probable etiology	Hepatitis B-associated cryoglobulinemic vasculitis Hepatitis B-associated vasculitis Syphilis-associated aortitis Drug-associated immune complex vasculitis Drug-associated ANCA-associated vasculitis Cancer-associated vasculitis	

Table D5.4 Classification of vasculitis – based on vessel size

Aorta and large-to-medium sized arteries	Giant cell temporal arteritis Takayasu's arteritis
Medium-sized arteries	Polyarteritis nodosa Kawasaki's disease
Medium-sized arteries and small vessels	Granulomatosis with polyangiitis Microscopic polyangiitis Eosinophilic granulomatosis with polyangiitis
Small vessels	Henoch-Schönlein purpura Mixed cryoglobulinemia Leukocytoclastic vasculitis Urticarial vasculitis

Table D5.5 Antigenic targets in non-blistering cutaneous disorders

Antigenic target	Disease association/s	Relevance
ANA	SLE (95%) Subacute LE (80%) DLE (25%)	Non-specific, low levels of positivity found normally in older people, more commonly in females
Anti-neutrophil elastase	Levamisole-induced vasculopathy ecchymosis and necrosis (LIVEN)	
B$_2$-glycoprotein 1	Lupus anticoagulant, thromboembolic events	
CCP	Rheumatoid arthritis, several autoimmune diseases	More specific than RF for rheumatoid arthritis
Centromere	Systemic sclerosis, scleroderma (57–82% in limited, 8% in diffuse),	Specific for CREST, associated with a high incidence of pulmonary hypertension
dsDNA	SLE (40–60% of cases), MCTD (low titers) DLE (low titers) Rheumatoid arthritis (low titers) Progressive systemic sclerosis (low titers) Sjogren's syndrome (low titers) Dermatomyositis (low titers)	Relatively specific for SLE, high titers associated with an increased risk of lupus nephritis, titers correlate with disease activity

Table D5.5 Antigenic targets in non-blistering cutaneous disorders (*cont.*)

Antigenic target	Disease association/s	Relevance
Histone	Drug-induced lupus (95% cases), SLE	Drugs commonly implicated include procainamide, hydralazine
Jo-1	Polymyositis	Often associated with pulmonary fibrosis, not seen in dermatomyositis
MPO	Microscopic polyangiitis	
NMDAR	SLE	Presence correlates with neuropsychiatric manifestations
Nuclear RNP (U1RNP)	Mixed connective tissue disease (MCTD), SLE, associated with Raynaud's phenomenon	
Phospholipid	Thromboembolic events	
Pm-Scl	Polymyositis/scleroderma overlap	
RAP (SS-C)	Primary Sjogren's syndrome (5%)	
RF	Rheumatoid arthritis (higher the titer, the higher the specificity), several autoimmune diseases	Non-specific
SS-A (Ro)	Sjogren's syndrome, subacute cutaneous lupus, neonatal lupus with heart block, SLE with interstitial pneumonia	Constitutes a diagnostic marker for Sjogren's syndrome Helpful in ANA-negative lupus
SS-B (La)	Sjogren's syndrome, SLE	Constitutes a diagnostic marker for Sjogren's syndrome
ssDNA	Found in most systemic autoimmune diseases	No clinical utility
Scl-70	Scleroderma (70% in diffuse, 13% in limited)	Associated with a high incidence of pulmonary fibrosis
Serine protease	Wegener's granulomatosis (found in >80% of patients)	Specific for Wegener's, correlates with disease activity
Sm	SLE (20–30%)	Helpful in RNP negative subset of LE Highly specific for SLE, serves as a disease marker for SLE
Thyroglobulin	Autoimmune thyroiditis	
TSH receptor	Graves's disease	

ANA = Antinuclear antibody; CCP = Cyclic citrullinated peptide; DLE = Discoid lupus erythematosus; dsDNA = Double stranded deoxyribonucleic acid; Jo 1 = Histidyl tRNA synthetase; NMDAR = N-methyl-D-aspartate receptor; RNP = Ribonucleoprotein; Pm-Scl = Polymyositis-scleroderma overlap syndrome-associated autoantigen; RF = Rheumatoid factor; Scl-70 = Topoisomerase 1; SLE = Systemic lupus erythematosus; Sm = Smith antigen

1. **B. Senile purpura is a common non-inflammatory purpura.**

   It typically presents clinically as expansile ecchymosis on the extensor aspect of the forearms and hands of the elderly. Histopathologic features include an abundance of extravasated erythrocytes in the superficial dermis in a background of marked solar elastosis.

2. **A. Livedo reticularis is a clinical feature of several unrelated entities characterized histopathologically by vascular occlusive diseases.**

   Clinically, livedo reticularis presents as a mottled bluish discoloration of the skin occurring in a net-like pattern. Synonyms include livedo racemosa and livedo annularis. While livedo reticularis usually occurs on exposure to cold, with time it can become permanent. Clinical diagnosis is typically confirmed by laboratory data in support of the underlying disorder.

3. **D. Protein C is a vitamin K dependent plasma glycoprotein.**

   Protein C is readily converted to active protein C (APC) by a complex of thrombin and thrombomodulin on the surface of endothelial cells. In the presence of another vitamin K dependent protein (protein S), APC inactivates factors Va and VIII and thus plays an important anticoagulant role. Congenital deficiency is usually inherited as an autosomal dominant trait. Acquired deficiency may occur in a wide variety of settings (ulcerative colitis, infections and anticoagulant therapy) and can predispose to warfarin-induced necrosis.

4. **A. Protein S is *not* a serine protease.**

   Protein S, like protein C, is a vitamin K dependent factor. However it is unique among the vitamin K dependent factors in that it is not a serine protease. Protein S is produced by a wide variety of cells that include hepatocytes, endothelial cells and megakaryocytes. In platelets it is present within α granules and is released in the environment of a forming hemostatic plug where it is most needed. Degradation of factors Va and VIII by APC (see above) requires a phospholipid surface, supplied by platelets and protein S. Deficiency of protein S, like that of protein C, can predispose to warfarin-induced necrosis.

5. **B** Warfarin necrosis typically occurs within 3 to 5 days of initiation of warfarin therapy.

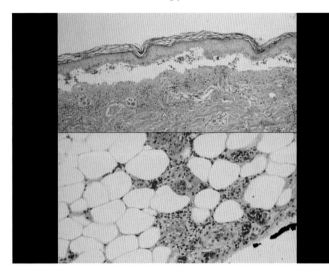

Warfarin necrosis manifests clinically as sharply demarcated foci of purpuric necrosis. It tends to occur more commonly in obese females. Cutaneous lesions are extremely tender and painful and have a predilection for "fatty" areas such as the breasts, thighs and buttocks. Warfarin necrosis is related to protein C deficiency – a vitamin K dependent protein with potent anticoagulant activity. It can also result from protein S deficiency as well as factor V Leiden mutation. Histopathologic features include fibrin-platelet thrombi in small vessels in the deep dermis and subcutis with variable amounts of extravasated erythrocytes superficially.

6. **D.** The primary event in atrophie blanche is an occlusive vasculopathy.

   The occlusive thrombi in atrophie blanche are believed to be due to the increased tendency of platelets to aggregate. This is thought to be due to decreased fibrinolytic activity of the blood. Other associations include an elevated level of fibrinopeptide A, protein deficiency, factor V Leiden mutation, prothrombin mutations and essential cryoglobulinemia – all conditions leading to a hypercoagulable state.

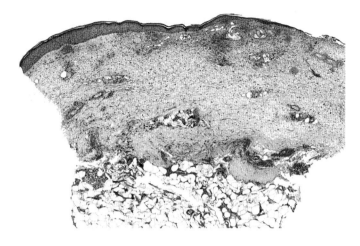

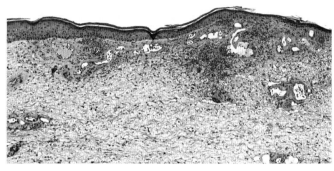

7. **C.** Livedoid vasculopathy is a synonym for atrophie blanche. Other synonyms for atrophie blanche include livedoid vasculitis, segmental hyalinizing vasculitis, and painful purpuric ulcers with reticular patterning on the lower extremities. Atrophie blanche is thought to be due to decreased fibrinolytic activity of the blood and can be associated with a number of entities (detailed above) resulting in the hypercoagulable state. It can be seen in association with livedo reticularis. Histopathologic features vary with the age of the lesion. In early lesions, hyaline thrombi may be seen in small vessels in the superficial and mid dermis with PAS positive material deposition in vessel walls. In established lesions, there is thickening of vessel walls, neovascularization and epidermal atrophy and/or ulceration.

8. **A.** Disseminated intravascular coagulation (DIC) is typically an acquired disorder.

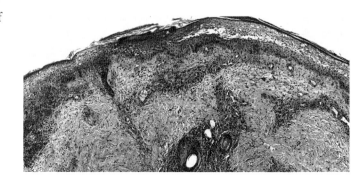

DIC may be encountered in a variety of different clinical situations (Table D5.1). In most cases it is associated with the exposure of tissue factor or thromboplastin-like material with resulting activation of coagulation pathways at the level of factor X (Figure D5.1). In patients with DIC, protein C concentrations are significantly decreased. Cutaneous lesions are not always present, typically noted in 70% of cases and, in select instances, may be the initial manifestation of DIC. Histopathologic features vary with the age of the lesion. In early lesions, hyaline thrombi may be seen in small vessels in the superficial dermis, while in older lesions epidermal necrosis, subepidermal bullae, an abundance of extravasated erythrocytes, necrosis of eccrine glands, and the pilosebaceous unit are noted.

9. **D.** Fibrinogen is decreased in acute disseminated intravascular coagulation (DIC).

    Laboratory findings in DIC are reflective of a consumptive coagulopathy as well as the presence of plasmin. Findings vary with stage of the disease:
    In acute DIC, activated partial thromboplastin time (APTT), prothrombin time (PT) and thrombin times (TT) are prolonged, and platelets, anti-thrombin (AT) III, protein C and fibrinogen decreased, and fibrin/fibrinogen degradation products (FDPs) and D-dimer increased. *In chronic DIC*, platelet counts are decreased only slightly, and the coagulation assays (APTT, PT and TT) within normal limits. Fibrin/fibrinogen degradation products (FDPs) and D-dimer are increased and, AT III decreased.

10. **A.** Type I cryoglobulins are cold-insoluble monoclonal proteins.

    Type I by virtue of being a monoclonal is not associated with circulating immune complexes (CICs) and is usually seen in association with multiple myeloma, Waldenström's macroglobulinemia and chronic lymphocytic leukemia. Type II are mixed polyclonal and monoclonal antibodies (present polyclonal IgG complexed to an unknown antigen and subsequently bound as CICs to a monoclonal IgM antibody with rheumatoid factor activity). Types II and III cryoglobulins are associated with hepatitis C infection as well as chronic Epstein-Barr virus infections. Type III are also mixed with IgG or IgA complexed to polyclonal rheumatoid factor as CICs.

11. **B.** Vasculitis is a feature of type III cryoglobulinemia.

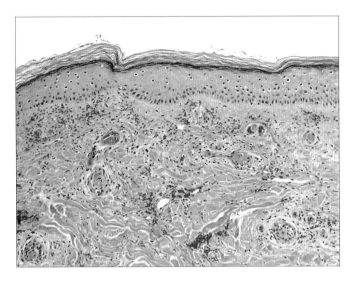

Type I monoclonal cryoglobulinemia accounts for approximately 25% of all cases of cryoglobulinemia and is characterized histopathologically by fibrin thrombi occluding small vessels in the superficial dermis and extravasated erythrocytes.

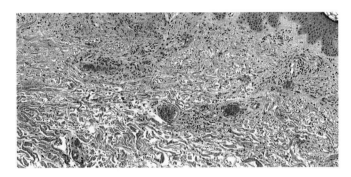

The histopathologic features of mixed (types II and III) cryoglobulinemia are those of an acute vasculitis with fibrinoid necrosis of vessel walls and leukocytoclasia.

12. **A.** Image shown is that of an occlusive vasculopathy. Senile purpura is a non-inflammatory purpura and not an occlusive vasculopathy.

    Senile purpura is characterized by an abundance of extravasated erythrocytes in the background of marked sun-damage. Entities characterized by an occlusive vasculopathy include protein C/S deficiency, factor V Leiden deficiency, atrophie blanche, warfarin necrosis, disseminated intravascular coagulation (DIC), purpura fulminans, cryoglobulinemia (type I), cholesterol emboli, antiphospholipid syndrome, factor

V Leiden mutation and Sneddon's syndrome (late stage) (Table D5.2).

13. **C.** The lupus anticoagulant is not diagnostic for systemic lupus erythematosus (SLE).

    The lupus anticoagulant may be seen in several clinical states and is *not* diagnostic for systemic lupus erythematosus (SLE). The name itself is a misnomer because the vast majority of patients actually do not have SLE. The lupus anticoagulant (LA) is a circulating IgG/IgM or both that interferes with one or more of the *in vitro* phospholipid dependent tests of coagulation. Clinical conditions associated with LA are several and include autoimmune disease (such as SLE and rheumatoid arthritis), drugs (chlorpromazine, procainamide, hydralazine, quinidine, phenytoin and antibiotics), infections (bacterial, viral and protozoa), and hematopoietic malignancies (such as lymphoma and hairy cell leukemia). While most inhibitors of coagulation are associated with clinical bleeding, the LA is paradoxically associated with an increased risk of thrombosis.

14. **B.** Stasis dermatitis is not a cutaneous manifestation of the lupus anticoagulant (LA).

    Cutaneous manifestations of LA include thrombophlebitis, Raynaud's phenomenon, subungual splinter hemorrhages, Sneddon's syndrome and livedo reticularis.

15. **E.** Factor VIII levels are normal in the work-up of the lupus anticoagulant.

    Factor VIII deficiency is observed in hemophilia A and is not an observation associated with work-up of the lupus anticoagulant. The laboratory diagnosis of LA requires 3 distinct steps:

    Step 1: Identification of an abnormal screening test (including prothrombin time, activated partial thromboplastin time)
    Step 2: Proof that the abnormality is the result of an inhibitor
    Step 3: Demonstration that the inhibitor is phospholipid dependent

16. **B.** Small-medium sized vessels at the junction of the dermis and subcutis are affected in Sneddon's syndrome.

    Sneddon's syndrome is characterized by widespread livedo reticularis and ischemic cerebrovascular manifestations related to damage of small as well as medium-sized vessels. Histopathologic findings are not specific and multiple deep biopsies are required to make a definitive diagnosis. Biopsy of a "white" area rather than a "red" area increases the sensitivity of the skin biopsy findings which are characteristically observed in small-medium sized vessels at the junction of the deep dermis

and the subcutis. Endothelitis is the initial change and is followed by partial or complete occlusion of the vessel involved.

17. **A.** Diagnostic features of leukocytoclastic vasculitis (LCV) are best seen in a lesion of 18–24 hours duration.

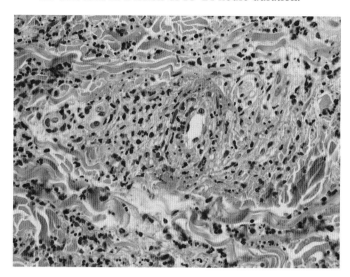

Leukocytoclastic vasculitis is a dynamic process in which changes characteristically involve post-capillary venules and include leukocytoclasia and fibrinoid necrosis. While eosinophils are not typically seen in early lesions, they may be present in older lesions. Other histopathologic features include reactive endothelial cell atypia and extravasation of erythrocytes. Fibrin thrombi within vessels is a feature of an occlusive vasculopathy.

18. **D.** Direct immunofluorescence findings are more often positive and thus informative in a biopsy of lesional *rather than* non-lesional skin in vasculitis.

    Direct immunofluorescence findings in vasculitis include the following:
    Early lesions: Fibrinogen, IgM and C3
    Fully developed lesions: Fibrinogen, IgG and albumin
    Late lesions: Fibrinogen with/without C3

    Serology is unhelpful in vasculitis

19. **D.** In the 2012 Chapel Hill Consensus Conference criteria, Henoch-Schönlein purpura is best described as an immune-complex small-vessel vasculitis.

    Henoch-Schönlein purpura (HSP) represents almost 10% of all cases of leukocytoclastic vasculitis (LCV), which it is believed to be a variant of. Some believe it to be associated with group A streptococcal infection (although controlled trials have yet to support a causal link). Diagnostic criteria include the following:

    - Palpable purpura

- Age of onset at or <20 years of age
- Bowel angina
- Biopsy findings of LCV, i.e. leukocytoclasia and fibrinoid necrosis of vessel walls and direct immunofluorescence findings

A diagnosis of HSP is made if any two of the above criteria are present. Henoch-Schönlein purpura is *not* synonymous with IgA-associated vasculitis but is a subcategory of it. Also see Table D5.3.

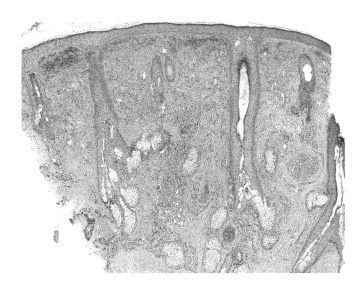

20. **C.** Kawasaki's disease is a medium vessel vasculitis.

Kawasaki's disease is an acute febrile illness affecting infants and children and characterized by cutaneous and mucosal erythema with edema and subsequent desquamation and cervical lymphadenitis. It is complicated by coronary artery aneurysms in a fifth of affected patients. Also see Table D5.3 and Table D5.4. Biopsy of cutaneous lesions is infrequently performed and typically shows non-specific features.

21. **B.** Leukocytoclasia and fibrinoid necrosis of vessel walls are *not* features of urticarial vasculitis.

Urticarial vasculitis presents clinically as urticarial wheals and/or angioedema often with associated purpura.

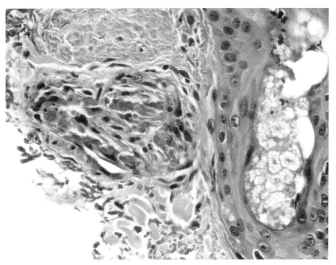

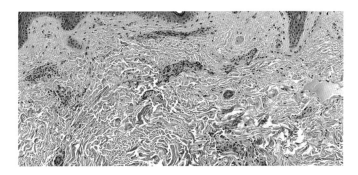

Histopathologically it represents a variant of lymphocytic vasculitis and is characterized by a perivascular infiltrate that is eosinophil-rich. Degranulating eosinophils as well as eosinophils transgressing vessel walls may be seen. The superficial plexus is typically involved and varying degrees of papillary dermal edema may be observed. Leukocytoclasia and fibrinoid necrosis of vessel walls are features of leukocytoclastic vasculitis.

22. **E.** A mixed pattern of an occlusive vasculopathy and leukocytoclastic vasculitis is typically seen in levamisole-induced vasculopathy, ecchymosis and necrosis (LIVEN).

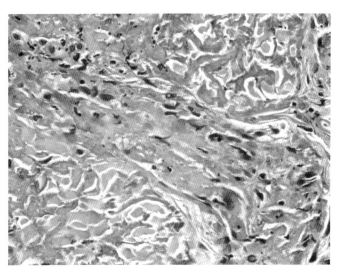

Other entities that demonstrate a mixed pattern, i.e. an occlusive vasculopathy as well as leukocytoclastic vasculitis, include:
- Septic vasculitis
- Vasculitis secondary to herpes
- Mixed cryoglobulinemia (beneath the area of ulceration)

All other entities listed fall under the umbrella of vascular occlusive disease.

23. **C.** Early lesions of erythema elevatum diutinum (EED) are characterized by a leukocytoclastic vasculitis.

Early lesions typically demonstrate a moderately dense perivascular neutrophil-rich infiltrate, reactive endothelial cell atypia, abundant apoptotic debris and fibrinoid necrosis of vessel walls.

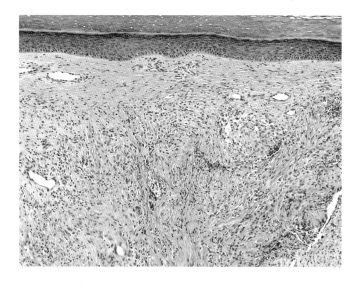

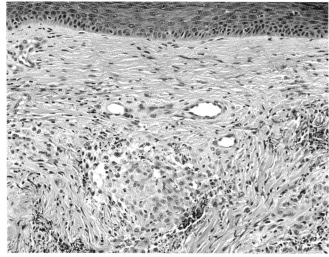

The acute histopathologic findings in EED contrast sharply with the chronic clinical course. Histopathologic changes vary with age of the lesion and late lesions are characterized by variable fibrosis with a somewhat

fasciculated fibroblast proliferation that resembles dermatofibroma at scanning magnification. However, at higher magnification, microscopic foci of an acute vasculitis with a neutrophilic infiltrate can be seen within the fibrosis and throughout the dermis.

24. **A.** Image shown is that of granuloma faciale in which extrafacial involvement is quite uncommon.

Granuloma faciale, an uncommon entity, typically manifests as a papulonodular "rash" on the face. Solitary lesions are not entirely uncommon and are often biopsied to "rule out a neoplasm." Histopathologic features include a dense polymorphous infiltrate composed of eosinophils, neutrophils, lymphocytes and histiocytes beneath a narrow uninvolved grenz zone which extends along the pilosebaceous unit. Reactive endothelial cell atypia and fibrinoid necrosis of vessels may be seen (the latter is uncommon though).

25. **C.** Leukocytoclastic vasculitis is not included in the 2012 Chapel Hill Consensus Conference definitions of anti-neutrophil cytoplasmic antibody-associated vasculitis (AAV).

The 2012 Chapel Hill Consensus Conference definitions of anti-neutrophil cytoplasmic antibody-associated vasculitis (AAV) include the following (Table D5.3):
- Granulomatosis with polyangiitis
- Microscopic polyangiitis
- Eosinophilic granulomatosis with polyangiitis

26. **A.** Proteinase 3 (PR3)-specific anti-neutrophil cytoplasmic antibodies (ANCA) are most often associated with granulomatosis with polyangiitis.

The diagnostic utility of ANC testing depends upon the assays used and the clinical setting. Serologic screening for ANCAs specific for proteinase 3 (PR3) and myeloperoxidase (MPO) is the gold standard. Also see Table D5.5.

27. **B.** Myeloperoxidase (MPO) ANCAs are seen predominantly in patients with microscopic polyangiitis.

Whereas PR3-ANCA and MPO-ANCA are highly specific for an anti-neutrophil cytoplasmic antibody-associated vasculitis (AAV), they have very little diagnostic value for non-vasculitic conditions.

28. **D.** Macular arteritis, depicted in the image shown, is best regarded as a latent form of polyarteritis nodosa.

Macular arteritis, described in 2013, clinically presents as erythematous and hyperpigmented plaques and/or papules in a reticulated pattern on the lower limbs and has an indolent chronic clinical course. Histopathologic features include varying degrees of lymphocytic infiltration and disruption of the arterial wall, concentric luminal fibrin deposition and fibrointimal scarring (endarteritis obliterans). It is believed to represent the chronic/healed end of the spectrum of polyarteritis nodosa.

29. **E.** Image shown is that of polyarteritis nodosa (PAN) for which serology is non-diagnostic.

    Cutaneous PAN has a chronic relapsing course and is usually ANCA-negative. Since the pathology involves vessels near the subcutis, doing a deep biopsy is key. Diagnostic histopathologic findings vary with age of the lesion and include the following:

    Early stage – Marked thickening of vessel walls, particularly the intima and a perivascular infiltrate composed of neutrophils and eosinophils and apoptotic debris (leukocytoclasia)

    Late stage – Luminal thrombi and/or aneurysms, perivascular infiltrate of lymphocytes

    End stage – Intimal and mural fibrosis leading to obliteration of the vessel

    A characteristic feature of PAN is the presence *of lesions at all stages of development within the same biopsy.*

30. **A.** Pruritic urticarial papules and plaques of pregnancy (PUPPP) is synonymous with polymorphous eruption of pregnancy.

    The designation used for this specific pregnancy-related dermatosis in the USA is PUPPP while the nomenclature used for exactly the same dermatosis in Europe is polymorphous eruption of pregnancy. Thus, they are the same entity. PUPPP typically has its onset in the third trimester of pregnancy and is characterized by intensely pruritic eruption of papules and plaques that has a predilection for the striae distensae on the abdomen. The rash is more common in primigravidas, does not typically recur with subsequent pregnancies, usually resolves spontaneously or with delivery and has no adverse effect on fetal outcome.

31. **E.** Direct immunofluorescence is usually negative in pruritic urticarial papules and plaques of pregnancy (PUPPP), a feature that is helpful in differentiating it from herpes gestationis.

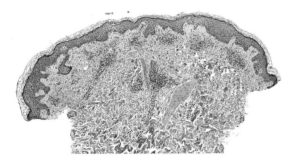

PUPPP is classified as a lymphocytic vasculitis (Table D5.2). Histopathologic features, shown in the image above, are not entirely specific and typically involve vessels in the superficial plexus, epidermal changes in the form of spongiosis and parakeratosis in a third of cases, and a perivascular infiltrate that contains lymphocytes and eosinophils.

32. **A.** Herpes gestationis, like pruritic urticarial papules and plaques of pregnancy (PUPPP), occurs in the last trimester of pregnancy.

    Herpes gestationis or pemphigoid gestationis is an uncommon vesicobullous dermatosis of pregnancy that typically manifests clinically with urticarial plaques and papules in a periumbilical distribution. It usually recurs in subsequent pregnancies and may be associated with other autoimmune disease particularly Graves's disease. Histopathologic features of herpes gestationis include papillary dermal edema (that can be so marked as to produce "teardrop-shaped" papillae), and an inflammatory infiltrate composed of lymphocytes, histiocytes and eosinophils.

33. **C.** The direct immunofluorescence (DIF) findings shown in conjunction with the clinical presentation are diagnostic of herpes gestationis.

    Positive DIF revealing C3 and sometimes IgG in a linear pattern along the basement membrane zone is a helpful differentiating feature from pruritic urticarial papules and plaques of pregnancy (PUPPP) (in which DIF is typically negative).

34. **B.** Erythema annulare centrifugum (EAC) is clinically self-limiting.

    While a variety of agents (infections, drugs and malignancies) have been implicated in the etiopathogenesis of EAC, in most cases the etiology is unknown.

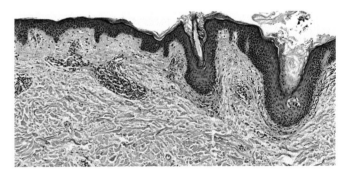

Two distinct types are recognized histopathologically:

Superficial type: Epidermal changes are evident in the form of pityriasiform spongiosis and the inflammation tends to involve the superficial plexus

Deep type: Vessels in the superficial as well as the deep plexus are involved

In both types, the perivascular infiltrate is well demarcated and has the characteristic "coat-sleeve" distribution. Despite the density of the perivascular infiltrate and the presence of cells transgressing vessel walls, there is no fibrinoid necrosis – so it is a "pseudovasculitis." Direct immunofluorescence is of no utility as a histopathologic adjunct.

35. **D.** Pityriasis lichenoides et varioliformis acuta (PLEVA/Mucha-Habermann disease) is best classified as a lymphocytic vasculitis.

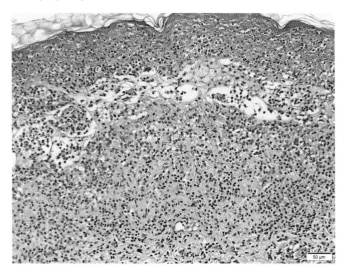

Histopathologic findings of PLEVA, shown in the image above, typically encompass *three distinct reaction patterns*: a lymphocytic vasculitis (Table D5.2), interface dermatitis with numerous individually necrotic, dyskeratotic keratinocytes at all levels of the epidermis and lichenoid dermatitis with an infiltrate that is composed predominantly of lymphocytes.

36. **B.** Pityriasis lichenoides chronica (PLC) represents one end of a self-limiting dermatosis with pityriasis lichenoides et varioliformis acuta (PLEVA) at the other.

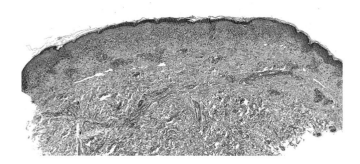

Pityriasis lichenoides is a self-limiting dermatosis of unknown etiopathogenesis with a spectrum of clinical and histopathologic changes. At one end is PLEVA, clinically characterized by hemorrhagic papules and nodules and histopathologically by a lymphocytic vasculitis and an interface and lichenoid dermatitis (see above). At the other end is PLC, clinically characterized by a scaly, red/brown maculopapular rash and histopathologically by a lymphocytic vasculitis and interface dermatitis. Overall, the density of the infiltrate in PLC is less than that observed in PLEVA. Despite the unifying features of lymphomatoid papulosis and PLEVA in terms of clinical presentation (hemorrhagic and ulcerating papulonodular lesions) and presence of CD30+ atypical lymphocytes, they are pathogenetically distinct entities.

37. **D.** Majoccchi's granuloma is not a variant of pigmented purpuric dermatosis.

Clinical variants of pigmented purpuric dermatosis (PPD) include the following:

Schamberg's disease (progressive pigmentary dermatosis) – The most common type, clinically presents as pin-head sized macules with a reddish-brown ("cayenne pepper") color with a predilection for the pretibial region and ankles

Majocchi's disease – Is essentially an annular form of Schamberg's disease with a perifollicular distribution

Gougerot-Blum disease – Clinically presents as lichenoid papules and macules, usually in association with Schamberg's disease

Lichen aureus – Clinically presents as grouped macules or lichenoid papules with a predilection for the head and neck area

Purpuric contact dermatitis – The least well known and a form of allergic contact dermatitis clinically presents as purpuric and hemorrhagic areas distributed in clothed areas

Majoccchi's granuloma is the clinical term used for a nodular lesion of the lower leg with a predilection for females and showing a histopathologic picture consistent with a granulomatous perifolliculitis. Fungi that have been implicated are several and include *Trichophyton rubrum, Microsporum canis, T. violaceum, T. tonsurans, T. mentogrophytes* and *Aspergillus fumigatus.*

38. **C.** Hemosiderin deposits would not be present in an early lesion of pigmented purpuric dermatosis (PPD).

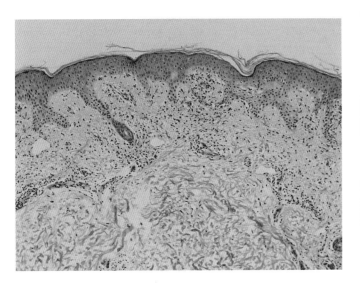

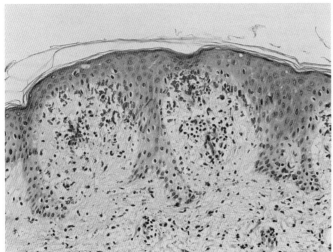

Histopathologic features of an early lesion of PPD include a band-like infiltrate composed of lymphocytes of the T helper phenotype (CD4+), a lymphocytic vasculitis and extravasated erythrocytes. While epidermotropism is typically not a feature of an early lesion of PPD, there are several reports indicating of an overlap between the histopathologic picture of early PPD and that of an early lesion of mycosis fungoides.

39. E. The inflammatory infiltrate in perniosis is not merely superficial.

Infiltrates filling the papillary dermis are best characterized by the mnemonic LUMP – which stands for *l*ichenoid dermatitis, *u*rticarial pigmentosa, *m*ycosis fungoides and *p*igmented purpuric dermatosis.

Histopathologic features of perniosis include a superficial and deep perivascular and periadnexal lymphocytic infiltrate, lymphocytic vasculitis, papillary dermal edema, +/− interface change and extravasated erythrocytes.

40. C. Lymphocytic vasculitis is a feature of Degos disease (malignant atrophic papulosis).

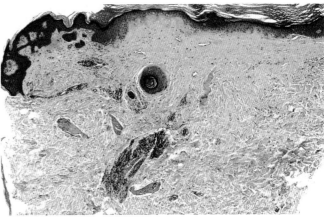

Histopathologic features of a well-developed lesion of Degos disease include epidermal atrophy with an underlying wedge-shaped area of ischemia, lymphocytic vasculitis involving vessels in the mid and deep dermis (Table D5.2), fibrin thrombi, reactive endothelial cell atypia and increased dermal mucin.

41. E. No single histopathologic feature is of utility in differentiating primary perniosis from lupus-related perniosis.

Both primary perniosis and lupus-related perniosis exhibit similar histopathologic findings, albeit to varying degrees, of interface change (albeit more widespread in lupus-related perniosis), a lymphocytic vasculitis involving superficial and deep vessels with "fluffy edema" of endothelial cells, a perivascular and periadnexal lymphocytic infiltrate, papillary dermal edema and extravasated erythrocytes.

42. A. Histopathology of pyoderma gangrenosum varies with age of the lesion.

Pyoderma gangrenosum is a clinically distinct, rapidly evolving, chronic and severely debilitating disease characterized by one or more necrotic ulcers with an undermined violaceous edge. *Histopathology characteristically varies with age of the lesion.*

Early lesions: Typically show an intradermal microabscess characteristically in a perifollicular distribution
Advanced lesions: Demonstrate a perivascular lymphoplasmacytic infiltrate, reactive endothelial cell atypia, fibrinoid extravasation and a lymphocytic and/or leukocytoclastic vasculitis that involves small vessels in the superficial and deep dermis; the vasculitis is not primary but believed to be reactive and secondary to the adjacent inflammation

43. D. Cryoglobulinemia is *not* characterized by a lymphocytic vasculitis.

Monoclonal cryoglobulinemia presents as an occlusive vasculopathy while polyclonal (mixed) cryoglobulinemia presents as a leukocytoclastic vasculitis.

Entities characterized by a lymphocytic vasculitis include collagen vascular disease, pruritic urticarial papules and plaques of pregnancy, erythema annulare centrifugum, erythema chronicum migrans, pityriasis lichenoides, pigmented purpuric dermatosis, malignant atrophic papulosis (Degos disease), perniosis, infections (Rickettsial, viral) and polymorphic light eruption (Table D5.2).

44. **C.** Approximately 80% of patients with Wegener's granulomatosis have circulating antibodies to serine protease 3.

    Associations of other antibodies listed are as follows (Table D5.5):

    - Anti-neutrophil elastase – Levamisole-induced vasculopathy ecchymosis and necrosis (LIVEN)
    - Myeloperoxidase – Microscopic polyangiitis
    - Histone – Drug-induced lupus primarily
    - Smith – Systemic lupus erythematosus

45. **E.** Necrotizing angiitis is a histopathologic defining feature of Wegener's granulomatosis (WG).

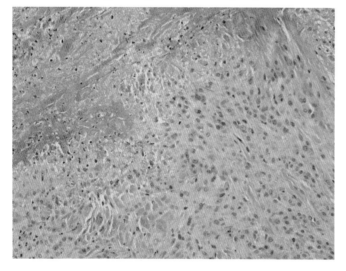

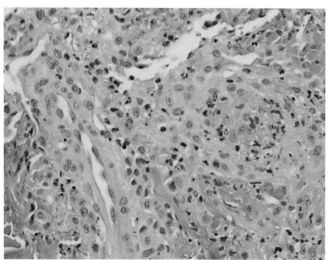

Other histopathologic changes in WG, shown in the image above, include extravascular, angiocentric granulomas and a palisaded lymphohistiocytic infiltrate. The palisade is typically best developed in older lesions. Primary septal panniculitis is not a typical histopathologic feature of WG. While the inflammatory process may "spill over" into the adjacent panniculus, the primary target antigen in WG is a medium-sized vessel and not the septal panniculus.

46. **C.** Antibody titers to serine protease 3 correlate with disease activity in Wegener's granulomatosis (WG).

    Circulating antibodies to serine protease 3 are found in >80% of patients with WG and are specific for WG. While antibodies to myeloperoxidase are also seen occasionally in WG, they are not specific to Wegener's but are more commonly associated with microscopic polyangiitis.

47. **E.** Antibodies to serine protease 3 are *not* included in the American College of Rheumatology (ACR) criteria for Wegener's granulomatosis (WG).

    Briefly, ACR criteria for WG include the following:
    - Nasal/oral inflammation
    - Abnormal chest X-ray
    - Urinary sediment
    - Granulomatous inflammation on biopsy

    For purposes of classification, a patient is said to have WG if *at least two of the above 4 criteria* are present. The presence of any 2 or more yields a sensitivity of 88% and a specificity of 92% for a diagnosis of WG.

48. **C.** Extravascular granulomas are a histopathologic feature of Churg-Strauss syndrome (CSS, allergic granulomatosis).

    Other histopathologic findings observed include necrotizing angiitis involving small/medium-sized vessels, interstitial eosinophils (including the presence of degranulating eosinophils) and a palisaded lymphohistiocytic infiltrate.

49. **E.** Hepatic infiltrates are *not* included in the American College of Rheumatology (ACR) criteria for a diagnosis of Churg-Strauss syndrome (CSS).

    The ACR criteria for the classification of CSS include:
    - Asthma
    - Eosinophilia (>10% of the peripheral count)
    - Mono/poly neuropathy (typically in a glove/stocking distribution and attributed to systemic vasculitis)
    - Pulmonary infiltrates (non-fixed, attributable to systemic vasculitis)
    - Paranasal sinus abnormality
    - Extravascular eosinophils

    For purposes of classification, a patient is said to have CSS if *at least 4 of the above 6 criteria* are present.

50. **E.** The image shown is that of Churg-Strauss syndrome (CSS).

Briefly, histopathologic findings observed in CSS include extravascular granulomas, necrotizing angiitis involving small/medium-sized vessels, interstitial eosinophils (including the presence of degranulating eosinophils) and a palisaded lymphohistiocytic infiltrate.

51. **B.** Image shown is that of Sweet's syndrome in which lesions are typically painful.

Sweet's syndrome is characterized by painful nodular plaque-forming inflammatory papules and mamillated plaques most commonly on the head and neck area and upper extremity. Truncal lesions are uncommon. It typically affects individuals from 30–60 years of age, women more than men. Other features include arthralgia, fever and peripheral leukocytosis.

52. **B.** Leukocytoclastic vasculitis is not a feature of Sweet's syndrome.

Histopathologic features of Sweet's syndrome include a dense infiltrate composed predominantly of neutrophils confined predominantly to the upper half of the dermis, leukocytoclasia and papillary dermal edema. True vasculitis, i.e. fibrinoid necrosis of vessel walls, is not a feature of Sweet's syndrome and when present should lead to other diagnostic considerations. *Histiocytoid Sweet's syndrome* is the term used for an infiltrate composed of histiocytoid-like cells in early lesions of Sweet's syndrome. These cells are not neoplastic but represent immature myeloid cells. The infiltrate in this variant tends to be deeper with involvement of the deep dermis and subcutis in contrast to that observed in regular Sweet's syndrome. Histopathologic hallmarks of vasculitis, i.e. fibrinoid necrosis of vessel walls and leukocytoclasia, are seen in the other entities listed and include mixed cryoglobulinemia, erythema elevatum diutinum, Henoch-Schönlein purpura and microscopic polyangiitis (other entities enumerated in Table D5.2).

53. **E.** The pathergic lesion in Behcet's syndrome is characterized histopathologically by a neutrophil-rich dermal infiltrate.

Other neutrophilic dermatoses include familial Mediterranean fever, Sweet's syndrome, Behcet's disease ("pathergic" lesion), rheumatoid neutrophilic dermatoses, bowel-associated dermatosis-arthritis syndrome, abscess-forming neutrophilic dermatosis and amicrobial pustulosis of the folds (Table D5.2).

54. **D.** Cutaneous collagenous vasculopathy shown in the image is a microangiopathy.

Cutaneous collagenous vasculopathy is a very rare entity first described in 2000, manifesting clinically with acquired, progressively diffuse, cutaneous telangiectases. Histopathologically, it is distinct. Superficial dermal vessels are characterized by a thick hyaline collagenous wall. Its cause is unknown.

D6 Granulomatous Reaction Patterns Questions

1. Biopsy of a yellowish brown papular rash on the central part of the face and around the eyelids in a patient with no prior significant medical history. The most likely diagnosis is:

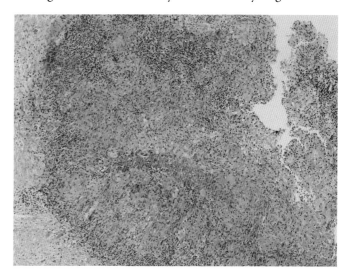

   A. Lupus miliaris disseminatus faciei
   B. Perioral dermatitis
   C. Actinic granuloma of O'Brien
   D. Idiopathic facial aseptic granuloma
   E. Granulomatous cutaneous T-cell lymphoma

2. Necrobiosis is typically seen in:
   A. Actinic granuloma
   B. Granuloma annulare
   C. Crohn's disease
   D. Sarcoidosis
   E. Granulomatous cutaneous T-cell lymphoma

3. The best-fit diagnosis is:

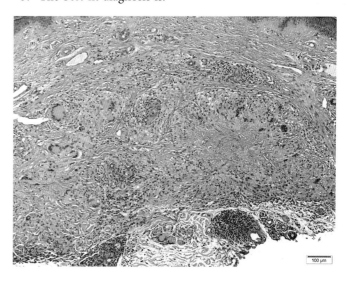

   A. Giant cell granuloma
   B. Granuloma annulare
   C. Crohn's disease
   D. Elastofibroma dorsii
   E. Granulomatous cutaneous T-cell lymphoma

4. Increased interstitial mucin is a feature of:
   A. Giant cell granuloma
   B. Granuloma annulare
   C. Crohn's disease
   D. Elastofibroma dorsii
   E. Granulomatous cutaneous T-cell lymphoma

5. This is an example of:

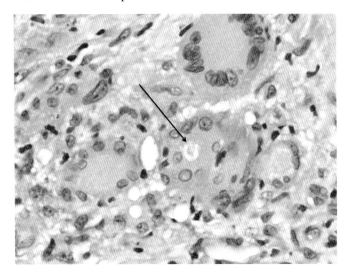

   A. Schaumann body
   B. Michelis-Gutmann body
   C. Asteroid body
   D. Dutcher body
   E. Russell body

6. This is an example of;

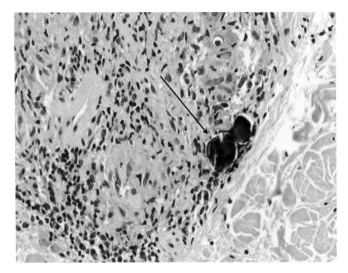

   A. Schaumann body
   B. Michelis-Gutmann body
   C. Asteroid body
   D. Dutcher body
   E. Russell body

7. Sarcoidal granulomas may be a feature of:
   A. Muir-Torre syndrome
   B. Cowden syndrome
   C. Brooke-Spiegler syndrome
   D. Wiskott-Aldrich syndrome
   E. Blau syndrome

8. Which of the following is not a Group I mycobacterium:
   A. *Mycobacterium marinum*
   B. *Mycobacterium kansasi*
   C. *Mycobacterium simiae*
   D. *Mycobacterium scrofulaceum*

9. Mycobacteria classified as "rapid growers" include:
   A. *Mycobacterium marinum*
   B. *Mycobacterium kansasi*
   C. *Mycobacterium simiae*
   D. *Mycobacterium scrofulaceum*
   E. *Mycobacterium chelonae*

10. Entities classified under "tuberculids" include:
   A. Lichen scrofulosorum
   B. Tuberculoid leprosy
   C. Borderline leprosy
   D. Sarcoidosis
   E. Lepromatous leprosy

11. The most likely diagnosis for this biopsy of a "pendular rash" in the flexural areas is:

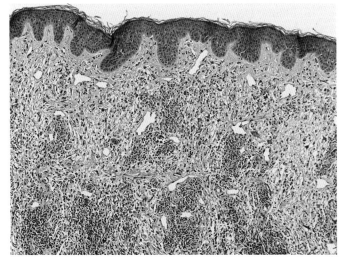

   A. Miliaria crystallina
   B. Necrobiosis lipoidica
   C. Lupus miliaris
   D. Granulomatous slack skin
   E. Hailey-Hailey disease

12. Lupus miliaris disseminatus faciei is believed to be related to which of the following:
    A. Lupus
    B. Miliaria
    C. Rosacea

13. The triad of Melkersson-Rosenthal syndrome includes:
    A. Iridocyclitis, facial nerve palsy, oropharyngeal granulomas
    B. Facial nerve palsy, fissured tongue, cheilitis granulomatosa
    C. Necrotizing vasculitis, cheilitis granulomatosa, iridocyclitis
    D. Apthous stomatitis, iridocyclitis, necrotizing granulomas
    E. Fissured tongue, necrotizing vasculitis, facial nerve palsy

14. The histopathologic triad of granuloma annulare includes:
    A. Caseating granulomas, increased dermal mucin, elastophagocytosis
    B. Necrotizing vasculitis, suppurative granulomas, necrobiosis
    C. Necrobiosis, granulomas, increased dermal mucin
    D. Elastophagocytosis, flame figures, granulomas
    E. Increased dermal mucin, vasculitis, caseating granulomas

15. The most likely diagnosis is:

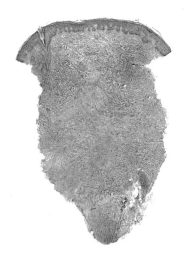

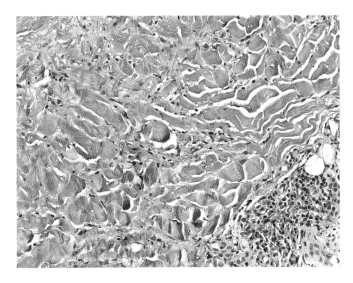

    A. Granuloma annulare
    B. Wegener's granulomatosis
    C. Necrobiotic xanthogranuloma
    D. Necrobiosis lipoidica
    E. Rheumatoid nodule

16. Which of the following best describes the typical clinical presentation of the above:
    A. Well-demarcated plaques on the shins
    B. Psoriasiform plaques on sun-exposed surfaces
    C. Painful, tender nodules on the lower legs
    D. Palpable purpura on the lower extremities
    E. Grouped papules on the abdomen

17. Deep/subcutaneous granuloma annulare:
    A. Is a marker for internal malignancy
    B. Typically involves the torso
    C. Is more common in children
    D. Is associated with a paraproteinemia
    E. Is associated with arthritis

18. Necrobiotic xanthogranuloma is typically associated with:
    A. Arthritis
    B. Perforation
    C. Emperipolesis
    D. Elastophagocytosis
    E. Paraproteinemia

19. "Red" granulomas include all of the following EXCEPT:
    A. Necrobiosis lipoidica
    B. Necrobiotic xanthogranuloma
    C. Rheumatoid nodule
    D. Granuloma annulare
    E. Churg-Strauss syndrome

20. Which of the following is NOT a dematiaceous fungus:
    A. *Fonsecaea pedrosoi*
    B. *Cladosporium carrioni*
    C. *Phialophora compacta*
    D. *Blastomyces dermatitidis*
    E. *Exophiala jeanselmei*

21. The best-fit diagnosis is:

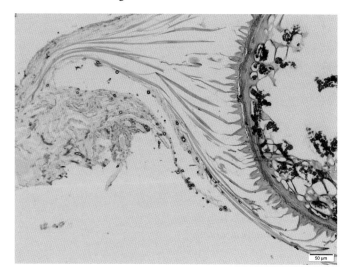

    A. Sporotrichosis
    B. Phaeohyphomycosis
    C. Chromomycosis
    D. Coccidiomycosis
    E. Paracoccidiomycosis

22. The best-fit diagnosis is:

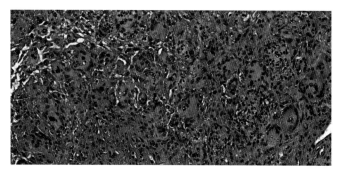

    A. Sporotrichosis
    B. Phaeohyphomycosis
    C. Chromomycosis
    D. Coccidiomycosis
    E. Paracoccidiomycosis

23. The best-fit diagnosis is:

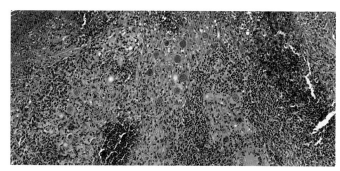

    A. Sporotrichosis
    B. Phaeohyphomycosis
    C. Chromomycosis
    D. Coccidiomycosis
    E. Paracoccidiomycosis

24. The organism above (based on question 23) is endemic in:
    A. Mississippi
    B. Africa
    C. India
    D. Mexico

25. The best-fit diagnosis is:

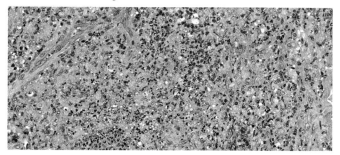

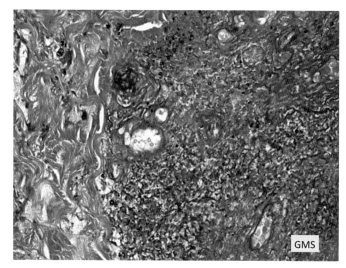

A. Sporotrichosis
B. Phaeohyphomycosis
C. Chromomycosis
D. Coccidiomycosis
E. Paracoccidiomycosis

26. Broad-based buds, lack of endospores and lack of a capsule are typical of:
    A. Sporotrichosis
    B. Phaeohyphomycosis
    C. Blastomycosis
    D. Coccidiomycosis
    E. Paracoccidiomycosis

27. Which of the following is NOT caused by *Bartonella*:
    A. Malakoplakia
    B. Cat scratch disease
    C. Bacillary angiomatosis
    D. Verruca peruana
    E. Trench fever

28. The best-fit diagnosis for this elbow "cyst" is:

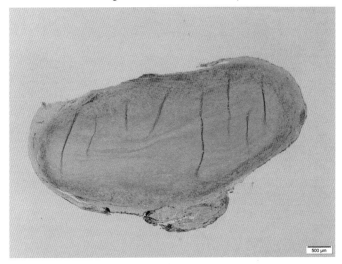

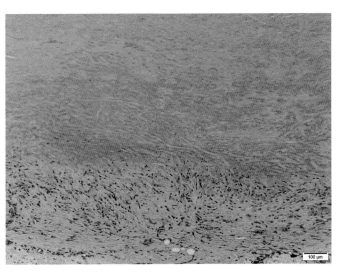

A. Granuloma annulare
B. Necrobiosis lipoidica
C. Rheumatoid nodule
D. Actinic granuloma
E. Necrobiotic xanthogranuloma

29. This is an example of:

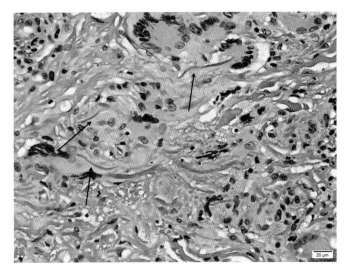

A. Emperipolesis
B. Elastoclasis
C. Necrobiosis
D. Leukocytoclasia
E. Calcinosis cutis

30. Which of the following is NOT a synonym for annular elastolytic giant cell granuloma:
    A. Granuloma annulare
    B. Actinic granuloma of O'Brien
    C. Giant cell elastophagocytosis
    D. Miescher's granuloma of the face
    E. Annular necrobiosis lipoidica

D6 Granulomatous Reaction Patterns
Answers

Table D6.1 Clinical and histopathologic features of key granulomatous dermatoses

Entity	Clinical features	Associations	Histopathologic features	Image
Sarcoidosis	More common in females, African-Americans, papules and plaques *symmetrically* distributed on the head and neck, upper trunk and extremities	Systemic sarcoidosis	"Naked" granulomas composed of epithelioid histiocytes with admixed multinucleate giant cells and sparse lymphocytes	
Granuloma annulare	More common in females, papules coalescing into plaques, extremities	Diabetes mellitus, malignancy	Necrobiosis, palisaded lymphohistiocytic infiltrate, increased dermal mucin	
Necrobiosis lipodica	More common in females, plaques with elevated borders on anterolateral aspect of distal and lower extremities	Diabetes mellitus (*not all cases though*; is NOT peculiar to diabetes)	"Sandwich" appearance, tiered hyalinized and necrobiotic collagen with intervening inflammatory cells	

Table D6.1 Clinical and histopathologic features of key granulomatous dermatoses (*cont.*)

Entity	Clinical features	Associations	Histopathologic features	Image
				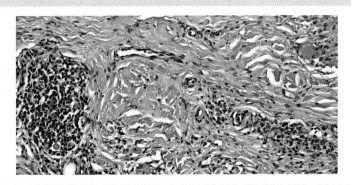
Annular elastolytic giant cell granuloma	More common in females, annular plaques on sun-damaged skin	Actinic damage	Non-caseating granulomas composed of multinucleate giant cells exhibiting elastophagocytosis, *variable loss of elastic fibers*	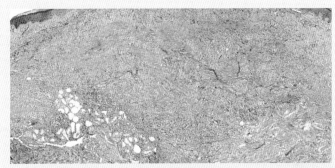
Crohn's disease	More common in females, dusky erythema on genital areas and lower greater than upper extremities	Intestinal Crohn's	Non-caseating granulomas in the dermis, occasionally in a perivascular distribution (*granulomatous perivasculitis*)	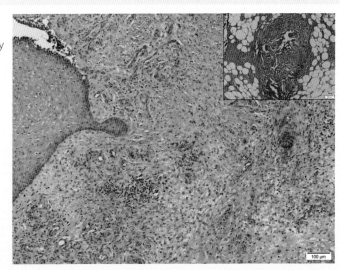
Rheumatoid nodule	More common in females, juxta-articular areas (elbows/hands/ankles/feet), firm, mobile subcutaneous nodules	Rheumatoid arthritis (occurs in 20% of patients)	Central area of homogeneous eosinophilic necrobiosis with a surrounding palisaded lymphohistiocytic infiltrate	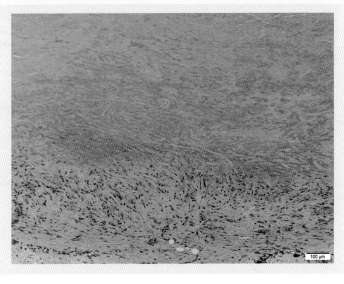

Table D6.2 "Red" and "blue" granulomas

Category	Entity	Key histopathologic features	Image
Blue granulomas	**Granuloma annulare**	Necrobiosis, palisaded lymphohistiocytic infiltrate, increased dermal mucin	
	Wegener's granulomatosis	Necrotizing vasculitis, palisaded lymphohistiocytic infiltrate forming granulomas	
	Rheumatoid vasculitis	Necrobiosis, palisaded lymphohistiocytic infiltrate, leukocytoclastic vasculitis	
Red granulomas	**Necrobiosis lipoidica**	"Sandwich" appearance, tiered hyalinized and necrobiotic collagen with intervening inflammatory cells	
	Necrobiotic xanthogranuloma	Palisaded lymphohistiocytic infiltrate, hyalinized collagen, necrobiosis, Touton-type multinucleate giant cells, cholesterol clefts, lymphoid follicles, plasma cell-rich infiltrate	

Table D6.2 "Red" and "blue" granulomas (*cont.*)

Category	Entity	Key histopathologic features	Image
	Rheumatoid nodule	Central area of homogeneous eosinophilic necrobiosis with a surrounding palisaded lymphohistiocytic infiltrate	
	Churg-Strauss syndrome	Eosinophil-rich perivascular and interstitial infiltrate, non-palisaded and palisaded granuloma, necrotizing vasculitis of superficial and mid-dermal vessels	

Table D6.3 Classification of mycobacteria other than *Mycobacterium tuberculosis* (MOTT)

Group	Classification	Species
I	**Photochromogens**	M. marinum M. kansasi M. simiae
II	**Scotochromogens**	M. scrofulaceum M. flavescens M. szulgai
III	**Nonchromogens**	M. ulcerans M. avium-intracellulare complex M. gastrii M. terrae M. xenopi M. hemophilum M. novum M. nonchromogenicum
IV	**Rapid growers**	M. fortuitum complex: M. fortuitum M. chelonae M. abscessus M. phlei M. vaccae M. smegmatis M. diernhoferi

1. **A.** In conjunction with the clinical presentation, the most likely diagnosis for the image shown is lupus miliaris disseminatus faciei.

   Lupus miliaris disseminatus faciei (LMDF) is an uncommon, chronic, inflammatory dermatosis characterized by red-to-yellow or yellow-brown papules of the central face, particularly on and around the eyelids. Lesions may occur singly or in crops. Spontaneous resolution after crusting or pustulation within 1–3 years is standard. Others believe it is a distinct entity because of its characteristic histopathology and occasional involvement of non-central facial areas. In 2000, a name change from LMDF to FIGURE (facial idiopathic granulomas with regressive evolution) was proposed. While the term LMDF is still widely used, the term FIGURE is now appearing in some publications. The cause is unknown, but suggestions have included infection by *Mycobacterium tuberculosis,* atypical mycobacteria, tuberculids, foreign body granuloma (particularly zirconium), reaction to cyst contents, and reaction to *Demodex folliculorum.* Histopathologic changes vary with age of the lesion:

   Early lesions: Show superficial perivascular and periappendageal lymphocytic infiltrates with a few histiocytes and neutrophils

   Fully developed lesions: Show round granulomas, typically with caseation necrosis

   Late lesions: Show fibrosis with scattered lymphocytes, histiocytes, and neutrophils and also may be perifollicular and may show epidermal thinning

2. **B.** Necrobiosis is typically seen in granuloma annulare.

   Other entities that demonstrate necrobiotic or collagenolytic granulomas include:

   - Necrobiosis lipoidica
   - Necrobiotic xanthogranuloma
   - Rheumatoid nodule

3. **A.** The best-fit diagnosis for the image shown is giant cell granuloma.

   Also known as annular elastolytic giant cell granuloma (AEGCG), this entity is characterized by smooth-surfaced annular plaques with raised red borders and central hypopigmentation, occurring mostly on sun-exposed areas of the head, neck, and upper extremities. Lesions are usually asymptomatic. A history of excessive sun exposure is typically associated. The term actinic granuloma (of O'Brien) is often used for the typical lesions of AEGCG on sun-damaged skin. Involvement of non-exposed areas may also occur in AEGCG. Histopathology of AEGCG, as shown in the image, indicates a granulomatous infiltrate composed for the most part of multinucleate giant cells exhibiting elastophagocytosis. Granuloma annulare (GA) is the main entity in the differential diagnosis, both clinically and histopathologically. The relationship between GA and AEGCG is controversial, and some consider AEGCG to be a form of GA. Individual lesions of AEGCG are clinically very similar to GA, but AEGCG *is more likely to occur in a photo-distributed pattern.* The histopathologic differences are most helpful in distinguishing the two entities. GA routinely demonstrates necrobiosis and mucin deposition, while AEGCG lacks both of these features. These histopathologic features, rather than elastophagocytosis, are most helpful in distinguishing AEGCG from GA. Elastophagocytosis is not specifically diagnostic of AEGCG. Elastophagocytosis is the phagocytosis of elastic fibers that can be seen microscopically in the cytoplasm of histiocytes, multinucleate giant cells, or both. Generally believed to be a characteristic feature of AEGCG, it can also be seen in mid-dermal elastolysis, select other cutaneous inflammatory conditions, cutaneous malignancies, infectious entities, and secondary to certain medications (also see answer 29).

4. **B.** Increased interstitial mucin is a feature of granuloma annulare.

   Mucin in granuloma annulare is hyaluronic acid and is visible in sections stained with hematoxylin and eosin as faintly basophilic stringy material. Its presence can be confirmed by staining with colloidal iron or Alcian blue at pH 2.5 (also see Table E2.1, Section E2).

5. **C.** The image shown is that of an asteroid body.

   Asteroid bodies (ABs) are striking cytoplasmic inclusions in giant cells of granulomas of many types including those of sarcoidosis, tuberculosis, leprosy, fungal infections, schistosomiasis, and lipoid and foreign body types. They vary in size from 5 to 30 μm and have up to 30 rays forming a star-like, spider, or umbrella pattern. The surrounding cytoplasm is vacuolated. There is controversy about their composition. Some believe the radiating spokes are composed of cytoplasmic filaments, and others believe they are composed of microtubular components. In any case, the pathophysiologic changes that produce the ABs are unknown.

6. **A.** Image shown is that of a Schaumann body.

   Schaumann bodies (SBs) are basophilic, lamellated, shell-like (conchoidal) bodies found in the cytoplasm of multinucleated giant cells of granulomas. Large SBs may be found extracellularly, as well. In addition, there is often a crystalline component that sometimes occurs alone. Entities characterized by SBs include:

   - Sarcoidosis (88% of cases)
   - Beryllium disease (62% of cases)
   - Active tuberculosis (6% of cases, found only in non-necrotizing granulomas and not in areas of caseation)

- Other (granulomas of Crohn's disease, hypersensitivity pneumonia, histoplasmosis, and lymph nodes draining cancer)

The basophilic component of the SB varies from 25 to 200 μm in diameter. Elemental analysis of the SB indicates the presence of calcium, phosphorus, and iron. In an electron microscopic study of early SBs, it appeared that the mineral salts were deposited on lamellated, phospholipid, myelin figures that develop in the cytoplasm of multinucleate giant cells. The crystals are colorless and brightly birefringent. They occur singly or in clumps. Size varies from 1–20 μm in diameter. Analysis suggests that they are composed of calcium oxalate. The crystals are soluble in water or formalin and tend to dissolve as the fixation time increases. When crystals occur alone, they should not be mistaken for foreign material such as talc or silica.

7. **E.** Sarcoidal granulomas may be a feature of Blau syndrome.

Blau syndrome is an inflammatory disorder that primarily affects the skin, joints, and eyes. Signs and symptoms begin in childhood, usually before the age of 4. Blau syndrome is inherited in an autosomal dominant pattern. Other names for this entity include early-onset sarcoidosis.

Granulomatous dermatitis is typically the earliest sign of Blau syndrome and is usually found on the torso, arms, and legs. Arthritis is another common feature of Blau syndrome. Most people with Blau syndrome also develop uveitis. Less commonly, Blau syndrome can affect other parts of the body, including the liver, kidneys, brain, blood vessels, lungs, and heart. Blau syndrome results from mutations in the *NOD2* gene.

8. **D.** *Mycobacterium scrofulaceum* is NOT a Group I mycobacterium.

M. scrofulaceum is a scotochromogen or Group II mycobacterium. Other members in this group include *M. flavescens* and *M. szulgai* (see Table D6.3).

9. **E.** Of the ones listed, *Mycobacterium chelonae* is the only one that is a rapid grower.

Other members in this category (Group IV) include (see Table D6.3):

M. fortuitum complex (*M. fortuitum, M. chelonae, M. abscessus*)
M. phlei
M. vaccae
M. smegmatis
M. diernhoferi

10. **A.** Lichen scrofulosorum is a tuberculid.

Tuberculids are a group of conditions involving recurrent eruptions of the skin, usually characterized by spontaneous involution and include:

- Erythema induratum
- Lichen scrofulosorum
- Papulonecrotic tuberculid
- Lupus miliaris disseminatus faciei (sometimes)

The characteristic symptom of lichen scrofulosorum, first recognized and described in 1868, is an eruption of miliary papules of pale yellow, brownish red or of the same color as the rest of the skin. Kaposi was the first to describe lichen scrofulosorum histologically. In his clinical description he classified the disease under the exanthems, since lichen scrofulosorum is an eruption of small papules usually present over the trunk, back and abdomen. Lichen scrofulosorum is a tuberculous entity consisting of small areas of lupus caused by tuberculous infiltrate, and is partly differentiated from lupus by the small dimension of the lesion. *It is believed to serve as the best example of a tuberculid.*

11. **D.** In conjunction with the clinical presentation, the most likely diagnosis for the image shown is granulomatous slack skin (GSS).

According to recent consensus at WHO/EORTC, GSS is classified as a rare subtype of mycosis fungoides with indolent clinical behavior. Clinically, GSS is characterized by the appearance of erythematous or violaceous painless plaques, with atrophic surface, sometimes with mild desquamation. It generally affects the axillary and inguinal regions. The size of the plaques increases slowly and progressively within a few years, leading to redundant folds of loose skin. Its clinical course is indolent and treatment is most often disappointing. In over 50% of cases, there is an association with Hodgkin's disease. Granulomatous mycosis fungoides (GMF) has been described as the main differential diagnosis for GSS. A multicentric recent study conducted by WHO/EORTC concluded that striking clinical differences exist between these two entities, but their histologic findings overlap. It is *therefore not possible to distinguish them only on a histopathologic basis.* The looseness of the skin in flexural areas is found only in GSS. The presence of elastophagocytosis is more characteristic of GSS; however, it can also be observed in GMF.

In terms of histopathology, GSS presents with a superficial lymphocytic infiltrate with admixed multinucleate giant cells some of which demonstrate elastophagocytosis. The reduction or absence of elastic fibers can be demonstrated by orcein stain. The infiltrate can sometimes span the entire dermis, even extending to the subcutaneous cellular tissue. Immunohistochemical studies demonstrate that the lymphocytic infiltrate has a predominance of CD4+, CD45RO+ and CD30+ cells with loss of pan T-cell markers such as CD3, CD5 and CD7.

12. C. Lupus miliaris disseminatus faciei (LMDF) is believed to be related to rosacea.

    Once considered a tuberculid because of the histology, LMDF is now considered by most to be an extreme variant of granulomatous rosacea. Others believe it is a distinct entity because of its characteristic histopathology and occasional involvement of non-central facial areas. Extrapolating from theories of the pathogenesis of other forms of rosacea, some suggest that LMDF is a reaction to *Demodex folliculorum*. While the usual distribution coincides with that of most rosacea cases, an association with *Demodex* has, to date, not been confirmed.

13. B. The triad of Melkersson-Rosenthal syndrome includes facial nerve palsy, fissured tongue, and cheilitis granulomatosa.

    Melkersson-Rosenthal syndrome is the term used when cheilitis occurs with facial palsy and plicated (fissured) tongue; this syndrome is occasionally a manifestation of Crohn disease or orofacial granulomatosis (OFG is the term used when there is no detectable evidence of Crohn disease). Histopathologic changes are not always conspicuous or specific in many cases of long duration; the infiltrate becomes denser and pleomorphic, and small, focal, non-caseating, sarcoidal granulomas are formed that are indistinguishable from Crohn disease or sarcoidosis.

14. C. The histopathologic triad of granuloma annulare (GA) includes necrobiosis, a palisaded lymphohistiocytic infiltrate forming granulomas and increased dermal mucin.

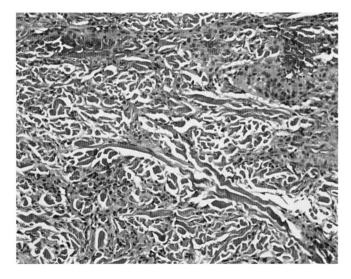

    While the histopathologic features of GA evolve with age of the lesion, the characteristic triad detailed above is present in most, if not all, lesions.

Early interstitial or incomplete granuloma annulare lesions show an interstitial pattern characterized by lymphocytes around vessels of the superficial and deep plexuses and by macrophages scattered between reticular dermal collagen bundles that are separated by mucin within which mast cells may be found.

Fully evolved granuloma annulare lesions and deep subcutaneous granuloma annulare nodules demonstrate palisaded granulomatous dermatitis or a septal and lobular panniculitis, respectively. Macrophages surround acellular necrobiotic areas in which collagen bundles are thinned, or they sometimes have a pale, homogeneous, light-blue appearance, the latter due to the presence of mucin. In many cases of subcutaneous granuloma annulare, and in some dermal infiltrates, the centers of granulomas contain degenerated, homogeneous-appearing collagen and are deeply eosinophilic. In some sections, necrotic small vessels in the centers of palisaded foci are surrounded by nuclear dust. Presence of fibrinogen can be shown by direct immunofluorescence in the centers of palisaded granulomas. In perforating lesions, necrobiotic material is extruded through focal perforations.

15. D. Image shown is that of necrobiosis lipodica (NL).

    Histopathologically, necrobiosis lipoidica presents with interstitial and palisaded granulomas that involve the subcutaneous tissue and dermis. At low magnification, lesions of necrobiosis lipoidica have a very characteristic appearance. The granulomas are arranged in a tier-like (layered) fashion and are admixed with areas of collagen degeneration. The granulomas are composed of histiocytes, lymphocytes, multinucleate giant cells, occasional plasma cells, and eosinophils. Reduction in the number of intradermal nerves is an additional feature of necrobiosis lipoidica. Thickening of vessel walls and reactive endothelial cell atypia, typical of vessels found in the middle to deep dermis, are characteristics shared with diabetic microangiopathy. Direct immunofluorescence findings of necrobiosis lipoidica include immunoglobulin M (IgM), IgA, C3, and fibrinogen in the thickened blood vessels. In non-diabetic patients with necrobiosis lipoidica, the vascular changes are not as prominent.

16. A. Necrobiosis lipoidica (NL) typically presents clinically as well-demarcated plaques on the anterior/lateral shins.

    Skin lesions of classic necrobiosis lipoidica begin as 1–3 mm, well-circumscribed papules that expand to form plaques with active, more indurated borders and waxy, strophic centers. Initially, these plaques are reddish brown but progressively become more yellow, shiny, and atrophic in appearance. Most cases of necrobiosis lipoidica occur on the pretibial area, but cases have been reported on the face, scalp, trunk, and upper extremities, where the diagnosis is more likely to be missed (atypical NL). Multiple telangiectatic vessels can be seen on the surface of the thinning epidermis. Ulceration at the site of trauma and subsequent infection are occasional complications of necrobiosis lipoidica. The Koebner phenomenon has been well established in patients with necrobiosis lipoidica.

17. **C.** Deep/subcutaneous granuloma annulare is more common in children.

    Deep/subcutaneous granuloma annulare is a disorder mainly in children in which deep dermal or subcutaneous nodules are distributed on the head and extremities. Histopathologic features are similar to those seen in granuloma annulare (GA) with a palisaded lymphohistiocytic infiltrate forming loose or well-formed granulomas surrounding foci of necrobiosis. Several labels such as subcutaneous granuloma annulare (SGA), deep GA, and pseudorheumatoid nodule have been applied to this entity. The etiology of childhood SGA remains unknown although proposed mechanisms and associations are numerous. Trauma appears to be the most probable association with SGA.

18. **E.** Necrobiotic xanthogranuloma (NXG) is typically always associated with a paraproteinemia.

    NXG is often accompanied by a monoclonal gammopathy of the immunoglobulin G-kappa (IgG-κ) type. NXG is characterized by firm yellow plaques and nodules, often occurring in a periorbital distribution.

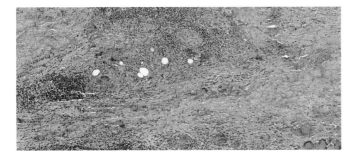

The histopathologic features of NXG are distinct. The epidermis may be atrophic or normal. NXG is always marked by a granulomatous inflammation in the dermis that can extend into the subcutaneous tissue. The granulomas are usually band-like and composed of foamy histiocytes, lymphocytes, foreign body-type multinucleate giant cells, and Touton giant cells alternating with foci of necrobiosis. Cholesterol clefts are usually visualized within the necrobiotic foci, but can be rare or absent. Nodular lymphoid aggregates are often reported in association with the granulomas. (For a list of other entities associated with a paraprotein, see Table D2.3, Section D2.)

19. **D.** Granuloma annulare is NOT a "red" granuloma.

    Granuloma annulare (GA) is a "blue" granuloma because of the foci of necrobiosis characteristic of GA. Other entities in this category include Wegener's granulomatosis and rheumatoid vasculitis (NOT rheumatoid nodule, which falls under the category of "red" granulomas). See Table D6.2.

20. **D.** *Blastomyces dermatitidis* is NOT a dematiaceous fungus.

    Subcutaneous dematiaceous fungal infections, which include chromoblastomycosis and phaeohyphomycosis, are a heterogeneous group of clinical entities caused by dematiaceous or pigmented fungi that are found in soil. These infections have a wide spectrum of clinical presentations that depend largely on the specific causative organism and on the integrity of the host's immune response. Chromoblastomycosis and phaeohyphomycosis are both caused by pigmented fungi and share a number of clinical features and causative organisms, yet are considered two distinct clinical entities.

    Other dematiaceous fungi include:
    - The dimorphic fungus *Sporothrix schenkii*
    - *Tinea nigra*
    - *Alternaria*

    Also see Section G, Table G7 and Table G8.

21. **B.** The best-fit diagnosis for the image shown is phaeohyphomycosis.

    Phaeohyphomycosis describes a heterogeneous group of fungal infections that are caused by over 100 species and 60 genera of dematiaceous fungi that are found in soil worldwide, with varied clinical presentations that are greatly influenced by the immune status of the host. Common causative agents of phaeohyphomycosis include fungi of the following genera:
    - *Exophiala*
    - *Wangiella*
    - *Bipolaris*
    - *Alternaria*
    - *Phialophora*

    The most common clinical presentations in immunocompetent hosts include localized cutaneous infection (superficial or subcutaneous), fungal sinusitis, allergic bronchopulmonary mycosis (similar to the presentation of allergic bronchopulmonary aspergillosis), and, rarely, fatal brain abscess. The subcutaneous lesions of phaeohyphomycosis typically result from direct inoculation *via* trauma to exposed skin, and, in immunocompetent patients, most commonly present as a single, inflammatory, cystic or indurated plaque. In immunocompromised patients, phaeohyphomycosis is increasingly being recognized as an opportunistic infection. In these individuals, the clinical presentation is variable and ranges from an isolated nodule to disseminated, indurated plaques, nodules, escars, and ulcers. In addition, immunocompromised patients are at risk for locally invasive phaeohyphomycosis, and, rarely, but often fatal, pneumonia or disseminated disease.

In terms of histopathology, the characteristic lesion, as evidenced in the figure, is a circumscribed cyst or chronic abscess in the deep dermis or subcutis. The wall is typically composed of compressed fibrous tissue with an adjacent granulomatous tissue reaction. A wood splinter or foreign body may be seen in the central cystic portion and brown filamentous hyphae may be seen in the wall, in the giant cells or even in the debris.

Also see Section G, Table G7 and Table G8.

22. **C.** Image shown is that of chromomycosis.

Chromoblastomycosis is a subcutaneous infection with highest prevalence in the tropics; it is typically seen in immunocompetent hosts and results from traumatic inoculation of skin by pigmented fungi. The principal causative agents are fungi of the following genera:

- *Fonsecaea* (tropical forests)
- *Cladophialophora* (dry climates)
- *Philalophora*

The disease is most commonly observed in agriculturists on the lower legs, which likely explains the observed propensity for men of lower socioeconomic status. Chromoblastomycosis typically presents with an asymptomatic papule or nodule that develops slowly over years into a localized verrucous plaque that expands and leaves behind a central sclerotic or keloidal scar. The lesion may have characteristic black dots on the surface, which represent the host's attempt at transepidermal elimination of fungal elements. The disease most often remains localized, but satellite lesions from autoinoculation and lymphatic spread have been documented. The diagnosis of chromoblastomycosis rests on identification of thick-walled, multiseptate, brown, sclerotic cells termed *medlar bodies, copper pennies,* or *muriform cells.* These pathognomonic features can be observed in tissue biopsy specimens or by direct microscopic examination of a scraping of black dots from the surface of the nodule with 10% potassium hydroxide. Identification of the causative fungal species can be achieved by tissue culture but is not reliably positive.

Also see Section G, Table G7 and Table G8.

23. **D.** The best-fit diagnosis for the image shown is coccidiomycosis.

Infection is typically transmitted by inhalation of airborne spores of *Coccidioides immitis* or *C. posadasii.*

The vast majority of coccidioidal infections result from airborne transmission. Pulmonary infection can result from inhalation of a single spore in humans, but high inoculum exposures are more likely to result in symptomatic disease. Inhaled *C. immitis* or *C. posadasii* arthroconidia (i.e., spores) are deposited into the terminal bronchiole.

Typically, the arthroconidia enlarge to form spherules, which are round double-walled structures measuring approximately 20–100 μm in diameter. The spherules undergo internal division within 48–72 hours and become filled with hundreds to thousands of offspring (i.e., endospores). Rupture of the spherules leads to the release of endospores, which mature to form more spherules. As an arthroconidium transforms into a spherule, the resulting inflammation results in a local pulmonary lesion. Extracts of *C. immitis* organisms react with complement, leading to the release of mediators of chemotaxis for neutrophils.

Some of the endospores are engulfed by macrophages, initiating the acute inflammation phase. If the infection is not cleared during this process, a new set of lymphocytes and histiocytes descend on the infection site, leading to granuloma formation with the presence of giant cells. This is the chronic inflammation phase. People with severe disease may have both acute and chronic forms of inflammation.

Also see Section G, Table G7 and Table G8.

24. **D.** Coccidiomycosis is endemic in Mexico.

Coccidioidomycosis is caused by *Coccidioides immitis*, a soil fungus native to the San Joaquin Valley of California, and by *C. posadasii*, which is endemic to certain arid-to-semiarid areas of the southwestern USA, northern portions of Mexico, and scattered areas in Central America and South America. Although genetically distinct, the 2 species are morphologically identical.

25. **A.** The best-fit diagnosis for the image shown is sporotrichosis.

Sporotrichosis is a subacute or chronic infection caused by the saprophytic dimorphic fungus *Sporothrix schenckii*. The characteristic infection involves suppurating subcutaneous nodules that progress proximally along lymphatic channels (lymphocutaneous sporotrichosis).

In lymphocutaneous sporotrichosis, the primary lesion develops at the site of cutaneous inoculation, typically in the distal upper extremities. After several weeks, new lesions appear along the lymphatic tracts. Patients with this form are typically afebrile and not systemically ill. The lesions usually cause minimal pain. The fixed cutaneous form is characterized by a painless violaceous or erythematous plaque that may ulcerate or become verrucous. This presentation should be considered when a wound fails to heal. There are no satellite lesions. The disseminated cutaneous form is usually seen in immunosuppressed individuals. This form of the disease can be the initial presentation of HIV infection or may develop as part of an immune reconstitution syndrome.

In terms of histopathology, sporotrichosis is characterized histopathologically by granulomatous inflammation with occasional asteroid bodies. The sporothrix may be present in the tissue as yeast-like forms, as elongate cells ("cigar bodies") or, albeit rarely, as hyphae. The "sporothrix asteroid" is the pathognomonic finding and is characterized by a blastospore surrounded by radiating strands of intensely basophilic, hyaline material.

Also see Section G, Table G7 and Table G8.

26. C. Blastomycosis is characterized by broad-based buds and lack of an endospore and capsule.

Blastomycosis is a fungal infection caused by inhalation of aerosolized conidia (spores) of *Blastomyces dermatitidis*. Clinical presentations occur across a wide spectrum, ranging from an asymptomatic, self-limited pulmonary infection to widely disseminated life-threatening disease.

Blastomycosis is endemic to the USA and Canada and most cases are clustered around the Mississippi and Ohio River Valley states and Canadian provinces around the Great Lakes. Within the USA, the most commonly affected states are Arkansas, Illinois, Kentucky, Louisiana, Mississippi, North Carolina, Tennessee, and Wisconsin. Exposure to soil is the common factor associated with contracting this disease. Blastomycosis is recognized increasingly in immunocompromised hosts, particularly in patients with acquired immune deficiency syndrome (AIDS).

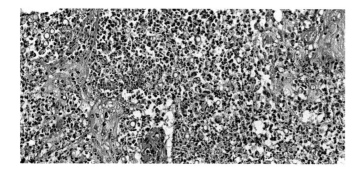

Microscopically, yeasts 8–20 μm in size, with single, broad-based buds, double refractile walls, and multiple nuclei, are extremely characteristic of *Blastomyces dermatitidis* (*B. dermatitidis* mold has a distinctive "lollipop" appearance with oval conidia, 2–4 μm in diameter at the tips of thin conidiophores). They also have thin septate hyphae, 1–2 μm in diameter.

Also see Section G, Table G7 and Table G8.

27. A. Malakoplakia is NOT caused by *Bartonella*.

Malakoplakia or malacoplakia is a rare inflammatory condition which makes its presence known as a papule, plaque or ulceration that usually affects the genitourinary tract. However, it may also be associated with other bodily organs. Microscopically it is characterized by the presence of foamy histiocytes with basophilic inclusions called Michaelis-Gutmann bodies.

Bartonella is a genus of Gram-negative bacteria. It is the only genus in the family Bartonellaceae. Facultative intracellular parasites, *Bartonella* species can infect healthy people, but are considered especially important as opportunistic pathogens. *Bartonella* species are transmitted by vectors such as ticks, fleas, sand flies, and mosquitoes. At least eight *Bartonella* species or subspecies are known to infect humans.

The best known ones are the following:

B. bacilliformis – Carrion's fever (Oroya fever, verruca peruana)

B. quintana –Trench fever, bacillary angiomatosis, endocarditis

B. clarridgeiae – Cat scratch disease

B. henselae – Cat scratch disease, bacillary angiomatosis, peliosis hepatitis, endocarditis, bacteremia with fever, neuroretinitis

28. C. In conjunction with the clinical presentation, the most likely diagnosis for the image shown is rheumatoid nodule.

The rheumatoid nodule is the most common cutaneous manifestation of rheumatoid arthritis (RA). Although nodules commonly are found on pressure points (such as the olecranon process), they may occur at other sites, including ones within internal organs of the body. Thus, bedridden patients can develop nodules on the occiput and ischial areas, and nodules occasionally form on the Achilles tendon and vocal cords. Rheumatoid "nodulosis" is characterized by multiple nodules on the hands and multiple subchondral bone cysts known as "geodes." These nodules tend to occur on extensor surfaces adjacent to joints, elbows, and fingers, as well as the forearm, metacarpophalangeal and proximal interphalangeal joints, occiput, back, heel, and other areas.

In terms of histopathology, the rheumatoid nodule is characterized by deeply eosinophilic foci of fibrinoid necrosis surrounded by a palisaded lymphohistiocytic infiltrate. The defining histopathologic features are typically seen in the deep dermis or even subcutis.

29. **B.** The image shown depicts elastoclasis or elastophagocytosis.

    Generally believed to be a characteristic feature of annular elastolytic giant cell granuloma (AEGCG), it can also be seen in mid-dermal elastolysis, select other cutaneous inflammatory conditions, cutaneous malignancies, infectious entities, and secondary to select medications (colony stimulating factor, nicorandil).

    Entities consistently exhibiting elastophagocytosis:

    - AEGCG
    - Mid-dermal elastolysis
    - Papillary dermal elastolysis
    - Granulomatous slack skin

    Entities inconsistently exhibiting elastophagocytosis:

    - Granuloma annulare
    - Lichen sclerosus
    - Sarcoidosis

    - Granulomatous mycosis fungoides
    - Atypical fibroxanthoma

30. **A.** Granuloma annulare is NOT a synonym for annular elastolytic giant cell granuloma.

    All of the other names listed are synonymous with annular elastolytic giant cell granuloma (AEGCG). This is considered a distinct entity characterized by the appearance of annular erythematous to skin-colored lesions preferentially on sun-exposed areas and histopathologically with a granulomatous reaction with elastolysis, phagocytosis of the elastic fibers, and multinucleate giant cells with absence or reduction of elastin fibers. While elastophagocytosis may be seen in several entities, albeit to varying degrees (see answer 29), the histopathologic hallmarks of AEGCG are the absence of collagen necrobiosis or mucin deposition.

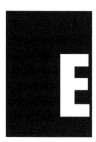

Disorders Involving the Dermis and/or Subcutis

E1 Collagen and Elastic Tissue Disorders
Questions

1. The most abundant collagen in the dermis is:
   A. Type I
   B. Type III
   C. Type IV
   D. Type V
   E. Type VII

2. The most likely diagnosis is:

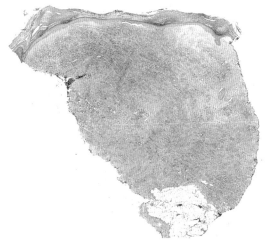

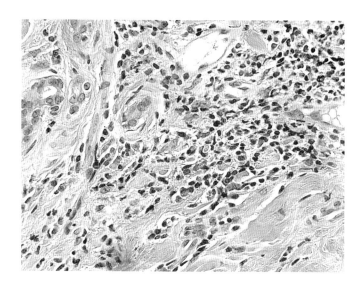

   A. Scleredema
   B. Scleromyxedema
   C. Nephrogenic systemic fibrosis
   D. Radiation dermatitis
   E. Scleroderma

3. The most likely diagnosis is:

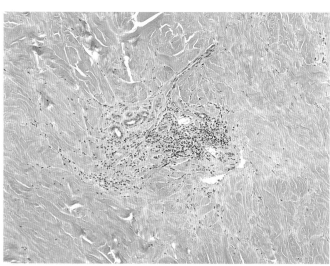

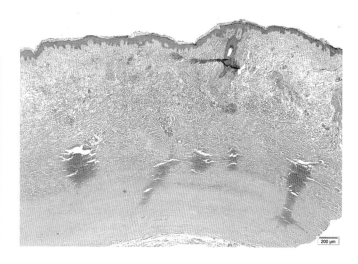

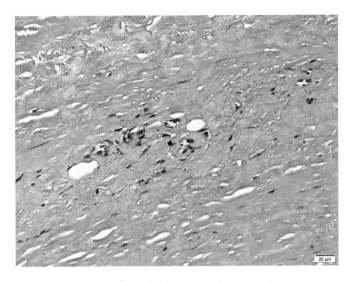

A. Exuberant dermal hypersensitivity reaction
B. Lymphomatoid papulosis
C. Churg-Strauss syndrome
D. Eosinophilic fasciitis
E. Nephrogenic systemic fibrosis

4. The best-fit diagnosis is:

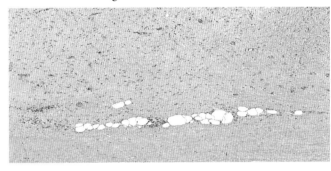

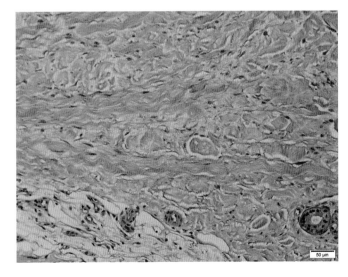

A. Scleromyxedema
B. Scleredema
C. Scleroderma

D. Nephrogenic systemic fibrosis
E. Reticular erythematous mucinosis

5. This (based on the image shown above) is most commonly associated with:
A. Infection
B. Hyperthyroidism
C. Renal disease
D. Stasis
E. Paraproteinemia

6. Lesional cells (based on the image shown above) are typically positive for:
A. CD30
B. CD31
C. CD34
D. CD43
E. CD45

7. "Tram-tracking" is typically associated with:
A. Necrobiotic xanthogranuloma
B. Nephrogenic systemic fibrosis
C. Scleromyxedema
D. Jessner's lymphocytic infiltrate
E. Reticular erythematous mucinosis

8. The most likely diagnosis is:

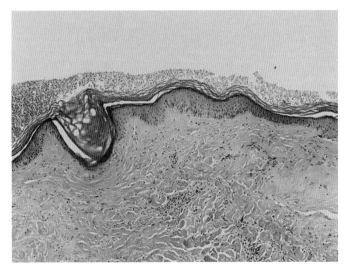

A. Lichen sclerosus
B. Lichen amyloidosus
C. Lichen planus
D. Lichen planus pemphigoides
E. Lichenoid drug eruption

9. The most likely diagnosis is:

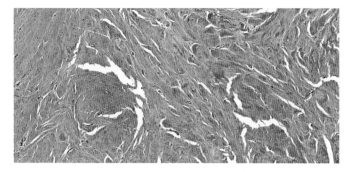

    A. Dermatomyofibroma
    B. Scleredema
    C. Collagenoma
    D. Scleroderma
    E. Keloid

10. This is most commonly associated with:

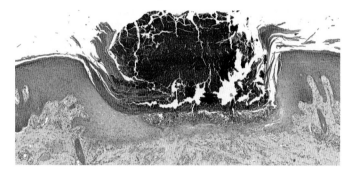

    A. Chemotherapy
    B. Hyperthyroidism
    C. Renal disease
    D. Stasis
    E. Paraproteinemia

11. The most likely location for this lesion is:

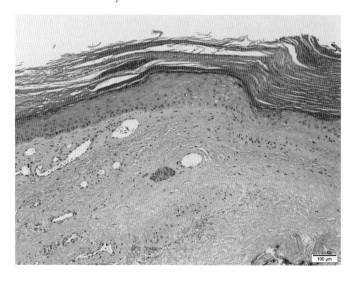

    A. Eye
    B. Ear
    C. Hand
    D. Foot
    E. Perineum

12. Buschke-Ollendorf syndrome is associated with disorders in:
    A. Elastic tissue
    B. Collagen
    C. Epidermal maturation
    D. Pigmentation
    E. Keratinization

13. The most likely diagnosis is:

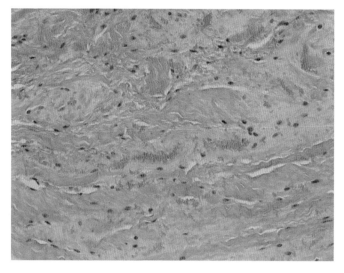

    A. Elastoderma
    B. Elastosis perforans serpiginosa
    C. Pseudoxanthoma elasticum
    D. Dermal elastosis
    E. Elastofibroma

14. The most likely location for this entity (based on the image shown above) is:
    A. Hand
    B. Foot
    C. Ear
    D. Back
    E. Abdomen

15. The drug most often implicated in this is:

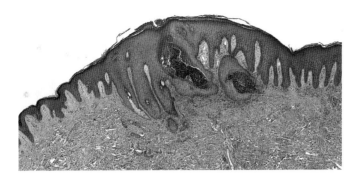

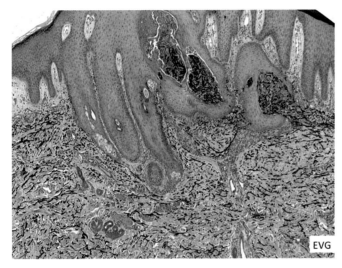

A. Vemurafenib
B. Cytarabine
C. Penicillamine
D. Vancomycin
E. NSAIDs

16. The most likely diagnosis is:

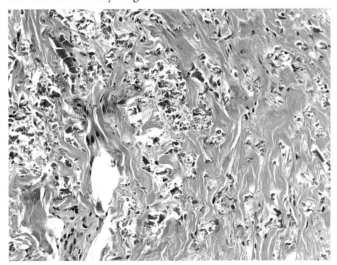

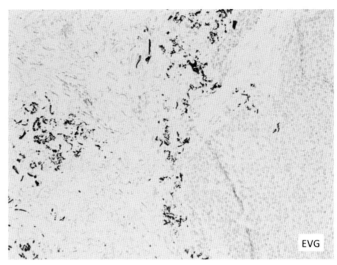

A. Focal dermal elastolysis
B. Elastosis perforans serpiginosa
C. Pseudoxanthoma elasticum
D. Mid dermal elastosis
E. Acrokeratoelastoidosis

17. Mutations in which of the following is associated with this (based on the image shown above):

A. *ABCB5*
B. *ABCC6*
C. *ABCF2*
D. *PTEN*
E. *MLH1*

E1 Collagen and Elastic Tissue Disorders
Answers

Table E1.1 Extracellular matrix components as antigenic targets in autoimmune disease with cutaneous involvement

Entity	Autoantigen	Cutaneous manifestations
Polychondritis, arthritis	Collagen II, IX	Chondritis of the ear
Bullous pemphigoid	BPAg1 (BP230, 80%), BPAg2 (BP 180, 30%)	Skin blisters
Cicatricial pemphigoid	BPAg2 (BP180) Epiligrin (laminin 332, 10%)	Skin blisters
Epidermolysis bullosa acquisita	Collagen VII	Skin blisters
Bullous systemic lupus erythematosus	Collagen VII	Skin blisters
Scleroderma	Fibrillin 1	Skin fibrosis

1. **A.** The most abundant collagen in the dermis is type I collagen.

    Type I collagen comprises about 80% of dermal collagen. Also known as alpha-1 type I collagen, it is a protein that in humans is encoded by the *COL1A1* gene. *COL1A1* encodes the major component of type I collagen, the fibrillar collagen found in most connective tissues, including cartilage. Mutations in the *COL1A1* gene are associated with the following conditions:

    - Ehlers-Danlos syndrome
    - Osteogenesis imperfecta
    - Osteoporosis

2. **E.** The most likely diagnosis for the image shown is scleroderma.

    Scleroderma refers to entities characterized by deposition of collagen in the skin as well as in other organs. Scleroderma may be localized (morphea and linear scleroderma) or systemic (diffuse, limited, mixed connective tissue disease, eosinophilic fasciitis and atrophoderma of Pasini and Pierini). Overproduction of collagen, particularly types I and III collagen, by fibroblasts in affected tissues is common to all forms of morphea, although the mechanism by which these fibroblasts are activated is unknown. Autoantibodies commonly present in all types of morphea include:

    Rheumatoid factor – Positive in 15–60% of morphea patients, most often children with linear morphea

    Antinuclear antibodies – Present in approximately 20–80% of morphea patients, typically with a homogeneous, speckled, or nucleolar pattern, prevalence is higher in patients with generalized, linear, and deep subtypes

    Anti-single-stranded DNA antibodies – Present in 25% of patients with plaque-type morphea, in 75% of those with generalized morphea, and in 50% of those with linear morphea; levels correlate with extensive, active disease and joint contractures

    Antihistone antibodies – Present in 47–87% of morphea patients overall and in 85% of those with generalized morphea, correlating with the number of plaque-type lesions and the total area affected, antibody titers may be related to the extent of involvement and the disease activity in linear scleroderma

    Antibodies to matrix metalloproteinase (MMP)-1 – Significantly elevated in 46% of morphea patients

    Antiphospholipid antibodies – Present in some morphea patients, IgM and IgG anticardiolipin antibodies are present in 60% and 25% of patients with generalized morphea, respectively, lupus anticoagulant can also be detected in approximately 50% of this subgroup of patients

    Antitopoisomerase II-alpha antibodies – Present in 76% of morphea patients

    Anti-Cu/Zn-superoxide dismutase antibodies – Present in 90% of morphea patients

    Histopathologic findings of morphea and systemic sclerosis are similar, with a fundamental process of thickening and homogenization of collagen bundles (depth of involvement is important for categorization into the morphea subtypes). The sclerotic process in superficial circumscribed morphea is centered in the lower reticular dermis, whereas other variants are characterized by replacement of the subcutaneous fat and underlying tissues by collagen.

    Changes in early inflammatory stage: Perivascular and interstitial, variably dense infiltrate of lymphocytes admixed with plasma cells and occasional eosinophils in the reticular dermis and/or the fibrous trabeculae of the subcutaneous tissues, reactive endothelial cell atypia, homogenization of dermal collagen.

    Changes in late sclerotic stage: Inflammatory infiltrate typically disappears, collagen bundles in the reticular dermis and subcutis become thick, closely packed, and hyalinized, loss of peri-eccrine adipocytes, replacement of subcutaneous fat by collagen (junction between deep dermis and subcutis well-demarcated and "almost a straight line"), paucity of blood, adnexal structures are progressively lost. Depending on the subtype, the process of sclerosis may extend into the fascia and even underlying muscle; in contrast, thickened collagen bundles are restricted to the dermis in superficial morphea.

Lichen-sclerosus-like change may be coexistent with select cases of morphea.

3. **D.** The most likely diagnosis for the image shown is eosinophilic fasciitis.

Eosinophilic fasciitis (EF), also called Shulman syndrome, is a rare, localized fibrosing disorder of the fascia of unknown etiology and pathophysiology. The cutaneous manifestations of eosinophilic fasciitis evolve as the disease progresses. In the acute inflammatory stage, cutaneous changes include erythematous swelling and non-pitting edema. These findings are later replaced by skin induration, and, eventually, fibrosis predominates. The affected skin is taut and firmly adherent to underlying tissues. Dimpling, *peau d'orange*, and venous furrowing, or the "groove sign," can be seen. Cutaneous manifestations are generally bilateral and symmetric. The upper extremity (proximal and distal to the elbow) and the lower extremity (proximal and distal to the knee) are most commonly involved. A concurrent localized lesion of morphea may be seen in 25% of patients. Characteristic laboratory findings of EF include:
- Peripheral blood eosinophilia (the degree of eosinophilia is variable over time, even in the absence of specific therapy)
- Hypergammaglobulinemia (characteristic and most often due to a polyclonal increase in IgG)
- Increased ESR

Histopathologic hallmarks include inflammation, edema, thickening, and sclerosis of the fascia. Acute findings include infiltration of deep fascia and adjacent subcutis with lymphocytes, plasma cells, histiocytes, and eosinophils. In the deeper portions of the panniculus, a similar infiltrate is found in the fibrous septa and at the periphery of the fat lobules. Deep in the fascia, the inflammatory infiltrate can extend into the epimysium, perimysium, and endomysium. In addition, vascular cuffing with lymphocytes and plasma cells is often evident. With disease progression, inflammatory changes are replaced by generalized sclerosis and thickening of the fascia and adjacent tissue layers.

4. **D.** Image shown is that of nephrogenic systemic fibrosis (NSF).

Unique histopathologic features of nephrogenic systemic fibrosis, first described in 2001, include thickened collagen bundles with surrounding clefts, mucin deposition, and a proliferation of fibroblasts and elastic fibers. Histopathologic findings most closely resemble those of scleromyxedema and vary with age of lesion.

Early lesions (within 20 weeks of clinical onset): Cellular dermal proliferation epithelioid or stellate spindled cells, proliferation can extend into and widen the subcutaneous fat lobule septa, spindle cells are diffusely arranged among thickened collagen bundles; clefts can encompass some spindle cells; most of the spindle cells are CD34/procollagen dual-positive cells that form a dense interconnecting network

Late lesions (>20 weeks of clinical onset): Typically have less prominent clefting, less mucin, and fewer CD34/procollagen-positive cells, calcification and sclerotic or "lollipop" bodies may be evident

5. **C.** Nephrogenic systemic fibrosis (NSF) is most commonly associated with renal disease.

NSF, also known as nephrogenic fibrosing dermopathy (NFD), is a disease of fibrosis of the skin and internal organs reminiscent but distinct from scleromyxedema. Nephrogenic systemic fibrosis always occurs (with the exception of one report in 2 transplant patients whose organ donors' histories were not noted) in patients with renal insufficiency that have had imaging studies (e.g., magnetic resonance angiography) with gadolinium, a contrast agent used in imaging studies. Gadolinium can be found in tissue samples of nephrogenic systemic fibrosis. The mechanism by which NSF occurs is not known, but it seems to involve a cell termed a circulating fibrocyte that is stimulated by gadolinium. Endothelin-1/endothelin receptor signaling plays a role in the calcification and fibrosis of nephrogenic systemic fibrosis.

Toll-like receptors (TLR), in particular TLR4 and TLR7, play a role in the development of nephrogenic systemic fibrosis. Nephrogenic systemic fibrosis manifests clinically with induration, thickening, and hardening of the skin with brawny hyperpigmentation and distinct papules and subcutaneous nodules. The skin can have a peau d'orange appearance, and plaques may have an amoeboid advancing edge. The skin is often shiny and hard to the touch. A woody consistency is typical. The extremities are the most common areas of involvement, followed by the trunk. The face is almost never involved. Yellow palmar papules resembling cutaneous calcinosis have been reported. In addition, yellow scleral plaques have been reported in patients with nephrogenic systemic fibrosis.

6. **C.** Lesional fibroblasts in nephrogenic systemic fibrosis (NSF) are CD34 positive.

CD34 is a 115 kDa transmembrane sialomucin encoded on a gene located on chromosome 1q32. It is expressed in activated bone marrow progenitor cells, which give rise to the hematopoietic and angioblastic lineages. While CD34 expression is lost during differentiation in the hematopoietic lineage, it is maintained in the angioblastic one. In addition, evidence exists supporting the idea that a subset of CD34 positive stromal cells derived from bone marrow and muscle represents a type of mesenchymal stem cell. For a detailed list of other CD34 positive entities, see Table E2.3, Section E2.

7. **B.** Tram-tracking is associated with nephrogenic systemic fibrosis (NSF).

In NSF, CD34 positive spindle or epithelioid cells are aligned in a reticular or parallel arrangement forming a complex network. CD34 dendritic cell processes form a "tram-track" arrangement around a central elastic fiber.

A clinicopathologic classification system has been developed for NSF based on the following:

Major clinical criteria: Patterned plaques, joint contractures, cobblestoning, marked induration
Minor clinical criteria: Puckering/linear banding, superficial plaque/patch, dermal papules, scleral plaques in those <45 years of age
Histopathologic criteria: Increased dermal cellularity, CD34+ cells with tram-tracking, thick and thin collagen bundles, preserved elastic fibers, septal subcutaneous involvement, osseous metaplasia

Identification of preserved elastic tissue is a finding that has value in excluding morphea/scleroderma, and therefore receives a score of 1 if it is absent; if present, it receives a neutral score of 0. A distinctive histopathologic finding consisting of small spicules of bone developing around elastic fibers ("lollipop lesion") has been observed in select cases evaluated to date. This feature is thought to represent a highly specific (but insensitive) histopathologic sign of NSF.

8. **A.** The most likely diagnosis for the image shown is lichen sclerosus.

Lichen sclerosus (LS) is a chronic inflammatory dermatosis that clinically presents as white plaques with epidermal atrophy and scarring. Lichen sclerosus has both genital and extragenital presentations and also goes by several names: balanitis xerotica obliterans (glans penis presentation) and kraurosis vulvae (older description of vulvar presentation). An increased risk of squamous cell carcinoma may exist in genital disease. Histopathologic findings include patchy or focally confluent squamatization of the basal layer, homogenization of the papillary dermis with an underlying lymphoid lichenoid inflammatory infiltrate. Of note, as the lesion ages, the lichenoid infiltrate gets pushed further down. Established lesions show hyperkeratosis, follicular plugging, epidermal attenuation and interface change. Vascular change predominantly in the form of lymphocytic vasculitis is often present.

9. **E.** The most likely diagnosis for the image shown is keloid.

A keloid is an abnormal proliferation of scar tissue that forms at the site of cutaneous injury. It does not regress and *grows beyond the original margins of the scar*. Keloids should not be confused with hypertrophic scars, which are raised scars that do not grow beyond the boundaries of the original wound and may reduce over time. The frequency of keloid occurrence in persons with highly pigmented skin is much (15 times) higher than in persons with less

pigmented skin. Histopathologic findings are distinct but vary with age of the lesion:

Early lesions: Abundant fibrillary collagen
Mature lesions: Broad, homogeneous, brightly eosinophilic bundles arranged in a haphazard array

Abundant mucopolysaccharides, particularly chondroitin-4-sulfate, are evident between bundles.

10. **C.** Perforating collagenosis shown in the image is commonly associated with renal disease.

The acquired form of perforating collagenosis usually occurs in patients with diabetes or chronic renal failure, especially those receiving dialysis. Clinically, perforating collagenosis presents as flesh-colored, umbilicated, dome-shaped papules or nodules as large as 10 mm in diameter with an adherent, keratinous plug. Lesions are most commonly found on the extensor surfaces of the limbs and the dorsa of the hands. Histopathology varies with age of the lesion.

Early lesions: Acanthosis and accumulation of basophilic collagen in the dermal papillae
Established lesions: Cup-shaped epidermal invagination filled with a plug composed parakeratotic and basophilic debris and collagen; vertically oriented collagen closely abutting the epidermis may be evident in the underlying dermis

11. **B.** Image shown is that of chondrodermatitis nodularis helicis which typically occurs on the ear.

Chondrodermatitis nodularis helicis (CNH), a common, benign, painful condition of the ear, more often affects middle-aged or older men and clinically presents as firm, tender, well-demarcated, round to oval nodules with a raised, rolled edge and central ulcer or crust. The name is a misnomer as there is no inflammation of the cartilage. The right ear is affected more commonly than the left. Lesions develop on the most prominent projection of the ear. The most common location is the apex of the helix. Distribution on the antihelix is more common in women. The precise cause of CNH is not certain; however, pressure, cold, actinic damage, and repeated trauma have each been implicated. Sleeping on the affected side as well as injury to the underlying cartilage and/or skin from pressure appears to be a primary etiologic factor. Histopathologic changes are similar to those seen in decubitus ulcers, but on a smaller scale. Within the central portion of a shave biopsy, the epidermis usually is invaginated and/or ulcerated with underlying papillary dermal fibrin deposits and an increased density of ectatic, endothelial cell-lined vessels in the superficial dermis.

12. **A.** Buschke-Ollendorf syndrome is associated with disorders in elastic tissue.

Buschke-Ollendorf syndrome is inherited as an autosomal dominant variant with incomplete penetrance. The dermal lesions are composed of collagen and elastin fibers and, in some instances, mucopolysaccharides. The cutaneous lesions are usually localized on the trunk, in the sacrolumbar region, and, symmetrically, on the extremities. Occasionally, the lesions may be found on the head. They present with slightly elevated and flattened yellowish papules and nodules grouped together forming plaques several centimeters in diameter. Histopathologic examination reveals numerous, variably thickened elastic fibers that are frequently fragmented.

13. **E.** Image shown is that of elastofibroma dorsii.

    Elastofibromas are slow-growing tumors in the region of inferior angle of the scapula, hence the name. Histopathologically, elastofibroma dorsii is characterized by thickened abnormal elastic fibers and is generally regarded as a reactive process, an unusual fibroblastic pseudotumor. Clinically elastofibromas usually present as a large, well-circumscribed tumor that most often does not adhere to the overlying skin. Histopathologic findings include a dermal unencapsulated tumor composed of branched and unbranched elastic fibers, eosinophilic collagen bundles, and scattered fatty tissue. The elastic fibers have a degenerated, beaded appearance or are fragmented into small globules or droplets arranged in a linear pattern.

14. **D.** Elastofibromas typically occur on the back.

    Elastofibroma is a rare, benign, slow-growing connective-tissue tumor that occurs most often in the subscapular area in elderly women. The etiology of elastofibroma remains unclear, although its prevalence is increased in persons who perform manual labor involving the shoulder girdle, suggesting that repeated trauma induces this process. While this theory provides an explanation for the right-sided preponderance, in up to 66% of cases the tumor is bilateral.

15. **C.** Penicillamine is the drug most often implicated in elastosis perforans serpiginosa, shown in the image.

    Elastosis perforans serpiginosa (EPS) is a rare condition affecting the skin elastic tissue. EPS is now a well-recognized potential complication of long-term penicillamine therapy. The acquired form secondary to long-term treatment with D-penicillamine (DPA) was first reported in 1972. The mechanism relates to the capacity of DPA to interfere with elastin cross-linking through the inhibition of a copper-dependent enzyme, the lysyl oxidase, or by formation of complexes with the collagen cross-linked precursors, impairing a normal maturation of elastic fibers. Iatrogenic EPS is extremely rare, even though DPA has been used for several conditions including cystinuria and rheumatoid arthritis. The majority of cases are associated with treatment for Wilson's disease, probably because copper chelating and elimination is pushed to the maximum, requiring constant high levels of the drug for years. Skin lesions actually appear after several years of drug intake and slowly regress after the drug discontinuation. In 30% of the cases it is associated with systemic diseases, such as Down syndrome, Ehlers-Danlos syndrome, osteogenesis imperfecta,

pseudoxanthoma elasticum, or Marfan syndrome. Histopathologic findings in EPS of any etiopathogenesis include broken and tortuous elastic fibers.

16. **C.** The most likely diagnosis for the image shown is pseudoxanthoma elasticum.

    Pseudoxanthoma elasticum (PXE) is a rare genetic disorder characterized by elastorrhexia, or progressive calcification and fragmentation, of elastic fibers primarily affecting the skin, the retina, and the cardiovascular system. Cutaneous lesions typically begin in childhood or early adolescence, but due to their asymptomatic nature, diagnosis is delayed by an average of 9 years. Cutaneous findings are most frequently the first diagnostic sign of PXE, classically arising on the lateral aspect of the neck. The cutaneous manifestations of pseudoxanthoma elasticum are highly characteristic. The lesions usually develop in childhood or early adolescence and consist of small, yellow papules 1–5 mm in diameter in a linear or reticular pattern. The skin takes on a plucked chicken, Moroccan leather, or cobblestone appearance. Typically, these changes are first noted on the lateral part of the neck and later involve the antecubital fossae, the axillae, the popliteal spaces, the inguinal and periumbilical areas, the oral mucosa involving the lower lip, cheek, and palate, and the vaginal and rectal mucosae. As the disease progresses, the skin of the neck, the axillae, and the groin may become soft, lax, and wrinkled, hanging in folds. The extent of these changes is usually limited. The characteristic ocular manifestations of pseudoxanthoma elasticum are angioid streaks of the retina, which are slate gray to reddish brown curvilinear bands that radiate from the optic disk. Histopathologic findings include basophilic elastic fibers (due to calcium deposition). The fibers are fragmented, swollen, and clumped in the middle and deep reticular dermis. Similar calcification is noted in the tunica media and intima of the blood vessels.

17. **B.** Mutations in *ABCC6* are associated with pseudoxanthoma elasticum (based on question 16).

    Pseudoxanthoma elasticum is associated with mutations in the *ABCC6* gene, which encodes an ATP-binding cassette transporter protein recently localized to the mitochondria-associated membrane (MAM). The gene is expressed predominantly in the liver and kidney; however, pseudoxanthoma elasticum most commonly involves the elastic fibers of the mid and deep reticular dermis of skin, the Bruch membrane of the eye, and the blood vessels. The disease's manifestations are primarily due to an underlying metabolic disorder.

    Major diagnostic criteria of pseudoxanthoma elasticum include the following:

    Skin – Yellow papules/plaques on the lateral neck or body, skin biopsy showing increased calcification with clumping of elastic fiber taken from affected skin

Eye – Peau d'orange changes, angioid streaks (confirmed by angiography)

Genetics – Presence of a pathogenic mutation of both alleles of *ABCC6*, a first-degree relative who meets criteria for definitive pseudoxanthoma elasticum

Minor diagnostic criteria include the following:

Eye – One angioid streak shorter than one disk diameter, "comets" in the retina, one or more "wing signs" on the retina

Genetics – A pathogenic mutation in one allele of the *ABCC6* gene

E2 Cutaneous Mucinoses
Questions

1. The primary receptor for hyaluronan is:
   A. CD31
   B. CD34
   C. CD43
   D. CD44
   E. CD45

2. Primary mucinosis includes all of the following EXCEPT:
   A. Papular mucinosis
   B. Reticular erythematous mucinosis
   C. Pretibial myxedema
   D. Focal cutaneous mucinosis
   E. Granuloma annulare

3. Which of the following is NOT a characteristic of chondroitin sulfate:
   A. Colloidal iron positive
   B. Alcian blue, pH 2.5 positive
   C. Alcian blue, pH 0.5 positive
   D. PAS positive
   E. Hyaluronidase resistant

4. The best-fit diagnosis is:

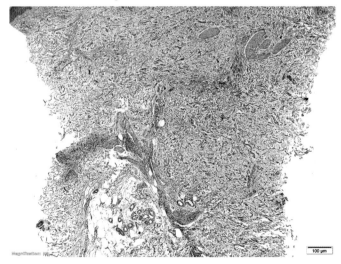

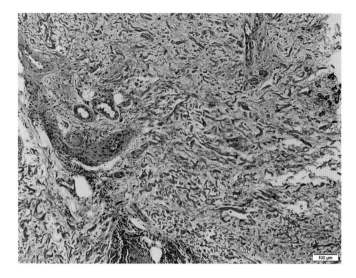

   A. Persistent papular mucinosis
   B. Scleromyxedema
   C. Pretibial myxedema
   D. Reticular erythematous mucinosis
   E. Scleredema

5. This is most commonly associated with (based on the image shown above):
   A. Paraproteinemia
   B. Hyperthyroidism
   C. Diabetes
   D. Stasis
   E. Renal disease

6. The best-fit diagnosis is:

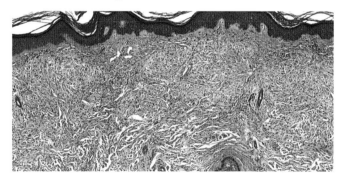

   A. Scleromyxedema
   B. Persistent papular mucinosis
   C. Pretibial myxedema
   D. Reticular erythematous mucinosis
   E. Scleredema

7. This is most commonly associated with (based on the image shown above):
   A. Renal disease
   B. Hyperthyroidism
   C. Diabetes
   D. Stasis
   E. Paraproteinemia

8. The best-fit diagnosis is:

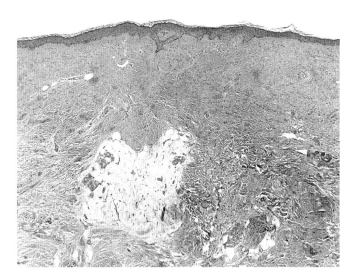

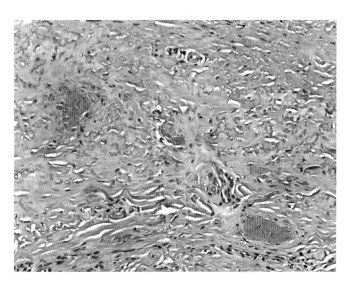

A. Scleromyxedema
B. Scleredema
C. Scleroderma
D. Nephrogenic systemic fibrosis
E. Reticular erythematous mucinosis

9. This is most commonly associated with (based on the image shown above):
A. Infection
B. Hyperthyroidism
C. Renal disease
D. Stasis
E. Paraproteinemia

10. Lesional cells in this entity (based on the image shown above) are typically positive for:
A. CD30
B. CD31
C. CD34
D. CD43
E. CD45

11. "Tram-tracking" is typically associated with:
A. Scleromyxedema
B. Nephrogenic systemic fibrosis
C. Scleroderma
D. Jessner's lymphocytic infiltrate
E. Reticular erythematous mucinosis

12. The best-fit diagnosis is:

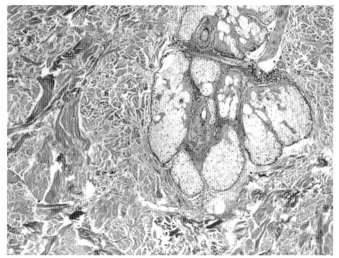

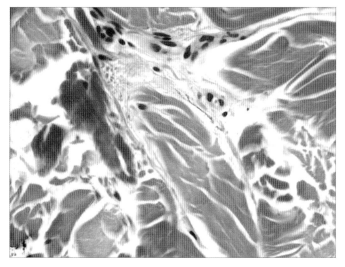

A. Scleredema
B. Nephrogenic systemic fibrosis
C. Scleroderma
D. Scleromyxedema
E. Reticular erythematous mucinosis

13. Cutaneous myxomas are a feature of all of the following EXCEPT:
A. NAME syndrome
B. LAMB syndrome
C. Carney's complex
D. Gardner's syndrome

14. The gene locus for Carney's complex is located on:
A. 4p
B. 10q

C. 11*q*

D. 12*q*

E. 17*q*

15. Components of Carney's complex may include all of the following EXCEPT:
    A. Atrial myxomas
    B. Neurofibromata
    C. Blue nevi
    D. Leiomyomata
    E. Ephilides

16. The best-fit diagnosis is:

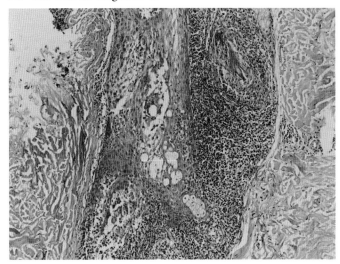

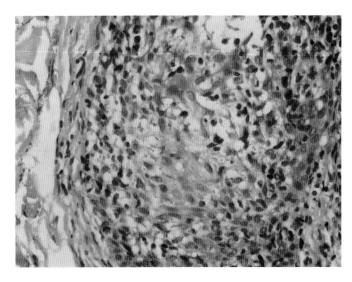

A. Infundibulofolliculitis
B. Apocrine miliaria
C. Follicular mucinosis
D. Atopic dermatitis (follicular lesion)
E. Eosinophilic folliculitis

17. Extracellular mucin may be seen in which of the following:
    A. Gardner's syndrome
    B. Hunter's syndrome
    C. Bloom's syndrome

D. Chediak-Higashi syndrome
E. Griscelli syndrome

18. Hunter's syndrome is linked to deficiency of:
    A. Iduronate sulfatase
    B. Urase
    C. Calcium pyrophosphatase
    D. Ferrochelatase
    E. Parathyroid hormone

19. The best-fit diagnosis is:

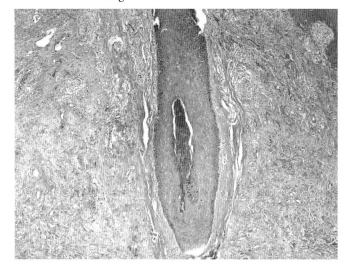

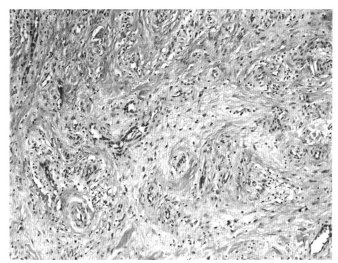

A. Focal mucinosis
B. Scleromyxedema
C. Digital mucous cyst
D. Reticular erythematous mucinosis
E. Superficial angiomyxoma

20. These may be a feature of (based on the image shown above):
    A. Gardner's syndrome
    B. Hunter's syndrome
    C. Bloom's syndrome
    D. NAME syndrome
    E. Griscelli syndrome

E2 Cutaneous Mucinoses
Answers

Table E2.1 Staining characteristics of mucopolysaccharides

Stain		Mucopolysaccharides	
		Non-sulfated (hyaluronic acid)	Sulfated (chondroitin sulfate, dermatan sulfate)
Colloidal iron		Positive	Positive
Alcian blue	pH 2.5	Positive	Positive
	pH 0.5*	**Negative**	**Positive**
Metachromasia with toluidine blue	pH 4.0	Positive	Positive
	pH < 2.0*	**Negative**	**Positive**
PAS		Negative	Negative
Hyaluronidase-sensitive*		**Positive**	**Negative**

* Differences shown in bold type

Table E2.2 Primary mucinoses – clues

Entity	Amount/primary site of mucin deposition	Other key histopathologic clues	Image
Pretibial myxedema	++/mid and lower dermis	Minimal interstitial cellular fibroblast proliferation	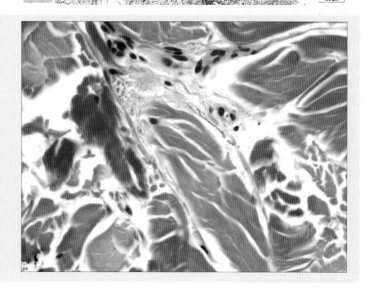
Scleredema	+/mid dermis	Thickened collagen bundles Splaying of collagen by interstitial mucin	

Table E2.2 Primary mucinoses – clues (*cont.*)

Entity	Amount/primary site of mucin deposition	Other key histopathologic clues	Image
Scleromyxedema	Minimal mucin	Prominent CD34 positive fibroblast proliferation	
Nephrogenic systemic fibrosis	Minimal mucin	Prominent CD34 positive fibroblast proliferation Involvement of subcutis Tram-tracking Lollipop bodies	
Focal cutaneous mucinosis	++/superficial dermis	Collarette, sharply circumscribed, deep	

Table E2.2 Primary mucinoses – clues (*cont.*)

Entity	Amount/primary site of mucin deposition	Other key histopathologic clues	Image
Reticular erythematous mucinosis	++/pandermal	Perivascular and periadnexal lymphocytic infiltrate	
Mucocele	++/mid dermis	Unremarkable minor salivary glands adjacent	
Cutaneous myxoma	++/deep dermis	Sharply circumscribed	

Table E2.2 Primary mucinoses – clues (*cont.*)

Entity	Amount/primary site of mucin deposition	Other key histopathologic clues	Image
Angiomyxoma	++/mid dermis	Vascular component Epithelial elements Neutrophils (early lesions)	
Follicular mucinosis	++/intrafollicular	Perifollicular lymphocytic infiltrate	

Table E2.3 CD34 positive proliferations – "a quick recap"

Lineage	Entity	Key histopathologic features
Fibroblastic, fibrohistiocytic and myofibroblastic	Dermatofibrosarcoma protuberans	Fascicles/whorls/storiform proliferation of bland spindled cells Infiltration of subcutis
	Giant cell fibroblastoma	Fascicles/whorls/storiform proliferation of bland spindled cells with admixed multinucleate giant cells Infiltration of subcutis
	Myxoinflammatory fibroblastic sarcoma	Proliferation of bizarre "Reed-Sternberg"-like cells ("ganglion-like nuclei") Admixed inflammatory infiltrate
	Solitary fibrous tumor	Proliferation of bland spindled cells Prominent vascularity

Table E2.3 CD34 positive proliferations – "a quick recap" (cont.)

Lineage	Entity	Key histopathologic features
	Giant cell angiofibroma	Proliferation of bland spindled and multinucleate giant cells
		Prominent vascularity with angiectoid spaces
	Nuchal-type fibroma	Variably cellular proliferation of bland spindled cells
	Sclerotic fibroma	Well-circumscribed, non-encapsulated
		Thick sclerotic collagen ("plywood-like")
		Acellular/hypocellular
	Superficial angiomyxoma	Variably cellular proliferation of bland spindled cells
		Epithelial elements
		Vascular and mucinous stroma
		Neutrophils (early lesions only)
	Superficial acral fibromyxoma	Variably cellular proliferation of bland spindled cells
		Vascular and mucinous stroma
	Spindle cell lipoma	Abundant adipose tissue
		Spindled fibroblast proliferation mainly involving septae
	Lipofibromatosis	Abundant adipose tissue
		Spindled fibroblast proliferation mainly involving septae of subcutis
	Cellular angiofibroma	Proliferation of short, spindled cells
		Thick small and medium-sized vessels
	Peri-cicatricial tissue	Proliferation of stellate, elongate cells
		"Squished" vessels
	Mammary-type extramammary myofibroblastoma	Fasciculated proliferation of spindled cells
Vascular	Kaposi's sarcoma	Closely packed proliferation of spindled cells
		Patchy host response with admixed plasma cells
	Angiosarcoma	Jagged vessels lined by multilayered hyperchromatic cells
	Epithelioid hemangioendothelioma	Well-circumscribed, dermal nodule
		Polygonal cellular proliferation
		Angiocentric growth pattern
	Kaposiform hemangioendothelioma	Poorly circumscribed, multifocal
		Nodules of vascular and cellular areas
		Hyalinized stroma
Neural	Neurofibroma	Bland spindled proliferation
		Mucinous stroma
		Admixed mast cells
	Perineurioma	Concentric perivascular cellular proliferation ("onion-skin" appearance)
	Solitary circumscribed neuroma	Unencapsulated, superficial dermal proliferation
		"Schwannoma-like"
Adipocytic	Spindle cell lipoma	Abundant adipose tissue
		Spindled fibroblast proliferation mainly involving septae
Follicular	Trichodiscoma	Well-circumscribed "neurofibroma-like" stromal component that envelopes the adnexal proliferation
	Fibrofolliculoma	
	Trichilemmoma	Peripheral palisading
		Clear cell differentiation
		Eosinophilic cuticle
Other	Pleomorphic hyalinizing angiectatic tumor of soft parts	Sheets and fascicles of plump, pleomorphic spindled cells
		Admixed clusters of ectatic vessels
		Vessels surrounded by hyaline material

1. **D. CD44 is the primary receptor for hyaluronan.**

The CD44 antigen is a cell-surface glycoprotein involved in cell–cell interactions, cell adhesion and migration. In humans, the CD44 antigen is encoded by the *CD44* gene on chromosome 11. CD44 has been referred to as HCAM (homing cell adhesion molecule), Pgp-1 (phagocytic glycoprotein-1), Hermes antigen, lymphocyte homing receptor, ECM-III, and HUTCH-1. CD44 is a receptor for hyaluronic acid and can also interact with other ligands, such as osteopontin, collagens, and matrix metalloproteinases (MMPs). CD44 function is controlled by its post-translational modifications.

Other antigens listed:

CD31 – Platelet endothelial cell adhesion molecule (PECAM-1) is a protein encoded by the *PECAM1* gene found on chromosome 17; used primarily to demonstrate the presence of endothelial cells in tissue sections.

CD34 – Hematopoietic progenitor cell antigen CD34 is encoded by the *CD34* gene; cells expressing CD34 (CD34 positive cells) are normally found in the umbilical cord and bone marrow as hematopoietic cells, a subset of mesenchymal stem cells, endothelial progenitor cells, endothelial cells of blood vessels but not lymphatics (except pleural lymphatics), mast cells, a subpopulation of dendritic cells (which are factor XIIIa-negative) in the interstitium and around the adnexa of dermis of skin, as well as cells in soft tissue tumors like dermatofibrosarcoma protuberans, gastrointestinal stromal tumor, solitary fibrous tumor and some malignant peripheral nerve sheath tumors (also see Table E2.3).

CD43 – Leukosialin, also known as sialophorin or CD43 (cluster of differentiation 43), is a transmembrane cell surface encoded by the *SPN* (sialophorin) gene and is a major sialoglycoprotein on the surface of human T lymphocytes, monocytes, granulocytes, and some B lymphocytes. It is important for immune function and involved in T-cell activation; defects are associated with the development of Wiskott-Aldrich syndrome. It also appears in about 25% of intestinal MALTomas. Although present in >90% of T-cell lymphomas, it is *generally less effective* at demonstrating this condition than CD3; however, it may be useful as part of a panel to demonstrate B-cell lymphoblastic lymphoma, since the malignant cells in this condition are often CD43 positive, and may be difficult to stain with other antibodies. It stains granulocytes and their precursors and is therefore also an effective marker for myeloid tumors.

CD45 – Protein tyrosine phosphatase, receptor type C (PTPRC) is also known as CD45 antigen and was originally called leukocyte common antigen (LCA); various isoforms of CD45 exist, including CD45RA, CD45RB, CD45RC, CD45RAB, CD45RAC, CD45RBC, CD45RO, CD45R (ABC). Expression is not restricted to B-cells and can also be expressed on activated T-cells, on a subset of dendritic cells and other antigen-presenting cells.

2. **E. Granuloma annulare (GA) is NOT a primary mucinosis.**

Primary mucinoses are subdivided into 2 broad categories: degenerative inflammatory mucinoses and hamartomatous-neoplastic mucinoses. The former category is further subdivided into dermal or follicular – depending upon where the mucin accumulation is located (also see Table E2.2). While increased mucin is a feature of granuloma annulare, it is not classified as a primary mucinosis. The classic histopathologic triad of GA includes a palisaded lymphohistiocytic infiltrate surrounding foci of necrobiosis and increased dermal mucin.

3. **D. Chondroitin sulfate is PAS negative.**

Chondroitin sulfate is a sulfated glycosaminoglycan (GAG) composed of a chain of alternating sugars (*N*-acetylgalactosamine and glucuronic acid). It is usually found attached to proteins as part of a proteoglycan. Its other properties (listed in Table E2.1) include positivity with colloidal iron, Alcian blue (pH 2.5 and 0.5), metachromasia with toluidine blue (pH 4.0 and <2.0) and resistance to hyaluronidase.

4. **C. The best-fit diagnosis for the image shown is that of pretibial myxedema (PTM).**

The characteristic histopathologic features consist of the deposition of mucin (glycosaminoglycans) throughout the reticular dermis, sometimes with extension into the subcutis with attenuation of collagen fibers. Mucin may appear as individual threads and granules. With extensive deposition of mucin, the collagen fibers are frayed, fragmented, and widely separated. Stellate fibroblasts are often observed, but the number of fibroblasts is not increased (as observed in scleromyxedema). The mucin is hyaluronic acid that stains blue with Alcian blue at a pH of 2.5 and stains with colloidal iron; metachromasia is shown with toluidine blue stain.

The precise cause of PTM remains uncertain. A leading theory proposes that fibroblasts are stimulated to produce abnormally high amounts of glycosaminoglycan under the influence of cytokines due to exposure to thyrotropin receptor antibody (TRAB) and antigen-specific T-cells. TRAB binding sites are found in the plasma membranes of fibroblasts derived from the skin of patients with PTM. TRAB is present in the serum of most patients with PTM (80–100%), but it has also been found in the serum of patients without PTM.

Skin lesions or areas of non-pitting edema appear on the anterior or lateral aspects of the legs or in sites of old or recent trauma in patients with Graves's disease.

5. **B.** Pretibial myxedema (PTM) is most commonly associated with hyperthyroidism.

PTM or, more appropriately, thyroid dermopathy is a term used to describe localized lesions of the skin resulting from the deposition of hyaluronic acid, usually as a component of thyroid disease. Thyroid dermopathy occurs rarely. Although PTM is most often confined to the pretibial area, it may occur anywhere on the skin, especially the ankle, dorsum of the foot, knees, shoulders, elbows, upper back, pinnae, nose, and neck. It is nearly always associated with autoimmune thyroid disease, i.e. Graves's disease. The onset of PTM most commonly occurs 1–2 years after the diagnosis of Graves's disease, but it may occur before or after the onset of thyrotoxicosis. PTM in the absence of Graves's disease is uncommon. Most patients who develop PTM also have Graves's ophthalmopathy, with the onset of dermopathy typically following the onset of ophthalmopathy by 6–12 months. The natural history of PTM is not well defined.

6. **A.** The best-fit diagnosis for the image shown is that of scleromyxedema.

Scleromyxedema is the *most distinctive* of all the primary mucinoses in that it is characterized by interstitial deposits of mucin as well as an interstitial cellular proliferation as shown in the image. Lesions have large depositions of mucin in the dermis. Numerous plump stellate CD34 positive fibroblasts proliferate throughout the dermis. The mucin stains with periodic acid-Schiff and Alcian blue at pH 2.5 but not pH 0.4, and it metachromatically stains with toluidine blue at pH 3.0. The mucin has been identified as hyaluronic acid, a non-sulfated acid mucopolysaccharide.

7. **E.** Scleromyxedema is most associated with a paraproteinemia.

Serum protein immunoelectrophoresis generally reveals the presence of a serum paraprotein (usually IgG) with lambda light chains. Few patients may have myeloma or Waldenström's macroglobulinemia. However, when myeloma is present, the patient generally has a poor prognosis. The association between this paraprotein and the mucin deposition is not clear, and the protein does not directly stimulate fibroblast proliferation. Paraprotein levels have not been shown to correlate with disease severity, response to therapy, or disease progression. The etiology is unknown; however, the disease is commonly associated with plasma cell dyscrasia. The basic defect is hypothesized to be a fibroblast disorder, which causes the increased mucin deposition in the skin. The cytokines interleukin (IL)-1, tumor necrosis factor (TNF)-alpha, and TNF-beta may play a role.

The terms lichen myxedematosus, papular mucinosis, and scleromyxedema are used interchangeably to describe the same disorder. A spectrum of disease appears to exist, with the more localized, less severe forms, which are generally called lichen myxedematosus or papular mucinosis, and the more sclerotic, diffuse form, which is referred to as scleromyxedema with both ends exhibiting similar if not identical histopathologic features of fibroblast proliferation and mucin deposition in the dermis, in the absence of thyroid disease. Sclerotic features, systemic involvement, and monoclonal gammopathy are absent in localized lichen myxedematosus. For lichen myxedematosus, the prognosis is a chronic course with little tendency for spontaneous resolution. Scleromyxedema usually has a poorer prognosis than the other forms. Patients with this form present with more widespread progressive induration and decreased mobility of the face, fingers, and extremities. The primary lesions may involve widespread erythematous, indurated skin that resembles scleroderma, with diffuse tightness of the skin. The range of motion of the face, fingers, and extremities is decreased. The systemic manifestations include restrictive and obstructive pulmonary dysfunction, cardiovascular abnormalities, and polyarthritis. Obstructive and restrictive lung disease is often manifested by dyspnea on exertion. Patients are also noted to have cysts and urticarial lesions. Patients may report systemic symptoms, such as dysphagia or weakness, and symptoms that resemble those of organic brain disease. For a list of other cutaneous disorders associated with a monoclonal gammopathy, also see Section D2, Table D2.3.

8. **D.** The best-fit diagnosis for the image shown is that of nephrogenic systemic fibrosis (NSF).

Unique histopathologic features of nephrogenic systemic fibrosis, first described in 2001, include thickened collagen bundles with surrounding clefts, mucin deposition, and a proliferation of fibroblasts and elastic fibers.

Early lesions (within 20 weeks of clinical onset) demonstrate reticular, dermal, large, and epithelioid or stellate spindled cells. These cells can extend into and widen the subcutaneous fat lobule septa. The spindle cells are diffusely arranged among thickened collagen bundles. Clefts can encompass some spindle cells. Most of the spindle cells are CD34/procollagen dual-positive cells that form a dense interconnecting network.

Late lesions (>20 weeks of clinical onset) typically have less prominent clefting, less mucin, and fewer CD34/procollagen-positive cells. Calcification and sclerotic or "lollipop" bodies have also been described in select patients with long-standing disease.

9. **C. Nephrogenic systemic fibrosis (NSF) is most commonly associated with renal disease.**

   NSF, also known as nephrogenic fibrosing dermopathy (NFD), is a disease of fibrosis of the skin and internal organs reminiscent but distinct from scleroderma or scleromyxedema. Nephrogenic systemic fibrosis always occurs (with the exception of one report in 2 transplant patients whose organ donors' histories were not noted) in patients with renal insufficiency that have had imaging studies (e.g., magnetic resonance angiography) with gadolinium, a contrast agent used in imaging studies. Gadolinium can be found in tissue samples of nephrogenic systemic fibrosis. The mechanism by which NSF occurs is not known, but it seems to involve a cell termed a circulating fibrocyte that is stimulated by gadolinium. Endothelin-1/endothelin receptor signaling plays a role in the calcification and fibrosis of nephrogenic systemic fibrosis.

   Toll-like receptors (TLR), in particular TLR4 and TLR7, play a role in the development of nephrogenic systemic fibrosis. Evidence for a link between nephrogenic systemic fibrosis and gadolinium was first described in a case series of 13 patients, all of whom developed nephrogenic systemic fibrosis after being exposed to gadolinium. One case of nephrogenic systemic fibrosis developed 10 years after gadolinium exposure. Newer contrast agents like gadobenate dimeglumine carry a lower risk.

   Nephrogenic systemic fibrosis manifests clinically with induration, thickening, and hardening of the skin with brawny hyperpigmentation and distinct papules and subcutaneous nodules. The skin can have a peau d'orange appearance, and plaques may have an amoeboid advancing edge. The skin is often shiny and hard to the touch. A woody consistency is typical. The extremities are the most common areas of involvement, followed by the trunk. The face is almost never involved. Yellow palmar papules resembling cutaneous calcinosis have been reported. In addition, yellow scleral plaques have been reported in patients with nephrogenic systemic fibrosis.

10. **C. Lesional fibroblasts in nephrogenic systemic fibrosis (NSF) are CD34 positive.**

    CD34 is a 115 kDa transmembrane sialomucin encoded on a gene located on chromosome 1q32. It is expressed in activated bone marrow progenitor cells, which give rise to the hematopoietic and angioblastic lineages. While CD34 expression is lost during differentiation in the hematopoietic lineage, it is maintained in the angioblastic one. In addition, evidence exists supporting the idea that a subset of CD34 positive stromal cells derived from bone marrow and muscle represents a type of mesenchymal stem cell. Other CD34 positive entities are detailed in Table E2.3.

11. **B. Tram-tracking is associated with nephrogenic systemic fibrosis (NSF).**

    In NSF, CD34 positive spindle or epithelioid cells are aligned in a reticular or parallel arrangement forming a complex network. CD34 dendritic cell processes form a "tram-track" arrangement around a central elastic fiber.

    A clinicopathologic classification system has been developed for NSF based on the following:

    Major clinical criteria: Patterned plaques, joint contractures, cobblestoning, marked induration
    Minor clinical criteria: Puckering/linear banding, superficial plaque/patch, dermal papules, scleral plaques in those <45 years of age
    Histopathologic criteria: Increased dermal cellularity, CD34+ cells with tram-tracking, thick and thin collagen bundles, preserved elastic fibers, septal subcutaneous involvement, osseous metaplasia

    Identification of preserved elastic tissue is a finding that has value in excluding morphea/scleroderma, and therefore receives a score of 1 if it is absent; if present, it receives a neutral score of 0. A distinctive histopathologic finding consisting of small spicules of bone developing around elastic fibers ("lollipop lesion") has been observed in select cases evaluated to date. This feature is thought to represent a highly specific (but insensitive) histopathologic sign of NSF.

12. **A. The best-fit diagnosis for the image shown is that of scleredema.**

    Histopathologic features of scleredema, depicted in the image, include a thickened dermis with increased spaces between large collagen bundles. The space results from increased deposition of mucopolysaccharide (hyaluronic acid) in the dermis. The mucin is more prominent in the deep dermis. The preservation of periappendageal fat and absence of a fibroblast proliferation help differentiate this from scleroderma and nephrogenic systemic fibrosis respectively. Clinically, scleredema is an uncommon fibromucinous connective-tissue disease and is characterized by woody induration and hardening of the skin. The term scleredema is a misnomer because *neither sclerosis nor edema* is found on microscopic examination! There are three distinct clinical forms of scleredema, which are classified by their associated condition. Patients in all types report stiff or hard skin, although the rapidity of onset and locations of involvement differ based on the clinical subgroup.

    Type 1 – Associated with a history of an antecedent infection, this was historically referred to as scleredema adultorum. However, this is considered by some to be a misnomer because most pediatric patients fall into this group. Patients report a hardening of the skin a few weeks after a febrile illness, most commonly an upper or lower respiratory tract streptococcal infection. The condition usually clears spontaneously in 6 months to 2 years.

Type 2 – Associated with a blood dyscrasia, most commonly a plasma cell dyscrasia, this subtype has gammopathies, diagnosed on average 10 years after the onset of scleredema skin changes. IgG monoclonal gammopathy with a kappa light chain is most common, followed by an IgA type. Spontaneous remission is much less likely to occur than in the type 1 subgroup.

Type 3 – Associated with diabetes mellitus, this tends to occur more often in middle-aged males, often obese, with long-standing, often uncontrolled, diabetes mellitus. Subtle skin hardening of the upper back begins in an insidious manner, progressing slowly over many years to involve the upper back, neck, and shoulders with associated erythema; often, a pebbled appearance may evolve. Patients typically experience a more protracted course that is refractory to therapy. Control of the hyperglycemia does not improve the scleredema.

Scleredema presents as ill-defined, woody, non-pitting, indurated plaques. Erythema, hyperpigmentation, and/or a peau-d'orange appearance of the affected areas may be present. The taut skin may appear shiny, and, when pinched, firmness is appreciated with noted wrinkling of overlying epidermis.

Scleredema is usually most evident in the upper part of the body, specifically the face, the neck, the trunk, and the extremities in types 1 and 2.

13. **D.** Cutaneous myxomas are NOT a feature of Gardner syndrome.

Carney complex and its subsets LAMB syndrome and NAME syndrome are autosomal dominant conditions comprising myxomas of the heart and skin, hyperpigmentation of the skin (lentiginosis), and endocrine overactivity.

The LAMB acronym refers to *l*entigines, *a*trial *m*yxomas, and *b*lue nevi.

NAME refers to *n*evi, *a*trial myxoma, *m*yxoid neurofibromas, and *e*phelides.

Gardner syndrome is genetically linked to band 5q21, the adenomatous polyposis coli (APC) locus. In 1951, Gardner described the occurrence of familial adenomatous polyposis (FAP) with the extracolonic manifestations of intestinal polyposis, desmoids, osteomas, and epidermoid cysts with pilomatrical change (i.e. Gardner syndrome). FAP and Gardner syndrome are believed to be variants of the same condition. Other cutaneous manifestations of Gardner syndrome include desmoid tumors, fibromas, lipomas (may be visceral, including intracranial), leiomyomas, neurofibromas and multifocal pigmented lesions of the fundus (seen in 80% of patients, may present shortly after birth and can be the

first marker of disease). More than half the patients with Gardner syndrome have dental anomalies.

14. **E.** The gene locus for Carney's complex is located on 17q.

Carney's complex is most commonly caused by mutations in the *PRKAR1A* gene on chromosome 17q23–q24, which may function as a tumor-suppressor gene. The encoded protein is a type 1A regulatory subunit of protein kinase A. *Inactivating germline mutations of this gene are found in 70% of people with Carney complex.*

15. **D.** Leiomyomata are NOT a feature of Carney's complex.

Cutaneous leiomyomas are benign soft-tissue neoplasms that arise from smooth muscle (arrector pili). The importance of multiple cutaneous leiomyomas lies in their association with uterine fibroids and papillary renal cell carcinoma in what is known as Reed syndrome, or hereditary leiomyomatosis and renal cell cancer (HLRCC), an autosomal dominant disorder. This disorder with variable penetrance is caused by a defect in fumarate hydratase secondary to a missense mutation. Fumarate hydratase is an enzyme in the tricarboxylic acid (Krebs) cycle that acts as a tumor suppressor.

16. **C.** The best-fit diagnosis for the image shown is follicular mucinosis.

Also known as alopecia mucinosa, follicular mucinosis was first reported by Pinkus in 1957. The characteristic histopathologic features, as evidenced in the image, include follicular degeneration with the accumulation of mucin within the follicles. Early lesions contain an abundance of mucin between the decaying root sheath cells or pooling in localized collections. The mucinous degeneration begins in the pilosebaceous units. A periappendageal, perivascular, or interstitial lymphocytic mixed inflammatory cell infiltrate often exists. In patients with chronic alopecia mucinosa, follicles are often distorted with variable disruption of follicular epithelia. *Histopathologic clues of concern for evolving mycosis fungoides* include the following:

Denser infiltrate, with more plasma cells, fewer eosinophils, less intrafollicular mucin and transgression of follicular epithelia by atypical lymphocytes with a high N:C ratio and a convoluted cytomorphology.

The dermatologic eruptions consist of follicular papules and/or indurated plaques with the face, the neck, and the scalp being the most frequently affected sites, although lesions may appear anywhere on the body. The presenting sign is hair loss in hair-bearing areas. Mycosis fungoides is recognized at the time of diagnosis in approximately 15–30% of patients with alopecia mucinosa. The alopecia that develops on hair-bearing skin is of the non-scarring type.

The 3 clinical variants of the disease include:

A primary disorder of young persons: Clinically consisting of focal cutaneous lesions typically limited to the head, the neck, and the shoulders. Most lesions spontaneously resolve between 2 months and 2 years. Pediatric cases comprise most of this type of alopecia mucinosa, with the remainder of patients being younger than 40 years.

A primary chronic alopecia mucinosa of older persons: Affects people older than 40 years. Lesions have a widespread distribution, and may persist or recur indefinitely.

Secondary alopecia mucinosa: Typically affects patients 40–70 years of age. Lesions are widespread and numerous. Alopecia mucinosa can occur secondary to benign disease, including inflammatory conditions, or may be associated with malignant disease, including mycosis fungoides, Kaposi sarcoma, and Hodgkin disease, with mycosis fungoides being by far the most common association. In most patients who exhibit both alopecia mucinosa and mycosis fungoides, these conditions appear to develop concomitantly; however, the concern exists that individuals exhibiting only alopecia mucinosa may also be at risk for subsequent development of lymphoma. Drug-induced alopecia mucinosa has been associated with the use of adalimumab and imatinib.

17. **B.** Extracellular mucin may be seen in Hunter's syndrome.

    Mucin is typically found within the interstitium of mid and lower dermis, typically splaying adjacent collagen bundles. Other histopathologic findings in Hunter's syndrome include the presence of metachromatic granules within the cytoplasm of fibroblasts.

    Mucopolysaccharidosis type II (MPS II), also known as Hunter syndrome, is a member of a group of inherited metabolic disorders collectively termed the mucopolysaccharidoses (MPSs). The MPSs are caused by a deficiency of lysosomal enzymes required for the degradation of mucopolysaccharides or glycosaminoglycans (GAGs). All of the MPSs are inherited in an autosomal recessive fashion, except for Hunter syndrome, which is inherited as X-linked recessive.

18. **A.** Hunter's syndrome is due to deficiency or absence of the lysosomal enzyme, iduronate 2-sulfatase deficiency (IDS).

    The cytogenetic location for the *IDS* gene is Xq28.

19. **E.** The best-fit diagnosis for the image shown is superficial angiomyxoma.

    Diagnostic histopathologic features of superficial angiomyxoma, depicted in the image shown, include a multilobulated, poorly circumscribed, vascular and

interstitial proliferation of scattered bland stellate and spindled cells predominantly involving the deep dermis and subcutis embedded in a myxoid stroma. Scattered neutrophils may be seen in early lesions and an entrapped epithelial component in 20–30% of cases. These may be in the form of a keratinous cyst or strands of squamous epithelium. The mucin is typically Alcian blue positive and hyaluronidase sensitive.

20. **D.** Superficial angiomyxomas may present as a component of NAME syndrome.

    Carney complex and its subsets LAMB syndrome and NAME syndrome are autosomal dominant conditions comprising myxomas of the heart and skin, hyperpigmentation of the skin (lentiginosis), and endocrine overactivity. The LAMB acronym refers to *l*entigines, *a*trial *m*yxomas, and *b*lue nevi. NAME refers to *n*evi, *a*trial myxoma, *m*yxoid neurofibromas, and *e*phelides. Testicular cancer, particularly Sertoli cell type, is associated with Carney syndrome. In some patients with cardiac myxoma(s), the cutaneous tumor(s) is often detected prior to diagnosis of the cardiac neoplasm and thus serves as an important marker.

E3 Cysts and Sinuses
Questions

1. Stratified squamous epithelial-lined cysts include all of the following EXCEPT:
   A. Steatocystoma
   B. Vellus hair cyst
   C. Dermoid cyst
   D. Trichilemmal cyst
   E. Median raphe cyst

2. Non-stratified squamous epithelial-lined cysts include all of the following EXCEPT:
   A. Hidrocystoma
   B. Bronchogenic cyst
   C. Thyroglossal duct cyst
   D. Pilonidal cyst
   E. Branchial cleft cyst

3. Non-epithelial-lined cysts include all of the following EXCEPT:
   A. Digital mucous cyst
   B. Pseudocyst of the auricle
   C. Ciliated cyst of the vulva
   D. Metaplastic synovial cyst
   E. Mucocele

4. The best-fit diagnosis is:

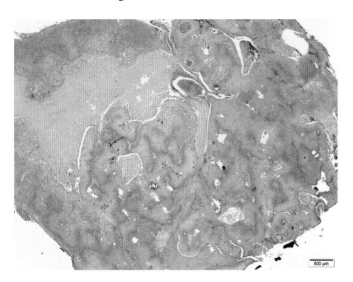

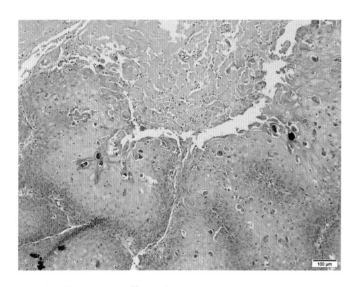

A. Squamous cell carcinoma
B. Proliferating trichilemmal cyst
C. Involuting keratoacanthoma
D. Malignant onycholemmal cyst
E. HPV-related epidermal cyst

5. The best-fit diagnosis is:

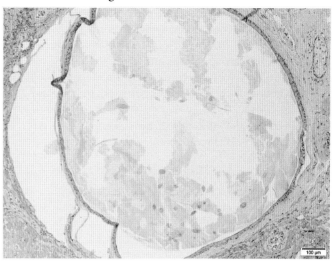

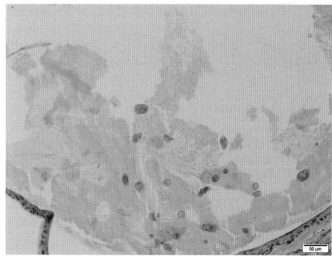

A. Vellus hair cyst
B. Hair matrix cyst
C. Pigmented follicular cyst
D. Median raphe cyst
E. Cystic teratoma

6. The best-fit diagnosis is:

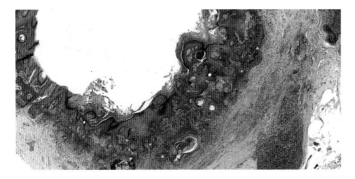

   A. Cystic sebaceoma
   B. Cystic teratoma
   C. Cystic hygroma
   D. Phaeohyphomycotic cyst
   E. Cystic panfolliculoma

7. Epidermal cysts with pilomatrical change are associated with:
   A. Darier's disease
   B. Muir-Torre syndrome
   C. Brooke-Spiegler syndrome
   D. Gardner syndrome
   E. Nevoid basal cell syndrome

8. The most likely diagnosis is:

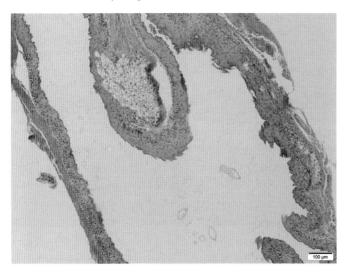

   A. Milium
   B. Dermoid cyst
   C. Steatocystoma
   D. Endosalpingosis
   E. Endometriosis

9. Activating mutations in which of the following is associated with this entity:

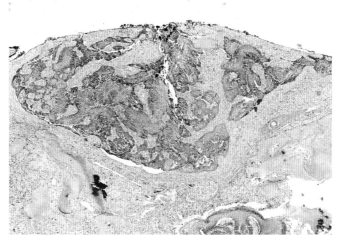

   A. *MEN1* gene
   B. β-catenin
   C. MMR proteins
   D. *CYLD* gene
   E. *MYB*

10. The best-fit diagnosis is:

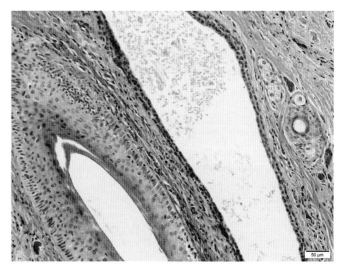

   A. Hidrocystoma
   B. Steatocystoma
   C. Mucocele
   D. Milium
   E. Keratocyst

11. The best-fit diagnosis is:

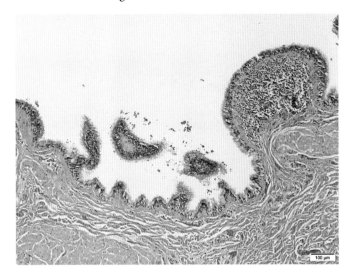

    A. Bronchogenic cyst
    B. Thyroglossal cyst
    C. Thymic cyst
    D. Dermoid cyst
    E. Cystic teratoma

12. Which of the following is true regarding the image shown above:
    A. Typically arise on the lower extremity
    B. Found along lines of embryonic fusion
    C. Strong predilection for the periorbital area
    D. Free-lying within the nail bed
    E. Found along the midline neck

13. These are typically located on the:

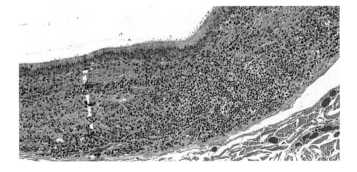

    A. Lower extremity
    B. Periorbital area
    C. Midline neck
    D. Lateral neck
    E. Midline face

14. The best-fit diagnosis is:

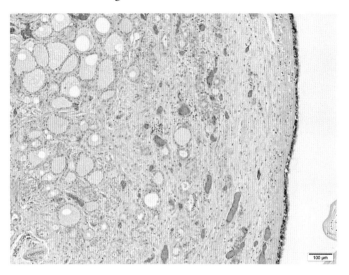

    A. Thymic cyst
    B. Dermoid cyst
    C. Thyroglossal cyst
    D. Pilonidal sinus
    E. Auricular pseudocyst

15. The best-fit diagnosis is:

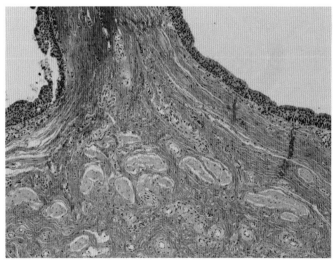

    A. Vellus hair cyst
    B. Median raphe cyst
    C. Pigmented follicular cyst
    D. Dermoid cyst
    E. Cystic teratoma

16. These (based on the image shown above) are typically located on the:
    A. Glans penis
    B. Periorbital area
    C. Midline neck
    D. Lateral neck
    E. Midline face

17. The best-fit diagnosis is:

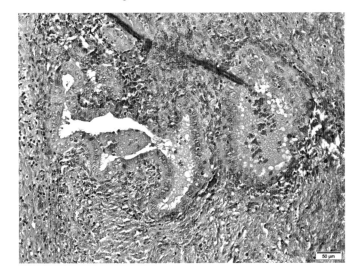

    A. Median raphe cyst
    B. Dermoid cyst
    C. Metastatic adenocarcinoma
    D. Endosalpingosis
    E. Endometriosis

18. The best-fit diagnosis is:

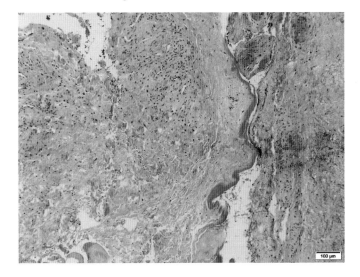

    A. Auricular pseudocyst
    B. Cutaneous endosalpingosis
    C. Cystic teratoma

D. Metaplastic synovial cyst
E. Cutaneous endometriosis

19. The best-fit diagnosis is:

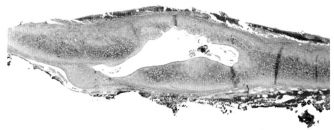

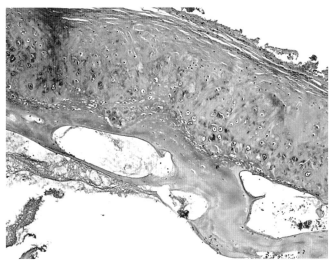

    A. Cystic teratoma
    B. Cutaneous endosalpingosis
    C. Auricular pseudocyst
    D. Metaplastic synovial cyst
    E. Cutaneous endometriosis

20. The typical site for these (based on the image shown above) is:
    A. Glans penis
    B. Periorbital area
    C. Midline neck
    D. Ear pinna
    E. Midline face

E3 Cysts and Sinuses
Answers

Table E3.1 Overview of cysts

Lining epithelia	Entity	Key histopathologic features	Image
Squamous	Epidermal inclusion cyst	Granular cell layer present, contains laminated keratin	
	Milium Trichilemmal (pilar) cyst	Similar to above, smaller Trichilemmal keratinization, no keratohyaline granules, contains eosinophilic compacted keratin	
	Proliferating trichilemmal cyst	Lobular proliferation of squamous cells *all within the confines of the cyst*, pre-existing pilar cyst typically present along one edge	

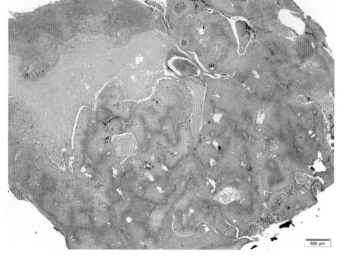

Table E3.1 Overview of cysts (*cont.*)

Lining epithelia	Entity	Key histopathologic features	Image
	Proliferating epidermal inclusion cyst	Multilocular, keratin-filled cystic spaces	
	Vellus hair cyst	Lumen contains keratin and numerous vellus hair shafts	
	Steatocystoma	Undulated lining, presence of mature sebaceous glands in wall	
	Pilonidal cyst	Tract, chronic inflammatory infiltrate, free, naked hair shafts within chronic abscess	

Table E3.1 Overview of cysts (*cont.*)

Lining epithelia	Entity	Key histopathologic features	Image
Non-stratified squamous	Hidrocystoma	Unilocular, cuboidal epithelial-lined	
	Bronchogenic cyst	Lined by ciliated/mucin-producing, pseudostratified columnar/cuboidal epithelium, smooth muscle and mucus glands in wall	
	Thyroglossal duct cyst	Ciliated epithelium, thyroid follicles in wall	

Table E3.1 Overview of cysts (*cont.*)

Lining epithelia	Entity	Key histopathologic features	Image
	Branchial cleft cyst	Lined by ciliated columnar epithelium, dense lymphoid infiltrate in wall	
	Cutaneous ciliated cyst **Median raphe cyst**	Ciliated cuboidal/ columnar epithelium Pseudostratified columnar epithelium with mucus cells	
	Omphalomesenteric cyst	Associated with Meckel's diverticulum, gastrointestinal mucosa adjoining cyst lining	
Non-lined	**Mucocele**	Cystic space containing mucin, adjacent unremarkable minor salivary glands	

Table E3.1 Overview of cysts (*cont.*)

Lining epithelia	Entity	Key histopathologic features	Image
	Digital mucous cyst	Myxoid pool with overlying attenuated epidermis	
	Ganglion cyst	Cystic cavity surrounded by compressed fibrous tissue	
	Metaplastic synovial cyst	Resembles hyperplastic synovium, partly hyalinized synovial villi	
	Pseudocyst of the auricle	Intracartiliginous cavity, may contain extravasated erythrocytes	

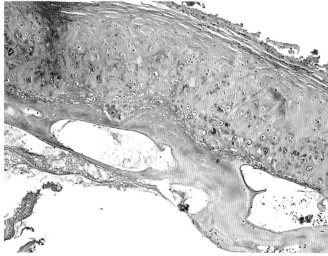

1. E. Median raphe cyst is NOT lined by stratified squamous epithelium.

   Median raphe cyst is lined by non-stratified, pseudostratified columnar epithelium with mucus cells. Other non-stratified squamous epithelial-lined cysts include:
   - Hidrocystoma
   - Bronchogenic cyst
   - Thyroglossal duct cyst
   - Branchial cleft cyst
   - Cutaneous ciliated cyst
   - Omphalomesenteric cyst

   Also see Table E3.1.

2. D. Pilonidal cyst is NOT lined by non-stratified squamous epithelium.

   Pilonidal cyst is lined by stratified squamous epithelium and surrounded by a mixed inflammatory cell infiltrate with admixed naked hair shafts. Other stratified squamous epithelial-lined cysts include:
   - Epidermal inclusion cyst, proliferating epidermal inclusion cyst, milium
   - Trichilemmal (pilar) cyst, proliferating trichilemmal cyst
   - Vellus hair cyst
   - Steatocystoma

   Also see Table E3.1.

3. C. Ciliated cyst of the vulva is lined by non-stratified squamous epithelium.

   Examples of non-epithelial-lined cysts include:
   - Mucocele
   - Digital mucous cyst
   - Ganglion
   - Metaplastic synovial cyst
   - Pseudocyst of the auricle

   Also see Table E3.1.

4. B. Image shown is that of a proliferating trichilemmal cyst.

   A proliferating trichilemmal cyst is a rare neoplasm arising from the isthmus region of the outer root sheath of the hair follicle. It is also commonly called a proliferating pilar tumor (PPT) or, less commonly, proliferating follicular-cystic neoplasm. It was first described by Wilson-Jones as a proliferating epidermoid cyst in 1966. It occurs most commonly on the scalp in women older than 50 years. *Most arise within a pre-existing pilar cyst.* They may be inherited in an autosomal-dominant mode, linked to chromosome 3.

   Even though they usually are benign in nature, malignant transformation with local invasion and metastasis has been described. A tentative stratification of this entity includes:

   Group 1 – Regarded as benign, has a circumscribed silhouette with "pushing" margins, modest nuclear atypia, and an absence of pathologic mitoses, necrosis, and invasion of nerves or vessels
   Group 2 – Similar to group 1 but believed to have the potential for locally aggressive growth and is categorized as a low-grade malignancy, manifests as irregular, locally invasive silhouettes with involvement of the deep dermis and subcutis
   Group 3 – Categorized as a high-grade malignancy, exhibits invasive growth patterns, marked nuclear atypia, pathologic mitotic forms, and geographic necrosis, with or without involvement of nerves or vascular structures, local and regional metastasis has been noted in 30% of cases

5. A. Image shown is that of a vellus hair cyst

   Histopathology shows a cystic structure in the mid dermis arising from the infundibulum of a hair follicle. The cysts contain multiple cross-sections of vellus hairs and layered laminated keratinous material. They are lined by stratified squamous epithelium 2–5 cells thick. A surrounding granulomatous reaction may be present, especially if the hairs disrupt the cyst wall.

   Eruptive vellus hair cysts (EVHCs) were first described in 1977 by Esterly and colleagues who reported 2 children with symmetrically distributed follicular papules or an "acneiform eruption" on the chest and flexor extremities. Although acquired or inherited in an autosomal dominant fashion, generally, they are isolated findings.

6. E. Image shown is that of a panfolliculoma.

   Panfolliculoma (PF) is an uncommon benign neoplasm with advanced follicular differentiation. It differentiates toward *all components of a hair follicle*. PF was first described by Ackerman *et al.* in 1993 in their textbook *Neoplasms with Follicular Differentiation*. Subsequently, varieties of PF such as epidermal PF, cystic panfolliculoma (CPF), and PF with sebaceous differentiation have been reported. PF demonstrates all the features of a benign neoplasm, namely circumscription and minimal or no cytological atypia. Differentiation toward all parts of a hair follicle, including infundibulum, isthmus, stem, and bulb/papilla are evident in all variants described to date (superficial, nodular and cystic). The cell components are germinative cells, matrical cells, cells with trichohyaline granules, pale/clear cells, and different corneocytes.

   The histopathologic differential diagnosis includes trichoblastoma and matricoma. Trichoblastoma consists of germinative cells mostly and contains almost no other components of the hair follicle while matricoma consists almost entirely of matrical cells and shadow cells and has no differentiation toward the other components of a hair follicle.

7. **D.** Epidermal cysts with pilomatrical change are associated with Gardner syndrome.

   Other cutaneous manifestations of Gardner syndrome include desmoid tumors, fibromas, lipomas (may be visceral, including intracranial), leiomyomas, neurofibromas and multifocal pigmented lesions of the fundus (seen in 80% of patients, may present shortly after birth and can be the first marker of disease). Gardner syndrome is genetically linked to band 5q21, the adenomatous polyposis coli (APC) locus. The *APC* gene located on chromosome 5 is the first mutation in the adenoma-to-carcinoma sequence and is believed to initiate the sequence.

8. **C.** Image shown is that of a steatocystoma simplex.

   These cysts, typically located in the mid dermis, are lined by a crenulated or wavy, homogeneous, eosinophilic horny layer collapsed around thin cystic spaces. The spaces hold varying amounts of keratin, vellus hairs, and sebum esters (latter of which often are removed by tissue processing). Walls are formed from several layers of epithelial cells, with embedded flattened lobules of sebaceous glands among the epithelial cells. Steatocystoma simplex is the sporadic solitary tumor counterpart to steatocystoma multiplex – an uncommon disorder of the pilosebaceous unit characterized by the development of numerous sebum-containing dermal cysts. Although steatocystoma multiplex has historically been described as an autosomal dominant inherited disorder, most presenting cases are sporadic. In the familial form of steatocystoma multiplex, mutations are localized to the keratin 17 (*K17*) gene in areas identical to mutations found in patients with pachyonychia congenita type 2 (PC-2). Based on this, some believe that steatocystoma multiplex is simply a variant of pachyonychia congenita type 2. Sporadic forms of steatocystoma multiplex have *not been shown* to be associated with *K17* mutations. Steatocystoma multiplex is associated with eruptive vellus hair cysts. Both diseases share overlapping clinical features, including age of onset, location, appearance of lesions, and mode of inheritance. Reports of hybrid lesions showing histologic features of both steatocystoma multiplex and eruptive vellus hair cysts exist. Given these similarities, some postulate that steatocystoma multiplex and eruptive vellus hair cysts are, in fact, variants of the same disease.

9. **B.** Image shown is that of a pilomatricoma which is associated with mutations in β-catenin.

   Catenin beta-1, also known as β-catenin, is a protein that in humans is encoded by the *CTNNB1* gene. β-catenin is a dual function protein, involved in regulation and coordination of cell–cell adhesion and gene transcription. β-catenin is a ubiquitous cytoplasmic protein that has a critical role in embryonic development and mature tissue homeostasis through its effects on E-cadherin-mediated cell adhesion and Wnt-dependent signal transduction. Mutations that alter specific β-catenin residues important for GSK-3β phosphorylation, or increase the half-life of the protein, have been identified in human cancer. Nuclear β-catenin has been shown to be highly conserved in other cutaneous matrical tumors including those with focal matrical differentiation such as matrical carcinomas, melanocytic matricomas, basal cell carcinomas with focal matrical differentiation as well as trichoepithelioma/trichoblastomas with focal matrical differentiation favoring a common tumorigenesis driven by Wnt pathway activation. Frequent β-catenin overexpression *without exon 3 mutations* has also been observed in select cutaneous B- and T-cell lymphomas.

10. **A.** Image shown is that of a hidrocystoma.

    Typically, hidrocystomas, eccrine or apocrine, appear as unilocular cysts, which usually contain a single cystic cavity composed of 1 or 2 layers of cuboidal cells. They are located within the mid dermal to superficial layers of the skin, especially around the eyes.

    The inherited disorders that are most commonly associated with the presence of multiple eccrine/apocrine hidrocystomas are the following:

    - *Goltz-Gorlin* (also known as Jessner-Cole syndrome, or focal dermal hypoplasia) tends to occur sporadically, with few familial cases having X-linked dominant transmission; it occurs mostly in females. Its cardinal features are microcephaly, midfacial hypoplasia, malformed ears, microphthalmia, periocular multiple hidrocystomas, papillomas of the lip, tongue, anus, and axilla, skeleton abnormalities, and mental retardation.
    - *Schopf-Schulz-Passarge* is an autosomal recessive syndrome characterized by multiple eyelid apocrine hidrocystoma, palmoplantar hyperkeratosis, hypodontia, and hypotrichosis. It is further characterized by hypotrichosis, cysts of the eyelids, and multiple periocular apocrine hidrocystomas.

    Graves's disease has also been associated with multiple eccrine hidrocystomas, possibly due to hyperhidrosis, which is seen in hyperthyroid patients, further supported by the disappearance of lesions after treatment of hyperthyroidism.

11. **A.** Image shown is that of a bronchogenic cyst.

    The lining of bronchogenic cysts is respiratory in origin, ciliated, with a pseudostratified columnar epithelium overlying a fibrous connective tissue wall containing seromucous subcutaneous glands and cartilage plates.

Bronchogenic cysts are rare congenital malformations of ventral foregut development. The majority of cases reported in the literature have been found in the pediatric population, few cases in adults. *A definitive diagnosis of bronchogenic cyst always requires histopathologic confirmation.*

12. **E.** Bronchogenic cysts are typically located in the midline area of the neck.

They are usually located in the mediastinum and intrapulmonary regions; localization in the cervical area is unusual. More common congenital anomalies are known to be initially seen in the upper triangles of the neck: thyroglossal duct cyst and branchial cleft cyst. Clinically, branchial cleft cysts are usually located higher and laterally on the side of the neck, while thyroglossal duct cysts are usually located midline on the anterior aspect of the neck, in close proximity to the hyoid bone.

13. **D.** Image shown is that of a branchial cleft cyst.

Most branchial cleft cysts are lined with stratified squamous epithelium with keratinous debris within the cyst. In a small number, the cyst is lined with respiratory (ciliated columnar) epithelium. Lymphoid tissue is often present outside the epithelial lining. Germinal center formation may be seen in the lymphoid component, but true lymph node architecture is not seen. In infected or ruptured lesions, inflammatory cells are seen within the cyst cavity or the surrounding stroma.

Branchial cleft cysts are congenital epithelial cysts, which arise on the lateral part of the neck from a failure of obliteration of the second branchial cleft in embryonic development. The second branchial arch usually grows caudally and, ultimately, covers the third and fourth arches. The buried clefts become ectoderm-lined cavities, which normally involute around week 7 of development. If a portion of the cleft fails to involute completely, the entrapped remnant forms an epithelium-lined cyst with or without a sinus tract to the overlying skin. A branchial cyst commonly presents as a solitary, painless mass in the neck of a child or a young adult. A history of intermittent swelling and tenderness of the lesion during upper respiratory tract infection may exist. Discharge may be reported if the lesion is associated with a sinus tract.

14. **C.** Image shown is that of a thyroglossal cyst.

Histopathologically, thyroglossal cysts have a variable number of components, including columnar, cuboidal, and/or non-keratinized stratified squamous epithelium. Ectopic thyroid tissue is present in varied proportion, with estimates ranging widely, from 1.5 to 62%.

Thyroglossal duct cysts occur with equal frequency in males and females and are the most common mass found in the midline of the neck in children. Thyroglossal duct cysts are the most common non-odontogenic cysts in the neck, representing approximately 70% of all congenital neck abnormalities. They occur as a result of anomalous development and migration of the thyroid gland during the fourth through eighth weeks of gestation. It is a cystic remnant along the course of the thyroglossal duct between the foramen cecum of the tongue base and the thyroid bed in the visceral space of the infra-hyoid region of the neck.

15. **B.** Image shown is that of a median raphe cyst.

Histopathologic features of a median raphe cyst, exemplified in the image shown, include a cystic cavity lined by a pseudostratified, columnar or stratified squamous cell epithelium, similar to urethral transitional epithelium. Of note, the lining epithelium varies according to the segment origin of the urethra of the lesion, i.e., stratified in the distal part (ectodermal origin) and columnar pseudostratified in the remainder of the urethra (endodermal origin). The luminal cells may present with what appears to be decapitation secretion.

Most are present from birth and remain undetectable until adolescence or adulthood, occurring as a solitary freely movable nodule on the ventral surface of the penis. Developmentally, cysts of the median raphe are thought to arise from embryologic developmental defects of the male urethra.

16. **A.** Median raphe cysts are typically located on the glans penis.

Cysts of the median raphe are midline-developmental cysts that can occur anywhere from the anus to the urinary meatus; when located on the border of the meatus they are also known as parameatal cysts. Several other terms including *mucus cyst of the penis, genitoperineal cyst of the medium raphe, hydrocystoma,* and *apocrine cystadenoma of the penile shaft* have been coined to describe the same lesion and should be regarded as synonymous.

17. **E.** The best-fit diagnosis for the image shown is cutaneous endometriosis.

Histopathologic features diagnostic for endometriosis, as evidenced in the image shown, include ectopic endometrial tissue formed by glandular structures and stroma. Immunohistochemistry can be of utility as the glandular tissue may be positive for hormonal receptors of estrogens (ER) and progesterone (PR).

Endometriosis is defined as the presence of normal endometrial mucosa (glands and stroma) abnormally implanted in locations other than the uterine cavity.

Endometriosis is an estrogen-dependent disease and, thus, usually affects reproductive-aged women. This condition has a prevalence rate of 20–50% in infertile women, but it can be as high as 80% in women with chronic pelvic pain. Based on etiology, there appear to be two types of endometriosis:

- *Secondary endometriosis*, is the most frequent form, and appears after surgical interventions on the abdomen or pelvis.

- *Primary or spontaneous endometriosis,* does not arise due to surgery, and affecting 0.5-1% of women suffering from endometriosis is most frequently located in the umbilicus. When affecting the skin, it can be located in both the dermis and the subcutis. The typical clinical presentation of secondary cutaneous endometriosis is as a nodule located on the scar of a previous surgical intervention. It will be a nodular mass, with variable color (erythematous, brownish or purplish) and with an increasing volume, occasionally with pain and bleeding coinciding with the menstrual cycle or previous to it (although there are some cases in which the symptoms are not directly related to the menstrual cycle and even asymptomatic). A specific standard has been described for the dermoscopy of these lesions known as "red atolls"; that is, homogeneous red pigmentation, uniformly distributed inside with more defined and more intensely colored small red globular structures. These "red atolls" correspond with the multiple irregular glands containing erythrocytes, and the homogeneous reddish mass surrounding these atolls corresponds with the myxoid vascular stroma with extravasated erythrocytes surrounding the glands.

18. **D.** Image shown is that of a metaplastic synovial cyst.

Histopathologic features, demonstrated in the image shown, include multiple villous structures resembling hyperplastic synovium projecting toward the center of the cavity with a lining that may be hypocellular or hypercellular and containing a mixture of fibroblastic, epithelioid, mononuclear inflammatory, and occasional multinucleate giant cells peripherally. The hypocellular regions may appear somewhat hyalinized and fibrin deposits may be seen.

This entity has also been referred to as synovial metaplasia of the skin. While the pathogenesis is unclear, surgical or non-surgical trauma is hypothesized to be the precipitating event in most cases reported to date.

19. **C.** Image shown is that of an auricular pseudocyst.

Histopathologically, pseudocysts of the auricle lack pathognomonic features, but are typically characterized by an intracartilaginous cavity containing extravasated erythrocytes and lacking an epithelial lining. They contain thinned cartilage and hyalinizing degeneration along the internal border of the cystic space. The epidermis and dermis overlying the pseudocyst are usually normal. However, a dermal perivascular lymphocytic infiltrate is commonly found, along with inflammatory cells within the cystic space. Eosinophilic degeneration and necrosis of the cartilage is also present in some areas in select cases.

20. **D.** Pseudocysts of the auricle typically present in the lateral or anterior surface of the pinna, usually in the scaphoid or triangular fossa.

Pseudocyst of the auricle was first reported by Hartmann in 1846 and first described in the English literature in 1966 by Engel. Historically, pseudocyst of the auricle has been addressed by many terms, including endochondral pseudocyst, intracartilaginous cyst, cystic chondromalacia, and benign idiopathic cystic chondromalacia. Pseudocysts usually present spontaneously or following repeated minor trauma. The observation that an auricular pseudocyst often results after repeated minor trauma, such as rubbing, minor sport injuries, ear pulling, sleeping on hard pillows, or wearing a motorcycle helmet or earphones, has led to the suggestion that these minor traumas may be the mechanism. In support of this traumatic etiology, elevated serum lactic dehydrogenase (LDH) values have been reported within the pseudocyst fluid. Contradicting this are other reports that pseudocysts are a variation of otoseroma.

E4 Cutaneous Appendageal Diseases Questions

1. Which of the following most accurately describes anagen:
   A. Is short
   B. Minimal regional variation
   C. Involves approximately 1% of scalp hairs at a given time
   D. Entry of follicles into this stage is a random process
   E. Is the phase of active hair production

2. Which of the following correctly describes catagen:
   A. Lasts for 2–6 years in scalp hairs
   B. Exhibits regional variation
   C. Involves approximately 90% of scalp hairs at a given time
   D. Is the involutionary phase of hair production
   E. Length of the hair shaft is directly proportional to length of the phase

3. This is commonly associated with:

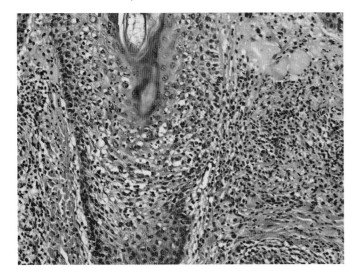

A. Halogenated aromatic compounds
B. *Pseudomonas* infection
C. Immunosuppression
D. *Pityrosporum* infection
E. Pregnancy

4. The most likely diagnosis is:

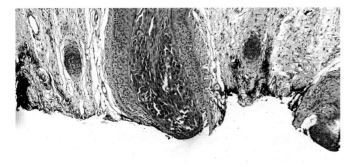

A. Dermatophyte folliculitis
B. Viral folliculitis
C. Pityrosporum folliculitis
D. Actinic folliculitis
E. Infundibulofolliculitis

5. This (based on the image shown above) is commonly associated with:
A. Immunosuppression
B. *Pseudomonas* infection
C. Halogenated aromatic compounds
D. *Pityrosporum* infection
E. Pregnancy

6. Hoffman's disease refers to:
A. Acne conglobata
B. Pediculosis capitis

C. Acne vulgaris
D. Perforating folliculitis
E. Dissecting cellulitis

7. The follicular occlusion triad refers to:
A. Pseudopelade, chloracne, actinic folliculitis
B. Acne necrotica, pseudofolliculitis, acne conglobata
C. Perforating folliculitis, acne fulminans, chloracne
D. Hidradenitis suppurativa, dissecting cellulitis, acne conglobata
E. Acne vulgaris, necrotizing folliculitis, chloracne

8. The most likely diagnosis is:

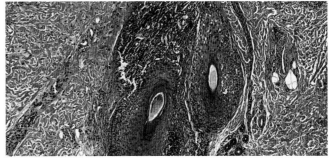

A. Majocchi's granuloma
B. Pityrosporum folliculitis
C. Inflamed cyst
D. Tinea pedis
E. Pityriasis versicolor

9. The causative organism (based on the image shown above) is:
A. *Tinea capitis*
B. *Tinea faciei*
C. *Malassezia furfur*
D. *Pityriasis versicolor*
E. *Candida albicans*

10. Which of the following refers to a hair shaft fracture:
A. Trichorrhexis nodosa
B. Trichostasis spinulosa
C. Trichodysplasia
D. Trichotillomania
E. Trichomegaly

11. Which of the following is NOT a scarring alopecia:
A. Traction alopecia
B. Folliculitis decalvans
C. Tufted-hair folliculitis
D. Pseudopelade
E. Androgenetic alopecia

12. The most likely diagnosis is:

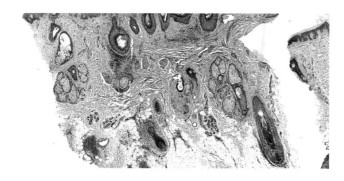

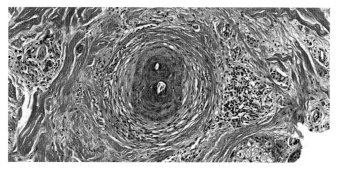

    A. Telogen effluvium
    B. Folliculitis decalvans
    C. Androgenetic alopecia
    D. Alopecia areata
    E. Lipedematous alopecia

13. Which of the following is a lymphocytic scarring alopecia:
    A. Telogen effluvium
    B. Folliculitis decalvans
    C. Pseudopelade of Brocq
    D. Alopecia areata
    E. Androgenetic alopecia

14. This may be secondary to:

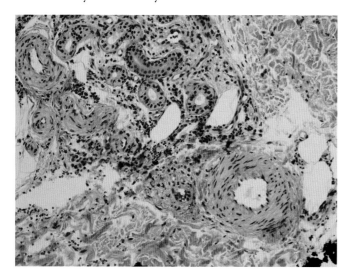

    A. A nutritional deficiency
    B. A storage disorder
    C. Chemotherapy
    D. An internal malignancy
    E. A genodermatosis

15. The drug most frequently associated with this (based on the image shown above) is:
    A. IVIg
    B. Rituximab
    C. Vemurafenib
    D. Imatinib
    E. Cytarabine

16. The most likely diagnosis is:

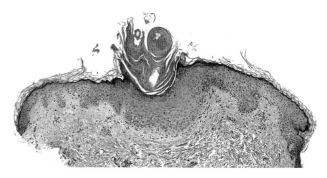

    A. Dilated pore
    B. Discoid lupus
    C. Apocrine miliaria
    D. Keratosis pilaris
    E. Trichostasis spinulosa

17. The most likely diagnosis is:

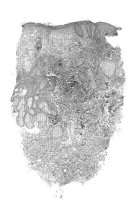

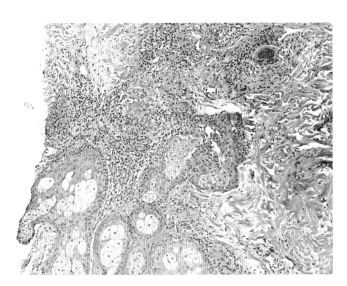

A. Miliaria crystallina
B. Chloracne
C. Rosacea
D. Lupus erythematosus
E. Keratosis pilaris

18. Biopsy from a papular rash around the eyelids. The most likely diagnosis is:

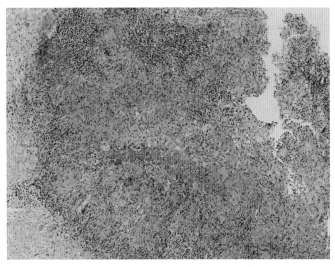

A. Lupus vulgaris
B. Lupus miliaris
C. Apocrine miliaria
D. Necrobiosis lipoidica
E. Acne fulminans

19. Fox-Fordyce disease primarily affects:
A. Apocrine glands
B. Eccrine glands
C. Sebaceous glands
D. Hair follicles
E. Elastic fibers

20. Sterile neutrophilic folliculitis is seen in:
A. Kyrle's disease
B. Fox-Fordyce disease
C. Bowen's disease
D. Degos disease
E. Behcet's disease

E4 Cutaneous Appendageal Diseases Answers

Table E4.1 Key histopathologic features of select scarring and non-scarring alopecias

Type		Entity	Key histopathology
Non-scarring		**Alopecia areata**	*Early*: Peribulbar lymphocytic infiltrate ("swarm of bees"), decreased terminal hairs, increased vellus hairs, eosinophils plus mast cells in the follicular stellae, multiple catagen hairs
			Long-standing disease: Decreased peribulbar inflammation, telogen hairs close to 100%, empty infundibula
			In all stages, a non-sclerotic fibrous tract extends along the site of the previous follicle into the subcutis
		Androgenetic alopecia	Progressive miniaturization, increased telogen and catagen hairs, Arão-Perkins bodies in streamers, perivascular inflammation containing mast cells
		Telogen effluvium	Telogen counts >25%
		Trichotillomania	Increased catagen hairs, presence of early and late anagen hairs, empty hair ducts, trichomalacia, pigment casts
		Drug-induced*	Increased telogen hairs, reversible scarring
Scarring	**Lymphocytic**	**Lupus erythematosus**	Loss of follicles and sebaceous glands, interface dermatitis extending along DEJ plus follicular epithelia, dermal mucin, perivascular and periadnexal inflammation with plasma cells, follicular plugging
		Lichen planopilaris	Loss of follicles and sebaceous glands, perifollicular myxoid fibrosis, peri-infundibular inflammation, interface dermatitis extending along follicular epithelia
		Central centrifugal alopecia	Loss of follicles and sebaceous glands, follicular miniaturization, premature desquamation of the IRS, compound follicles, PFF, naked hair shafts, streamers
		Alopecia mucinosa	Follicular degeneration with intrafollicular mucin, abundant mucin in early lesions, periappendageal, perivascular, or interstitial lymphocytic mixed inflammatory cell infiltrate
		Classic pseudopelade of Brocq	*Early lesions*: Loss of follicles and sebaceous glands, replacement by fibrous tracts containing elastic fibers (prominent perifollicular lamellar fibroplasia), moderate perifollicular (around the upper two-thirds) lymphocytic infiltrate
			Late/end-stage lesions: Minimal inflammation, follicular drop-out
	Neutrophilic	**Folliculitis decalvans**	Folliculitis, disruption of follicular epithelia, dense perifollicular mixed inflammatory infiltrate containing plasma cells
		Tufted folliculitis	Several closely set complete follicles with a common opening from which multiple hair shafts emerge
		Dissecting folliculitis	Dense, predominantly neutrophilic, mixed-cell perifollicular infiltrate, neutrophilic microabscesses in the dermis or subcutaneous tissue, follicular dilatation may be evident in early disease, granulomatous inflammation, scarring, and fibrosis common in advanced or late-stage disease
	Mixed	**Erosive pustular dermatosis**	Epidermal denudation, loss of follicles, granulation tissue
		Folliculitis keloidalis	Folliculitis, naked hair shafts, disrupted follicular epithelia, dense perifollicular mixed inflammatory infiltrate

* Thallium, excessive vitamin A, retinoids, cholesterol-lowering agents, anticonvulsants, antithyroid, EGF-R inhibitors, β-blockers
DEJ = Dermoepidermal junction; IRS = Inner root sheath; PFF = Perifollicular fibrosis

1. **E. Anagen is the phase of active hair production.**

   The terminal anagen hair extends from its bulb in the subcutaneous tissue to its point of emergence from the epidermis. At a given point, 80–90% of scalp hairs are in anagen. There is regional variation in the duration of anagen (2–6 years in the scalp, 1 year in the beard region, 2–6 months in the axilla and pubic region). The length of a hair shaft is directly proportional to the length of the anagen phase.

2. **D. Catagen is the involutionary phase of hair production.**

   When anagen ends, the hair goes into catagen, the intermediate stage between growth and rest, for 10–14 days. There is minimal regional variation in catagen which is a random process in humans (in contrast to animals). At a given time, approximately 1% of scalp hairs are in catagen.

3. C. Eosinophilic folliculitis, shown in the image, is associated with immunosuppression secondary to HIV infection.

Eosinophilic folliculitis has been classified as an AIDS-defining illness. In both children and adults, eosinophilic pustular folliculitis should be viewed as a possible cutaneous sign of immunosuppression. However, eosinophilic folliculitis may also develop in immunocompetent persons. Eosinophilic folliculitis is a non-infectious eosinophilic infiltration of hair follicles. Over the past 2 decades, the spectrum of eosinophilic folliculitis has expanded to pediatric populations, transplant recipients, and persons with HIV and hematopoietic disorders. The 3 variants of eosinophilic folliculitis include:

- Classic eosinophilic pustular folliculitis
- Immunosuppression-associated eosinophilic folliculitis (mostly HIV-related)
- Infancy-associated eosinophilic folliculitis

In patients with eosinophilic folliculitis, a CBC count reveals leukocytosis and eosinophilia.

Immunoelectrophoresis reveals elevated levels of IgE, low levels of IgG3, and low levels of IgA in pediatric eosinophilic folliculitis. Obtaining two punch biopsy specimens, to allow for both vertical and transverse sectioning, increases the sensitivity of finding the characteristic features of eosinophilic folliculitis. The infundibulum of the hair follicle manifests eosinophilic spongiosis and pustulosis. The infiltrate often extends to the adjacent sebaceous gland. Although most follicles are preserved, some follicular walls are destroyed by the inflammatory infiltrate which is typically composed of eosinophils with variable numbers of neutrophils and mononuclear cells. HIV-associated eosinophilic folliculitis has a more intense perivascular and diffuse inflammatory infiltration compared with that of the HIV-related pruritic papular eruption.

4. B. Image shown is that of viral-associated trichodysplasia.

Viral-associated trichodysplasia of immunosuppression is a rare cutaneous eruption that is characterized by follicle-centered shiny papules and alopecia with characteristic histopathologic findings of abnormally anagen follicles with excessive inner root sheath differentiation. Immunohistochemical staining for the polyomavirus middle T antigen typically demonstrates strongly positive staining of cellular inclusion within keratinocytes composing the inner root sheath, confirming the presence of polyomavirus. Scanning electron microscopy reveals small (35.6 nm), icosahedral, regularly spaced, intracellular viral particles within these inclusions, consistent with polyomavirus.

5. A. Viral-associated trichodysplasia is typically associated with immunosuppression.

Viral-associated trichodysplasia (VAT), a folliculocentric viral infection, was originally described in a patient receiving cyclosporine after kidney and pancreas transplantation. Since then, it has been reported under a variety of names (e.g. cyclosporine-induced folliculodystrophy, trichodysplasia spinulosa, pilomatrix dysplasia) as well as in association with other immunosuppressant agents that are used in cases of organ transplantation or as part of chemotherapy regimens. Both children and adults are known to have been affected by VAT, and it has been reported to occur after lung, heart, and kidney transplantations and in the setting of acute lymphocytic leukemia.

6. E. Hoffman's disease refers to dissecting cellulitis of the scalp.

Dissecting cellulitis of the scalp (DCS), also known as *perifolliculitis capitis abscedens et suffodiens* or Hoffman disease, is a chronic inflammatory disorder of the scalp characterized by boggy, suppurative nodules that are often associated with patchy hair loss. Histopathologic features of DCS vary according to stage of the disease and severity but characteristically include a dense, predominantly neutrophilic, mixed-cell perifollicular infiltrate. There may be neutrophilic microabscesses in the dermis or subcutaneous tissue. Follicular dilatation may be evident in early disease. Granulomatous inflammation, scarring, and fibrosis are common in advanced or late-stage disease.

7. D. The follicular occlusion triad refers to hidradenitis suppurativa, dissecting cellulitis of the scalp and acne conglobata.

Hidradenitis suppurativa typically involves apocrine gland-bearing areas such as the axillae, perineum, groin and pubic region. Acne conglobata develops in any hair-bearing areas such as the trunk, buttocks and proximal portion of the extremities. Dissecting cellulitis, as implied by the name, involves the scalp. *Follicular occlusion is a key pathogenic event in these three entities.*

8. B. The most likely diagnosis for the image shown is pityrosporum folliculitis.

The diagnosis of pityrosporum folliculitis is based on clinical suspicion of the classic presentation of pruritic papulopustules found in a follicular pattern on the back, chest, upper arms, and, occasionally the neck of young to middle-aged adults. They are rarely present on the face. An improvement in the lesions with empiric antimycotic therapy supports a clinical diagnosis of pityrosporum folliculitis. The basic lesion observed is that of folliculitis. The ostium of the hair follicles is dilated, partially disrupted with keratin plugging, cellular debris, and an inflammatory infiltrate including lymphocytes, histiocytes, and neutrophils. Some follicles may be cystic and ruptured. Single as well as aggregates of spores are noted within the follicle. *A key histopathologic clue is the presence of basophilic debris in the dermis adjacent to the partially disrupted follicle.*

9. **C.** The causative organism associated with pityrosporum folliculitis is *Malassezia furfur.*

   Yeasts, specifically *Malassezia furfur,* are the pathogenic agents in pityrosporum folliculitis. *M. furfur* has been linked to several skin diseases, including seborrheic dermatitis, folliculitis, confluent and reticulated papillomatosis, and pityriasis versicolor. In 1874, Malassez first described round and oval budding yeasts from scales of patients with seborrheic dermatitis. He coined the phrases "bottle bacillus of Unna" to describe the small oval cells in the scale and "spore of Malassez" to name the bud that is observed in association with the yeast. Saborouraud proposed the *Pityrosporum* genus in 1904 to describe the budding yeast cells without hyphal elements from normal skin. Later, in the 1900s, *Pityrosporum ovale* and *Pityrosporum orbiculare* were isolated. Pityrosporum folliculitis is caused by *Malassezia* species that are part of the cutaneous microflora and not by exogenous species.

10. **A.** Trichorrhexis nodosa refers to a hair shaft fracture.

    Trichorrhexis nodosa is characterized by small/beaded swellings along the shaft corresponding to sites that fracture easily. Scalp hair is typically involved. Other hair shaft fractures include the following:
    - Trichoschisis (clean transverse break of the hair shaft)
    - Trichoclasis (irregular transverse/oblique fracture with irregular borders and a partially intact cuticle)
    - Trichorrhexis invaginata (nodose swellings)
    - Trichoptilosis (longitudinal splitting)
    - Trichoteiromania (self-inflicted damage to hair)
    - Trichotemnomania (factitious, resulting from habit of cutting hair with scissors or razor)

11. **E.** Androgenetic alopecia is a non-scarring alopecia.

    Other causes of a non-cicatricial alopecia include:
    - Alopecia areata
    - Anagen effluvium
    - Dermatopathia pigmentosa reticularis
    - Telogen effluvium
    - Trichotillomania (trichotillosis)

    Also see Table E4.1.

12. **D.** The most likely diagnosis for the image shown is alopecia areata.

    Alopecia areata is a recurrent non-scarring type of hair loss that can affect any hair-bearing area and can manifest in many different patterns. The natural history of alopecia areata is unpredictable. Most patients have only a few focal areas of alopecia, and spontaneous regrowth usually occurs within 1 year. The condition is usually localized when it first appears and typically presents as a single patch (80% of cases). There is no correlation between the number of patches at onset and subsequent severity. While it can affect any hair-bearing area, and more than one area can be affected at once, it usually involves the scalp followed by the beard. While the exact pathophysiology of alopecia areata remains unknown, a widely accepted hypothesis is that alopecia areata is a T-cell-mediated autoimmune condition that occurs in genetically predisposed individuals. In terms of clinical presentation, the presence of smooth, slightly erythematous (peach color) or normal-colored alopecic patches is characteristic. *The presence of exclamation point hairs (i.e. hairs tapered near the proximal end) is pathognomonic* but is not always found. A positive result from the pull test at the periphery of a plaque usually indicates that the disease is active, and further hair loss can be expected. *The presence of yellow dots seen on dermoscopy is a specific feature of alopecia areata and has been reported to be present in 95% of patients, regardless of their disease stage.*

    In terms of histopathology, findings vary with disease stage as well as the biopsied site. Horizontal sections usually are preferred to vertical sections because they allow examination of multiple hair follicles at different levels.

    Expanding edge, active disease: The most characteristic feature is a peribulbar lymphocytic infiltrate ("swarm of bees"). A significant decrease in terminal hairs is associated with an increase in vellus hairs, with a ratio of 1:1 (normal is 7:1). Other helpful findings include pigment incontinence or the presence of eosinophils as well as mast cells in the follicular stellae, multiple catagen hairs, hyperkeratosis of the infundibulum, and pigment casts in the infundibulum. A shift occurs in the anagen-to-telogen ratio, which is not specific; in alopecia areata, 73% of hairs are found to be in the anagen phase and 27% in the telogen phase (normal ratio is approximately 90% anagen phase to 10% telogen phase hair follicles).

    Long-standing disease: Peribulbar inflammation minimal, the percentage of telogen-phase hairs can approach 100%, empty infundibula.

    In all stages, a non-sclerotic fibrous tract (representing the collapsed fibrous root sheath or stela) extends along the site of the previous follicle into the subcutis.

13. C. Pseudopelade of Brocq is a lymphocytic scarring alopecia.

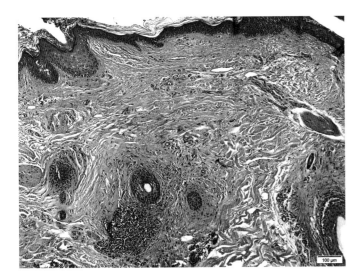

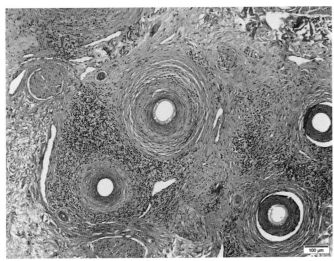

In 1888, Brocq used the term pseudopelade to describe a unique form of cicatricial alopecia resembling alopecia areata (*pelade* is the French term for alopecia areata). Over the last century, this condition has been a source of controversy and the current consensus is that it is an end-stage or clinical variant of various forms of cicatricial alopecia. The same pattern of alopecia can be found in end-stage discoid lupus erythematosus (DLE), lichen planopilaris (LPP), and other forms of cicatricial alopecia. Pseudopelade of Brocq is not a specific disease, but a pattern of cicatricial alopecia. If a definitive diagnosis of DLE, LPP, or another condition can be made based on clinical, histologic, or immunofluorescent features, then the term pseudopelade of Brocq should not be used. A primary form of traditional pseudopelade may exist, although this has yet to be established with certainty. Lesions of pseudopelade are randomly distributed,

irregularly shaped, and often cluster in patches on the scalp. The individual lesion is hypopigmented ("porcelain white") and slightly depressed (atrophic). Pseudopelade of Brocq lesions often are shaped irregularly (as opposed to the round or oval patches usually seen in alopecia areata). Absence of follicular ostia is noted with dermoscopy. The histopathologic findings vary with disease stage.

Early lesions: Loss of follicles and sebaceous glands, replacement by fibrous tracts containing elastic fibers (in horizontal sections manifests as prominent perifollicular lamellar fibroplasia), moderate perifollicular (around the upper two-thirds) lymphocytic infiltrate
Late/end-stage lesions: Minimal inflammation, follicular drop-out

14. C. Neutrophilic eccrine hidradenitis (shown in the image) is typically secondary to chemotherapy.

Neutrophilic eccrine hidradenitis (NEH), a self-limited process, was initially described in acute myelogenous leukemia (AML) patients undergoing chemotherapy. Patients with this uncommon, self-limited condition usually present with fever and non-specific cutaneous lesions. More than 70% of oncology patients who develop NEH do so after their first course of chemotherapy. NEH does not appear to portend a worse prognosis for the underlying malignancy when occurring in that setting. The cutaneous manifestations of NEH are highly variable and include lesions that may be solitary or multiple, erythematous or purpuric macules, papules, nodules, or plaques with the trunk or limbs most commonly involved. The cause of NEH is unknown and a direct toxic effect of chemotherapy and a paraneoplastic mechanism have both been proposed to explain NEH in the context of malignancy. Histopathologic findings include a dense neutrophilic infiltrate within and around eccrine glands, with necrosis of eccrine epithelial cells. Some severely neutropenic patients may have a paucity or absence of neutrophils, but *necrosis of eccrine glands is evident in all.*

15. E. Cytarabine is most frequently associated with neutrophilic eccrine hidradenitis (NEH).

NEH was first described in a patient with acute myeloid leukemia who had received cytarabine as chemotherapy. Other cytotoxic drugs associated with NEH include chlorambucil, cyclophosphamide, doxorubicin, lomustine, mitoxantrone, topotecan, and vincristine.

16. D. The most likely diagnosis for the image shown is keratosis pilaris.

Keratosis pilaris (KP), an extremely common benign condition, is a genetic disorder of keratinization of hair follicles of the skin that manifests as small, rough folliculocentric keratotic papules ("chicken bumps, chicken skin, or goose-bumps"), in characteristic areas of the body, particularly the outer-upper arms and thighs. Ulerythema ophryogenes (keratosis pilaris atrophicans faciei), an uncommon variant of keratosis pilaris, is characterized by follicular-based, small horny, red papules of the eyebrows and cheeks. The histopathologic triad in KP consists of epidermal hyperkeratosis, hypergranulosis, and plugging of individual hair follicles (the plug typically fills the infundibulum and protrudes above the surface).

17. C. The most likely diagnosis for the image shown is rosacea.

Rosacea is a common condition characterized by symptoms of facial flushing and a spectrum of clinical signs, including erythema, telangiectasia, coarseness of skin, and an inflammatory papulopustular eruption resembling acne. The National Rosacea Society classifies rosacea into the following subtypes:

- Erythematotelangiectatic type
- Papulopustular
- Phymatous
- Ocular

Histopathologic findings of rosacea depend on the subtype. Non-pustular lesions show a non-specific perivascular and perifollicular lymphohistiocytic infiltrate with admixed plasma cells and telangiectases. Papulopustular lesions demonstrate a more pronounced perifollicular granulomatous inflammation with caseating as well as non-caseating granulomas and perifollicular abscesses. *Demodex folliculorum* may be abundant in nearby follicles.

18. B. In conjunction with the clinical presentation, the most likely diagnosis for the image shown is lupus miliaris disseminatus faciei (LMDF).

Also known as acne agminata, LMDF manifests with inflammatory erythematous or flesh-colored papules distributed symmetrically across the upper part of the face, particularly around the eyes and the nose. The lesions tend to be discrete, and surrounding erythema is not a marked feature but may be present. These patients typically do not have a history of flushing. Histopathologic findings vary with disease stage.

Early lesions: Superficial perivascular and periappendageal lymphocytic infiltrates with a few histiocytes and neutrophils

Fully developed lesions: Granulomas with caseation necrosis

Late lesions: Fibrosis with scattered lymphocytes, histiocytes, and neutrophils, may also be perifollicular and may show an attenuated epidermis

19. A. Fox-Fordyce disease primarily affects the apocrine glands.

Fox-Fordyce disease is an infrequently occurring chronic pruritic papular eruption that localizes to areas where apocrine glands are found. Lesions are most often found in the axillae, where they tend to be bilateral. Lesions may also affect the periareolar, inframammary, and pubic areas. The primary lesion is a flesh-colored to reddish, smooth, dome-shaped, discrete, and follicular or perifollicular papule. Affected areas usually have many papules as the papules usually appear to affect every follicle in a given area. The observed pathophysiology is a keratin plug in the hair follicle infundibulum obstructing the apocrine acrosyringium and producing an apocrine anhidrosis. Histopathologically, a rupture of the apocrine excretory duct occurs, and spongiotic inflammation at the point of entry of the apocrine duct results. Follicular dyskeratosis and an orthokeratotic plug filling the dilated infundibulum may also be evident.

20. E. Sterile neutrophilic folliculitis may be seen in Behcet's disease.

The term sterile neutrophilic folliculitis was coined by Magro and Crowson for a distinctive cutaneous reaction pattern usually accompanying systemic diseases. Disease entities associated with a sterile neutrophilic folliculitis include:
- Inflammatory bowel disease
- Reiter's disease
- Hepatitis B infection
- Connective tissue disease

The clinical presentation is that of a folliculitis or vasculitis, predominantly on the arms, legs and the back with accompanying fever, malaise and arthritis. Histopathologic findings include a neutrophilic or suppurative folliculitis accompanied by a folliculocentric neutrophilic vascular reaction.

E5 Panniculitis
Questions

1. Which of the following is predominantly a lobular panniculitis:
   A. Scleredema adultorum
   B. Necrobiosis lipoidica
   C. Sclerema neonatorum
   D. Erythema nodosum
   E. Wegener's granulomatosis

2. Septal panniculitides include all of the following EXCEPT:
   A. Scleroderma
   B. Necrobiosis lipoidica

C. Sclerema neonatorum

D. Nephrogenic systemic fibrosis

E. Microscopic polyangiitis

3. The best-fit diagnosis is:

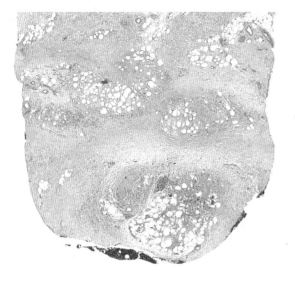

A. Erythema induratum

B. Lupus profundus

C. Scleroderma

D. Necrobiosis lipoidica

E. Erythema nodosum

4. Miescher's radial granuloma is a pathognomonic finding in:
   A. Necrobiosis lipoidica
   B. Sclerema neonatorum
   C. Nodular vasculitis
   D. Erythema nodosum
   E. Pancreatic panniculitis

5. Necrobiosis lipoidica is clinically characterized by:
   A. A depressed plaque with a shiny yellow/brown center
   B. A violaceous ulceration surrounded by a mottled ischemic zone
   C. An expansile ulcer with an undermined boggy border
   D. A circinate, confluent reddish-brown plaque
   E. Sharply demarcated area of necrosis

6. Histopathologic features characteristic of necrobiosis lipoidica are best appreciated at:
   A. The center
   B. The edge
   C. Perilesionally

7. Features of utility in differentiating necrobiosis lipoidica from granuloma annulare include:
   A. Presence of necrobiosis
   B. Density of the infiltrate

C. Presence of plasma cells

D. Presence of multinucleate giant cells

E. Presence of lipoid droplets

8. The best-fit diagnosis is:

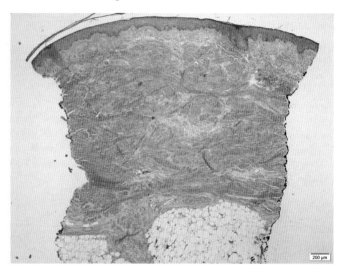

A. Scleredema

B. Scleroderma

C. Scleromyxedema

D. Necrobiosis lipoidica

E. Granuloma annulare

9. Nodular vasculitis is clinically characterized by:
   A. Violaceous perifollicular papules
   B. Expansile ulcer with an undermined boggy border
   D. Circinate, confluent reddish-brown plaques
   D. Tender erythematous nodules
   E. Non-inflamed purpuric plaques

10. The best-fit diagnosis is:

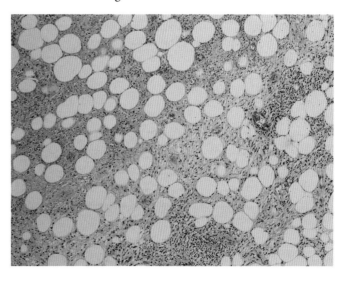

A. Polyarteritis nodosa
B. Superficial migratory thrombophlebitis
C. Neutrophilic panniculitis
D. Nodular vasculitis
E. Infection-induced panniculitis

11. This may be seen in all of the following EXCEPT:

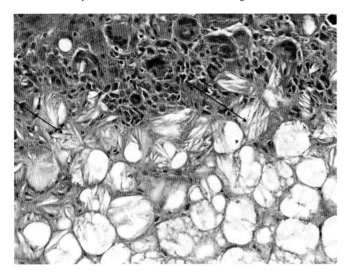

A. Sclerema neonatorum
B. Subcutaneous fat necrosis
C. Post-steroid panniculitis
D. Lipodermatosclerosis

12. Histopathologic features of α_1-antitrypsin deficiency include all of the following EXCEPT:
A. Septal panniculitis
B. Neutrophil-rich infiltrate
C. Liquefaction necrosis
D. "Skip" areas
E. Primary vasculitis

13. Feature/s of utility in differentiating α_1-antitrypsin deficiency from pancreatic panniculitis include:
A. Septal panniculitis
B. Neutrophil-rich infiltrate
C. Liquefaction necrosis
D. "Skip" areas
E. Dermal involvement

14. In the WHO/EORTC classification scheme, subcutaneous panniculitis-like T-cell lymphoma is:
A. γδ positive
B. CD4 positive
C. CD8 positive
D. CD30 positive
E. CD56 positive

15. The best-fit diagnosis is:

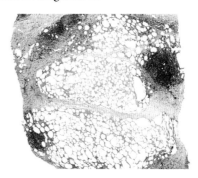

A. Panniculitis-like T-cell lymphoma
B. Lupus profundus
C. Extranodal NK/T-cell lymphoma
D. Hydroa vacciniforme-like lymphoma
E. Cytophagic histiocytic panniculitis

16. This is associated with:

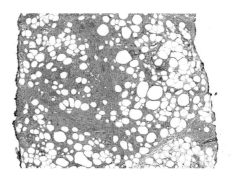

A. Venous stasis
B. Infection
C. Crohn's disease
D. Sarcoidosis
E. Cryoglobulinemia

17. The best-fit diagnosis is:

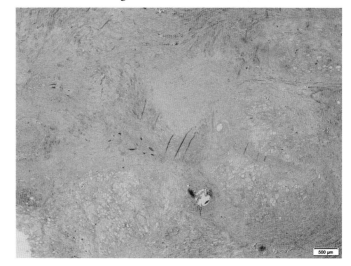

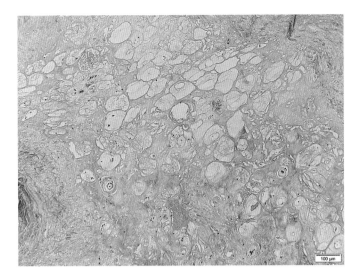

A. Encapsulated fat necrosis
B. Post-irradiation panniculitis
C. Pancreatic panniculitis
D. Total lipodystrophy
E. Subcutaneous fat necrosis

18. The best-fit diagnosis is:

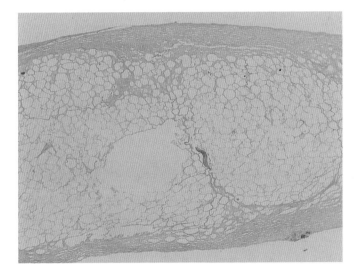

A. Encapsulated fat necrosis
B. Post-irradiation panniculitis
C. Pancreatic panniculitis
D. Total lipodystrophy
E. Subcutaneous fat necrosis

19. This may be associated with:

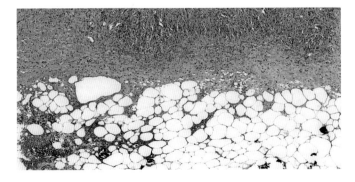

A. Childhood onset
B. Thyroid dysfunction
C. End-stage renal disease
D. Hypercholesterolemia
E. Addison's disease

20. Which of the following is INCORRECT regarding the cutaneous variant of this entity:

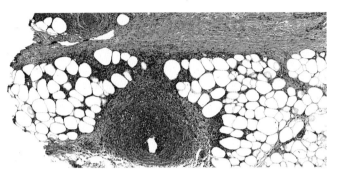

A. May be ANCA negative
B. Chronic relapsing course
C. Involves medium-sized vessels
D. Deep biopsy key
E. Serology diagnostic

21. This is best regarded as a latent form of:

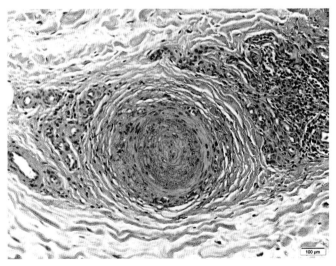

A. Granuloma faciale
B. Erythema elevatum diutinum
C. Urticarial vasculitis
D. Polyarteritis nodosa
E. Kawasaki syndrome

E5 Panniculitis
Answers

Table E5.1 Primary septal panniculitis – a histopathologic approach

Entity	Key histopathologic features	Image
Erythema nodosum	Lymphohistiocytic inflammatory infiltrate, Miescher's radial granuloma – *pathognomonic finding* (may not always be present though) *Early lesions*: Presence of neutrophils, edematous widening of septa with fibrinoid change *Late lesions*: Fibrotic thickening of septa	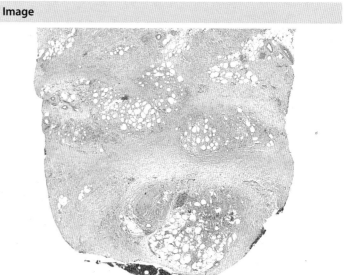
Necrobiosis lipoidica	Changes best seen at the edge Pandermal involvement, interstitial and palisaded granulomatous dermatosis with a characteristic "tiered" appearance at scanning magnification *Early lesions*: Superficial and deep perivascular and interstitial inflammatory infiltrate *Late lesions*: Minimal necrobiosis and more fibrosis	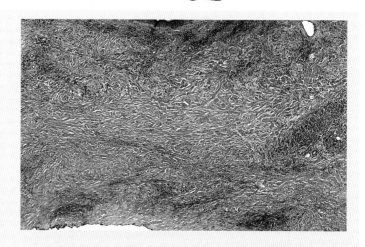
Scleroderma	Pandermal homogenization of dermal collagen, loss of peri-eccrine adipocytes; sharply demarcated junction between dermis and subcutis; atrophy of adnexae particularly the pilosebaceous units; arrectores pilorum are often hypertrophied Thickening of small vessel walls Lymphoplasmacytic inflammatory infiltrate – more diffuse in distribution in the deeper dermis, particularly prominent at the junction of the deep dermis and the subcutis	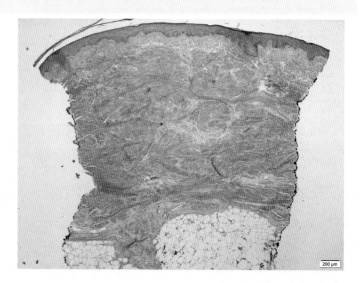

Table E5.1 Primary septal panniculitis – a histopathologic approach (*cont.*)

Entity	Key histopathologic features	Image
Nephrogenic systemic fibrosis	"Busy" dermis with thickened collagen, interstitial mucin and an interstitial reticular to parallel proliferation ("tram-track" configuration) of CD34 positive plump spindled cells Osseous sclerotic bodies/lollipop bodies with elastic fiber entrapment	
Microscopic polyangiitis	Neutrophilic vasculitis, RBC extravasation, fibrinoid degeneration of arterioles	

Table E5.2 Primary lobular panniculitis – a histopathologic approach

Entity	Key histopathologic features	Image
Nodular vasculitis	Inflammatory changes restricted to the lower dermis and subcutis Changes vary with the age of the lesion Vasculitis involving small deep vessels evident in 90% of cases (*not a requisite for the diagnosis*) Presence of both septal and lobular granulomatous inflammation characteristic	
Subcutaneous fat necrosis of the newborn (SFN) **Post-steroid panniculitis** **Sclerema neonatorum**	Fat necrosis, needle-shaped clefts within adipocytes, polymorphous inflammatory infiltrate Similar to SFN Similar to SFN but *no inflammation*	

Table E5.2 Primary lobular panniculitis – a histopathologic approach (*cont.*)

Entity	Key histopathologic features	Image
Cold panniculitis	Changes most marked at junction of deep dermis and subcutis Lymphohistiocytic infiltrate	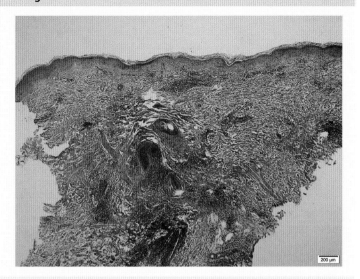
α₁-antitrypsin deficiency (AATD)	Predominantly lobular neutrophilic panniculitis in which the affected fat lobules are necrotic and replaced with an intense neutrophilic infiltrate "Skip areas" characteristic *Presence of extensive collagenolysis/ elastolysis resulting in "floating fat" separated from the surrounding reticular dermis and pannicular septa characteristic* Highly suggestive feature is the spread of neutrophils into the reticular dermis and septa of the subcutis	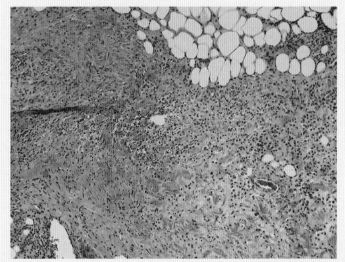
Pancreatic panniculitis	*Early lesions*: Enzymatic fat necrosis, ghost-like outline of fat, +/1 septal involvement, neutrophilic infiltrate, calcium deposition *Late lesions*: MNGCs, lipophages, hemosiderin deposits and fibrosis *Like AATD*: Neutrophil-rich infiltrate and the fat necrosis *Unlike AATD*: Does not exhibit "skip areas"	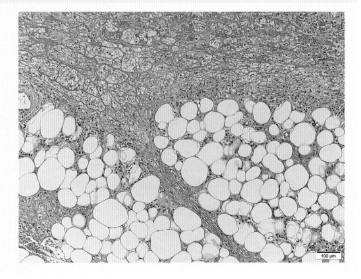

Table E5.2 Primary lobular panniculitis – a histopathologic approach (*cont.*)

Entity	Key histopathologic features	Image
Subcutaneous panniculitis-like T-cell lymphoma	Predominantly subcutaneous atypical lymphoid infiltrate, showing typical adipotropism and characteristically involving the lobules Extension of the atypical infiltrate into the reticular dermis common Neoplastic infiltrate composed of pleomorphic T-cells of variable size with irregular and often hyperchromatic nuclei Rimming of individual adipocytes by neoplastic CD3 positive, CD8 positive, CD4 negative T-cells, with expression of cytotoxic proteins (granzyme B, TIA-1, perforin T) common, although present sometimes focally Fat necrosis and karyorrhexis typical	
Lupus panniculitis	Epidermal changes of chronic discoid LE present >50% cases Predominantly lobular lymphocytic panniculitis in the absence of typical epidermal and dermal changes of lupus, 40–50% of cases Lymphoid follicles with peripheral plasma cells and germinal center formation, present in approximately 50% Nuclear fragmentation – clue to the diagnosis Hyaline sclerosis of lobules with focal extension into intralobular septa characteristic feature	
Lipodermatosclerosis	Histopathology varies with the age of the lesion *Early lesions*: Septal and lobular panniculitis with a predominantly lymphocyte-rich infiltrate with variable fat necrosis may be seen *Late lesions*: Septal fibrosis and fatty microcysts with membranocystic change Interstitial hemosiderin deposits often present in the dermis and may also be seen in the subcutis Blood vessels typically prominent in the septa in all stages of the disease process	

LE = Lupus erythematosus; MNGCs = Multinucleate giant cells

Table E5.3 Secondary panniculitis – a histopathologic approach

Entity	Key histopathologic features	Image
Post-irradiation panniculitis	Lobular lymphohistiocytic infiltrates with lipophages, plasma cells, and eosinophils, and septal sclerosis Ischemic fat necrosis common Enlarged fibroblasts (radiation fibroblasts) and endothelial cells (radiation vasculopathy) with hyperchromatic atypical nuclei often present	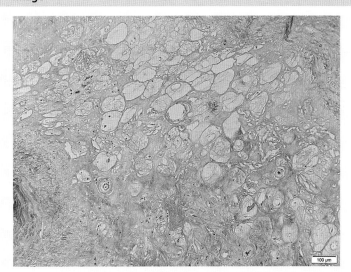
Cutaneous polyarteritis nodosa	Findings vary with age of the lesion *Early stage*: Marked thickening of vessel walls, particularly the intima and a perivascular infiltrate composed of neutrophils and eosinophils and apoptotic debris (leukocytoclasia) *Late stage*: Luminal thrombi and/or aneurysms, perivascular infiltrate of lymphocytes *End stage*: Intimal and mural fibrosis leading to obliteration of the vessel Characteristic feature is the presence *of lesions at all stages of development within the same biopsy*	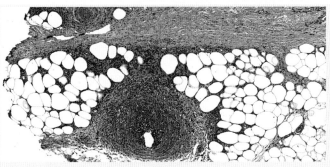
Superficial migratory thrombophlebitis	Varying degrees of lymphocytic infiltration and disruption of the arterial wall, concentric luminal fibrin deposition and fibrointimal scarring (endarteritis obliterans) *Believed to represent the chronic/healed end of the spectrum of polyarteritis nodosa*	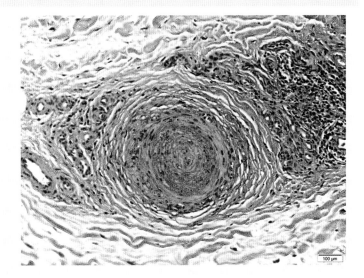

1. C. Sclerema neonatorum is an example of a lobular panniculitis.

    Sclerema neonatorum is a disease confined to the newborn period. While it can present at birth, onset within the first week of life is more common. Half the infants affected by sclerema neonatorum are premature, and the others are full term but have a serious underlying illness. They are often of low birth weight (<2500 g) and have cyanosis and low Apgar scores. Physical findings of sclerema neonatorum appear suddenly, first on the thighs and buttocks and then, spreading rapidly, often affecting all parts of the body except the palms, soles, and genitalia. The involved skin is pale, waxy, and firm to palpation. The skin cannot be pitted or pinched up because it is bound to underlying subcutaneous tissue, muscle, and bone. The affected infant often displays flexion contractures at the elbows, knees, and hips, temperature instability, restricted respiration, difficulty in feeding, and decreased spontaneous movement. Newborns may also present with mask-like facies or "pseudotrismus," an inability to completely open the mouth, secondary to the thickening of the skin over the face, arms, and hands.

    Despite the striking clinical presentation, histopathologic findings of sclerema neonatorum are subtle. The subcutaneous fat may appear normal or may have only sparse inflammation. The most consistent findings are edema, a thickening of the subcutaneous fibrous septa, and *a radial array of fine, needle-like clefts in the fat cells, representing former sites of fat crystals.* The lack of a granulomatous inflammation and the absence of fat necrosis help distinguish sclerema neonatorum from subcutaneous fat necrosis of the newborn (SCFN) since radially arranged needle-like clefts are common to both sclerema neonatorum and SCFN. Laboratory abnormalities associated with sclerema neonatorum correlate with the underlying disease process. Hypoglycemia, metabolic acidosis, respiratory alkalosis, hyperkalemia, hypocalcemia, and elevated blood urea are common, albeit non-specific, findings.

2. C. Sclerema neonatorum is NOT an example of a septal panniculitis.

    Entities commonly characterized by a septal panniculitis include:

    - Erythema nodosum
    - Necrobiosis lipoidica
    - Scleroderma

    Uncommon entities characterized by a septal panniculitis include nephrogenic systemic fibrosis, erythema nodosum migrans (subacute nodular migratory panniculitis) and microscopic polyangiitis. While some textbooks also include α_1-antitrypsin deficiency under this category, most authors (including myself) regard this

    entity as a lobular or a mixed septal-lobular panniculitis (also see Table E5.1 and Table E5.2).

3. E. Image shown is that of erythema nodosum.

    Erythema nodosum is the *best known example of a septal panniculitis*. While involvement of the septum is the primary pathology, "spill over" of the inflammatory infiltrate into the adjacent lobule/s is not uncommon. *However, the center of the lobule is spared allowing for a distinction from a primary lobular panniculitis.* Spill over into the adjacent deeper dermis may also be seen. The inflammatory infiltrate is typically composed of lymphocytes and histiocytes, although, albeit occasionally, eosinophils may be seen. Changes specific to the age of the lesion include the following:

    Early lesions: Presence of neutrophils, edematous widening of septa with fibrinoid change
    Late lesions: Fibrotic thickening of septa

    Vascular changes are not uncommon and are typically non-specific by the time the lesion is biopsied. They can include endothelial cell swelling (of small as well as large vessels), lymphocytic cuffing of small venules, and even vasculitis.

    In erythema nodosum migrans (subacute nodular migratory panniculitis), the septae are markedly thickened and fibrotic and inflammation is usually mild (although multinucleate giant cells and granulomas can be prominent at the septal border).

4. D. Miescher's radial granuloma is a pathognomonic finding in erythema nodosum.

    Miescher's radial granuloma consists of a radial array of histiocytes around a minute central slit. Although pathognomonic for erythema nodosum, it may not be seen in all biopsied lesions.

5. A. Necrobiosis lipoidica is clinically characterized by a depressed plaque with a shiny yellow/brown center and a well-demarcated edge.

    Since initial descriptions of necrobiosis lipoidica (NL) in isolated patients with diabetes, several cases of NL in non-diabetic patients have been described. Rollins and Winkelmann, in 1960, also described this condition in non-diabetic patients, and a renaming of the disorder was suggested to exclude diabetes from the title. *Today, the term necrobiosis lipoidica is used to encompass all patients with the same clinical lesions, regardless of whether or not diabetes is present.* The average age of onset for necrobiosis lipoidica is 30 years, but it can occur at any age although the disease tends to develop at an earlier age in patients with diabetes. It also shows a sex predilection, being 3 times more common in women than in men. Most cases of necrobiosis lipoidica occur on the pretibial area, but cases have been reported on the face, scalp, trunk, and upper extremities, where the diagnosis is more likely to be missed. Multiple telangiectatic vessels can be seen on the surface of the thinning epidermis. The Koebner phenomenon has been well established in patients with necrobiosis lipoidica, especially in patients with vasculitis at the site of trauma. In most patients, lesions of necrobiosis lipoidica are multiple and bilateral. The lesions may become painless because of cutaneous nerve damage (75% of cases), or they may be extremely painful (25% of cases).

6. **B.** Histopathologic features of necrobiosis lipoidica (NL) are *best* appreciated at the edge.

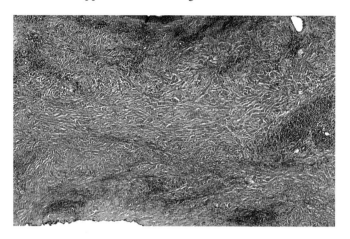

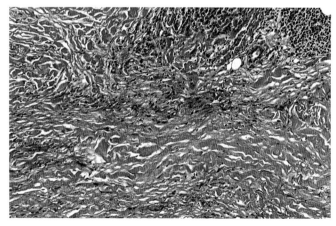

Histopathologic changes in NL involve the full thickness of the dermis and often the underlying panniculus. Histopathologically, necrobiosis lipoidica presents as an interstitial and palisaded granulomatous dermatosis *with a characteristic appearance at scanning magnification*. The granulomas are arranged in "tiers" or a layered fashion with admixed foci of necrobiosis. The granulomas are composed of histiocyte lymphocytes, occasional plasma cells, eosinophils and multinucleate giant cells. Reduction in the number of intradermal nerves is an additional

feature of necrobiosis lipoidica. Changes peculiar to the age of the lesion are the following:

Early: Are often not biopsied but when biopsied show a superficial and deep perivascular and interstitial inflammatory infiltrate which may involve the septum
Late: Minimal necrobiosis and more fibrosis (which again may involve the underlying subcutis)

Findings common to diabetic microangiopathy are the presence of thickened blood vessel walls and endothelial cell swelling of vessels in the mid to deep dermis. In non-diabetic patients with necrobiosis lipoidica, the vascular changes are not as prominent.

Direct immunofluorescence microscopy of necrobiosis lipoidica has demonstrated IgM, IgA, C3, and fibrinogen in the blood vessels (believed to be the cause of the vascular thickening).

7. **C.** The presence of plasma cells in lesions of necrobiosis lipoidica (NL) and the absence in lesions of granuloma annulare (GA) are helpful in distinguishing between these two entities.

Other helpful features include:
- The necrobiosis is more irregular and less complete in NL than GA
- While the presence of lipid in necrobiotic areas of NL was used in the past to distinguish lesions of NL from GA, subsequent studies have indicated that lipid droplets can also be seen in GA

8. **A.** Image shown is that of scleroderma.

Diagnostic histopathologic features of scleroderma involve the following:
Collagen – Pandermal homogenization of dermal collagen (in the author's personal experience, the junction between the deep dermis is sharply demarcated and a "straight line") with loss of peri-eccrine adipocytes
Adnexae – Atrophy of adnexae particularly the pilosebaceous units; typically eccrine glands appear higher in the dermis due to the deposition of collagen below; arrectores pilorum are often hypertrophied
Vessels – Thickening of small vessel walls
Inflammatory infiltrate – Composed of lymphocytes and plasma cells which is more diffuse in distribution in the deeper dermis and is particularly prominent at the junction of the deep dermis and the subcutis

Clinically, scleroderma can involve multiple organ systems. Skin manifestations of systemic sclerosis include:
- Progressive skin tightness and induration, often preceded by swelling and puffiness (edematous stage)
- Skin induration initially affects the fingers (sclerodactyly) and extends proximally

- Prominent pigmentary changes (hypopigmentation and hyperpigmentation)
- Pruritus
- Raynaud phenomenon is part of the initial presentation in 70% of patients with systemic sclerosis; 95% eventually develop it during the course of their disease; Raynaud phenomenon may precede obvious systemic sclerosis features by months or even years

9. **D.** Nodular vasculitis is clinically typically characterized by tender erythematous nodules.

The nodules are concentrated on the lower third of the legs, especially around the ankles. The nodules have a chronic, recurrent course and heal with ulcerations or depressed scars. Leg edema may be present. Common sites are the calves, although the shins are also sometimes involved. A past or present history of tuberculosis at an extracutaneous site occurs in about 50% of patients. Pulmonary tuberculosis is most common. Tuberculous cervical lymphadenitis is the next most common finding. *It is important to consider whether HIV infection is present when tuberculosis and nodular vasculitis are present.* Historically, in 1861, Bazin gave the name erythema induratum to a nodular eruption that occurred on the lower legs of young women with tuberculosis. In 1945, Montgomery *et al.*, while fully acknowledging the existence of tuberculosis-associated erythema induratum, coined the term nodular vasculitis to describe chronic inflammatory nodules of the legs that showed histopathologic changes similar to those of erythema induratum, that is, vasculitis of the larger vessels and panniculitis. Since then, erythema induratum and nodular vasculitis had been considered the same disease entity for a long time. However, nodular vasculitis is now considered a multifactorial syndrome of lobular panniculitis in which tuberculosis may or may not be one of a multitude of etiologic components. Therefore, erythema induratum/nodular vasculitis complex is classified into 2 variants:

- Erythema induratum of Bazin type (associated with tuberculosis)
- Nodular vasculitis or erythema induratum of Whitfield type (not associated with tuberculosis)

Morphologic, molecular, and clinical data suggest that erythema induratum and nodular vasculitis represent a common inflammatory pathway, that is, a hypersensitivity reaction to endogenous or exogenous antigens. One such antigen is the tubercle bacillus. Patients with erythema induratum have a positive tuberculin skin test result and a marked increase in their peripheral T lymphocyte response to purified protein derivative (PPD) of tuberculin, which can cause a delayed-type hypersensitivity reaction. Results from the enzyme-linked immunosorbent assay-based IGRA (QuantiFERON-TB Gold In-Tube, Cellestis; Victoria,

Australia) blood test for tuberculosis commonly are positive in patients with erythema induratum, again suggesting that erythema induratum is a hypersensitivity reaction to a systemic infection.

10. **D.** Image shown is that of nodular vasculitis.

Inflammatory changes in nodular vasculitis are usually restricted to the lower dermis and subcutis. As in all panniculitides, changes vary with the age of the lesion. The histopathologic features are not specific and overlap with other forms of panniculitis. Vasculitis is evident in 90% of cases and is not a requisite for the diagnosis. *The presence of both septal granulomatous inflammation and lobular granulomatous inflammation is, nonetheless, characteristic of nodular vasculitis* and contrasts with erythema nodosum (primarily septal) and polyarteritis nodosa (medium vessel vasculitis with minimal lobular inflammation). The location of vessels involved in descending order is as follows:

Small venules of the fat lobule
Both the venules of the fat lobule and veins of the connective-tissue septa
Only veins contained in connective-tissue septa
Veins and arteries contained in venules of the fat lobule and in the connective-tissue septa
Connective-tissue septa veins and arteries

Polymerase chain reaction provides rapid and sensitive detection of *Mycobacterium tuberculosis* in formalin-fixed, paraffin-embedded specimens. Polymerase chain reaction can be applied to differentiating nodular vasculitis from erythema induratum of Bazin because the demonstration of mycobacteria emerges as the only reliable criterion in erythema induratum of Bazin type. The diagnosis of erythema can be made with the help of polymerase chain reaction testing. The CDC states that interferon-gamma release assays (IGRAs) are whole-blood tests that can aid in diagnosing infection with *Mycobacterium tuberculosis*. Two IGRAs that the FDA has approved and are commercially available in the USA are the QuantiFERON-TB Gold In-Tube test (QFT-GIT) and the T-SPOT. *TB* test (T-Spot). The QuantiFERON test can confirm the presence of latent tuberculosis in association with erythema induratum.

In terms of significant laboratory findings, the erythrocyte sedimentation rate may be increased.

11. **D.** Image shown demonstrates needle-shaped clefts within adipocytes – a feature NOT noted in lipodermatosclerosis.

Entities characterized by needle-shaped clefts within adipocytes include:
- Sclerema neonatorum
- Subcutaneous fat necrosis of the newborn
- Post-steroid panniculitis

In contrast to adult fat, the subcutaneous fat of newborns is prone to crystal formation because of the higher content of saturated fatty acids such as palmitic and stearic acids and a relatively lower content of unsaturated fatty acids such as oleic acids. This results in a higher melting point of stored fats and promotes crystallization. Microsized crystals or type A crystals do not incite an inflammatory response and are not uncommon in infants at or below 6 months of age. Larger or type B crystals are typically arranged in rosettes and incite a granulomatous reaction. It is these crystals that are encountered in the 3 entities mentioned above.

12. **E.** Vasculitis is NOT a histopathologic feature of α_1-antitrypsin deficiency (AATD).

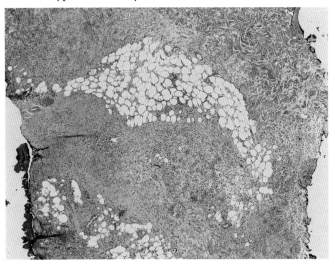

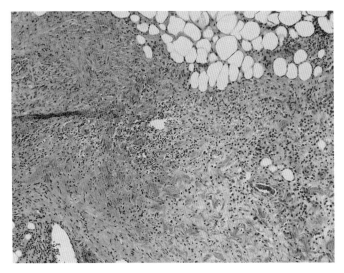

At its fully developed stage, AATD panniculitis is a predominantly lobular neutrophilic panniculitis in which the affected fat lobules are necrotic and replaced with an intense neutrophilic infiltrate. Such findings tend to be focal and sharply delineated, often juxtaposed with large areas of normal panniculus. Chronic inflammation at the

periphery of the acute inflammatory focus and focal collection of histiocytic cells may also be present. *A characteristic finding is the presence of extensive collagenolysis/elastolysis (i.e. collagen degradation/ loosening of elastic fibers), resulting in "floating fat" separated from the surrounding reticular dermis and pannicular septa.* Typically, there is no evidence of a primary vasculitis. An early pathologic change, considered as highly suggestive of this disease, is the spread of neutrophils into the reticular dermis and septa of the subcutis.

13. **D.** "Skip areas" are present in α_1-antitrypsin deficiency but NOT in pancreatic panniculitis.

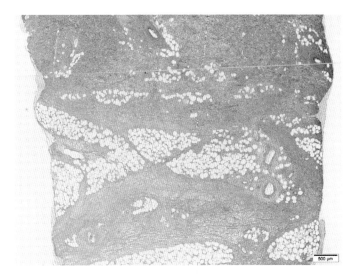

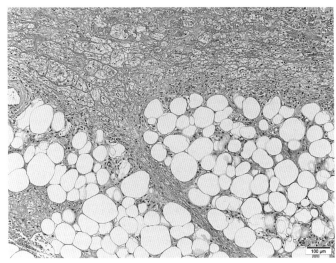

While both entities share the unifying features of a lobular panniculitis with a neutrophil-rich infiltrate and although the fat necrosis of α_1-antitrypsin deficiency resembles the ghost cells of pancreatic panniculitis, "skip areas" of normal uninvolved fat are not present in pancreatic panniculitis.

14. **C. In the WHO/EORTC classification scheme, subcutaneous panniculitis-like T-cell lymphoma is CD8 positive.**

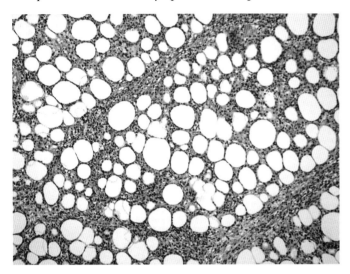

In the WHO classification, subcutaneous panniculitis-like T-cell lymphoma (SPTL) is defined as a distinct type of T-cell lymphoma with an aggressive clinical behavior. Histopathologically, it is characterized by a predominantly subcutaneous atypical lymphoid infiltrate, showing typical adipotropism and characteristically involving the fat lobules resembling a lobular panniculitis. Septal involvement is generally mild or absent and secondary. Mild to moderate extension of the atypical infiltrate into the reticular dermis, surrounding and occasionally infiltrating sweat glands and sometimes hair follicles and sebaceous glands, is often observed. However, infiltration of the superficial dermis and epidermis is uncommon as is angioinvasion or angiodestruction. The neoplastic infiltrate is composed of pleomorphic T-cells of variable size with irregular and often hyperchromatic nuclei. In most cases, there is a predominance of small- to medium-sized cells with only scattered large lymphoid cells with clear cytoplasm. Rimming of individual adipocytes by neoplastic T-cells is a common feature, although present sometimes focally. Fat necrosis and karyorrhexis are typically always present, although to a variable degree. In all cases, the neoplastic T-cells are admixed with small reactive lymphocytes and many histiocytes, which are frequently vacuolated because of ingested lipid material. However, multinucleate giant cells are uncommon, and well-defined granulomas are rare. Neutrophils and eosinophils are generally absent, apart from accumulating neutrophils in necrotic foci in select cases.

The immunophenotype of the neoplastic cells is CD3+, CD8+, CD4− T-cells, with expression of cytotoxic proteins (granzyme B, TIA-1, perforin) and loss of CD2, CD5, and/or CD7. Staining for CD45RA and CD45RO performed in a minority of cases, consistently shows expression of CD45RO and negative staining for CD45RA. CD30 is always negative, while CD56 is expressed by the minority of neoplastic T-cells. *Staining for betaF1 is typically positive in all cases confirming the alpha/beta T-cell phenotype.* Mib-1 staining shows a high proportion of proliferating cells, which are characteristically concentrated around fat cells. Clonal rearrangements of the TCR beta and gamma genes have been documented in 9 of 9 and 28 of 36 cases investigated, respectively in one series.

15. **B. Image shown is that of lupus profundus.**

Lupus profundus (LP) is an uncommon variant of lupus erythematosus (LE) that develops in 1% to 3% of patients with cutaneous LE. It may arise in patients with discoid LE or systemic LE, or as an isolated phenomenon. Lupus profundus is more common in women than men and most often presents as multiple subcutaneous nodules or plaques involving the upper arms, shoulders, buttocks, or face (areas that are uncommonly involved in other panniculitides). The surface of lesions may show classic features of discoid LE or appear completely normal. Ulceration may also be present. Regressing lesions often appear as depressed scars. Lipoatrophy in the shoulder region is so characteristic as to allow retrospective diagnosis of LP. *Typically patients with LP have a mild clinical form of lupus erythematosus.*

In greater than 50% of cases, histopathologic clues to the diagnosis in the form of typical changes of chronic discoid LE are present, including epidermal atrophy, interface changes, a thickened basement membrane, superficial and deep perivascular and periadnexal lymphocytic inflammation, and increased dermal mucin. In the remainder of cases, findings consist of a predominantly lobular lymphocytic panniculitis in the absence of typical epidermal and dermal changes of lupus. Lymphoid follicles with germinal center formation, which are rarely seen in other forms of panniculitis, are present in approximately 50% of cases and are highly characteristic of LP. Lymphoid follicles tend to extend interstitially between collagen bundles and into septa of the subcutis and often have many plasma cells at their peripheries. *The lymphocytic infiltrate may show nuclear fragmentation, another clue to the diagnosis of LP, which is rarely seen in other forms of lobular panniculitis. Finally, hyaline sclerosis of lobules with focal extension into intralobular septa is another characteristic feature and a useful clue to the diagnosis of LP when present.*

16. **A. Image shown is that of lipodermatosclerosis – a consequence of venous stasis and ischemia.**

Lipodermatosclerosis, also called hypodermitis sclerodermiformis and sclerosing panniculitis, refers to a skin change of the lower legs that often occurs in patients

who have venous insufficiency. Two-thirds of affected patients are obese. Affected legs typically have the following characteristics:
- Skin induration (hardening)
- Increased pigmentation
- Swelling
- Redness
- "Inverted champagne bottle" or "bowling pin" appearance

Histopathology varies with the age of the lesion:

In early lesions (uncommonly biopsied because of poor healing) – There is a septal and lobular panniculitis with a predominantly lymphocyte-rich infiltrate. Variable fat necrosis may be seen.

In late lesions (which is when the lesions are typically biopsied) – Demonstrate septal fibrosis and fatty microcysts with membranocystic change. The latter is a consequence of amorphous eosinophilic material lining the microcysts. Interstitial hemosiderin deposits are often present In the dermis and may also be seen in the subcutis. *Blood vessels are typically prominent in the septa in all stages of the disease process.*

17. **B.** Image shown is that of post-radiation panniculitis.

Sclerosing post-radiation panniculitis (post-radiation sclerodermoid panniculitis) occurs secondary to megavoltage radiation therapy, usually for treatment of breast cancer. Nodular lesions appear on the chest within several months (but sometimes several years or even longer than a decade) of megavoltage radiation therapy within the field of treatment.

In terms of histopathologic features, sclerosing post-radiation panniculitis exhibits a mostly lobular or mixed septal and lobular pattern with the combined presence of lobular lymphohistiocytic infiltrates with lipophages, plasma cells, and eosinophils, and septal sclerosis. Ischemic fat necrosis is also expected. Enlarged fibroblasts (radiation fibroblasts) and endothelial cells (radiation vasculopathy) with hyperchromatic atypical nuclei are often noted.

18. **A.** Image shown is that of encapsulated fat necrosis.

In encapsulated fat necrosis, the affected fat lobules appear encapsulated by a sclerotic fibrous capsule with a loss of nuclear adipocyte staining and variable superimposed lipophages, lipomembranous fat necrosis, or calcification.

19. **C.** Image shown is that of calciphylaxis – which is associated with end-stage renal disease.

Calciphylaxis (calcific uremic arteriolopathy) is a life-threatening variant of metastatic calcification that occurs almost exclusively in the setting of end-stage renal insufficiency. Its prevalence in patients in hemodialysis is almost 4%. Clinically, it presents with hard, tender, erythematous but cold necrotic plaques with subsequent eschar formation, usually on the lower extremities or abdomen. Most cases progress acutely, although more protracted, subacute presentation may also occur.

In terms of histopathologic features, the *sine qua non* of calciphylaxis is calcification of subcutaneous vessel walls. There is usually epidermal ulceration. *Peri-eccrine calcification, albeit noted rarely, is believed to be highly specific for calciphylaxis.* Variable findings include pandermal ischemic necrosis with secondary subepidermal clefting, sparse neutrophils, and vascular thrombosis.

Laboratory findings include elevated serum calcium and phosphate levels. Elevated parathyroid hormone levels are also expected. Exceptional cases in patients without renal insufficiency have been associated with metastatic breast cancer or Crohn's disease.

20. **E.** Image shown is that of polyarteritis nodosa (PAN) for which serology is non-diagnostic.

Cutaneous PAN has a chronic relapsing course and is usually ANCA-negative. Since the pathology involves vessels near the subcutis, doing a deep biopsy is key. Diagnostic histopathologic findings vary with age of the lesion and include the following:

Early stage – Marked thickening of vessel walls, particularly the intima and a perivascular infiltrate composed of neutrophils and eosinophils and apoptotic debris (leukocytoclasia)

Late stage – Luminal thrombi and/or aneurysms, perivascular infiltrate of lymphocytes

End stage – Intimal and mural fibrosis leading to obliteration of the vessel

A characteristic feature of PAN is the presence *of lesions at all stages of development.*

21. **D.** Macular arteritis, depicted in the image shown, is best regarded as a latent form of polyarteritis nodosa.

Macular arteritis, described in 2013, clinically presents as erythematous and hyperpigmented plaques and/or papules in a reticulated pattern on the lower limbs and has an indolent chronic clinical course. Histopathologic features include varying degrees of lymphocytic infiltration and disruption of the arterial wall, concentric luminal fibrin deposition and fibrointimal scarring (endarteritis obliterans). *It is believed to represent the chronic/healed end of the spectrum of polyarteritis nodosa.*

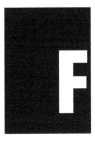

Depositional Diseases and Cutaneous Manifestations of Systemic Disease Questions

1. This is most likely related to deficiency of:

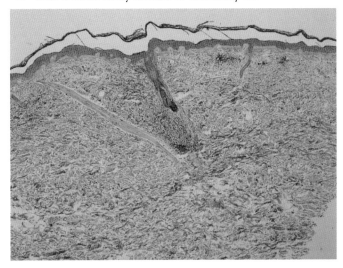

   A. Vitamin A
   B. Vitamin B₁₂
   C. Vitamin C
   D. Vitamin D
   E. Vitamin K

2. Gaucher's disease is due to mutations in which of the following genes:
   A. Glucocerebrosidase
   B. α-galactosidase
   C. Galactosylceramidase
   D. Sphingomyelinase
   E. Acid ceramidase

3. Niemann-Pick disease is due to deficiency of:
   A. Glucocerebrosidase
   B. α-galactosidase
   C. Galactosylceramidase
   D. Sphingomyelinase
   E. Acid ceramidase

4. The best-fit diagnosis is:

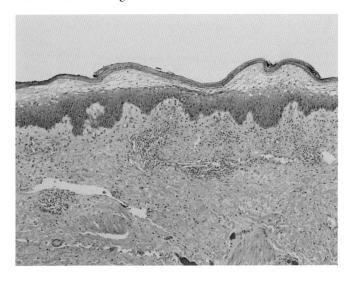

   A. Erythema multiforme
   B. Toxic epidermal necrolysis
   C. Acrodermatitis enteropathica
   D. Seborrheic dermatitis
   E. Subcorneal pustular dermatosis

5. This (based on question 4) is due to defects in:
   A. *MAN2B1*
   B. *MCOLN1*
   C. *ZIP4*
   D. *FUCA1*
   E. *SMPD1*

6. Necrolytic migratory erythema is a feature of:
   A. Acrodermatitis enteropathica
   B. Glucagonoma syndrome
   C. Hartnup disease
   D. Crohn's disease
   E. DRESS syndrome

7. Porphyria cutanea tarda is due to:
   A. Reduced activity of aminolevulinic acid (ALA)-synthase
   B. Reduced activity of ALA-dehydratase
   C. Reduced activity of porphobilinogen deaminase
   D. Reduced activity of uroporphyrinogen III cosynthase
   E. Reduced activity of uroporphyrinogen decarboxylase

8. "Caterpillar bodies" in porphyria cutanea tarda contain:
   A. Collagen I
   B. Collagen II
   C. Collagen IV
   D. Collagen VII
   E. Collagen IX

9. Ultrastructural features of porphyria cutanea tarda include:
   A. Oval/round juxtanuclear inclusions
   B. Farber bodies
   C. Reduplication of the basal laminae
   D. Vacuolation of endothelial cells
   E. Zebra bodies

10. The most likely diagnosis is:

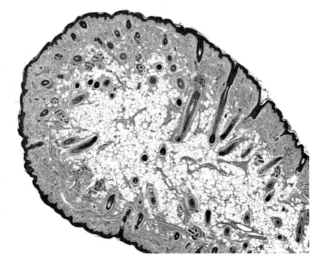

A. Eyelid skin
B. Accessory tragus
C. Accessory nipple
D. Eccrine hamartoma
E. Fibroepithelial polyp

11. The most likely diagnosis is:

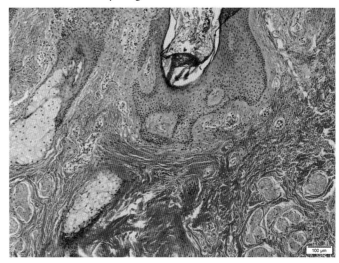

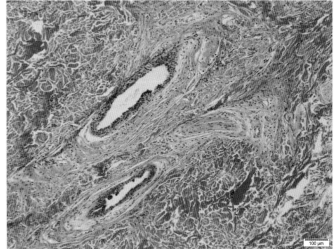

A. Accessory nipple
B. Accessory tragus
C. Becker's nevus
D. Pilar leiomyoma
E. Fibroepithelial polyp

12. The most likely diagnosis is:

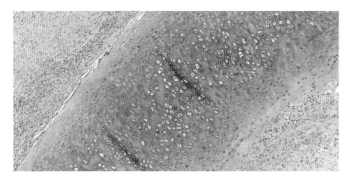

    A. Chondrodermatitis nodularis helicis
    B. Accessory tragus
    C. Osteoma cutis
    D. Calcinosis cutis
    E. Relapsing polychondritis

13. This may represent a cutaneous manifestation of:

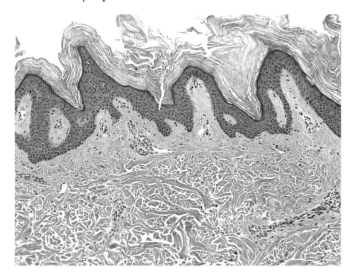

    A. A nutritional deficiency
    B. A storage disorder
    C. Metabolic disease
    D. An internal malignancy
    E. A genodermatosis

14. This may be secondary to:

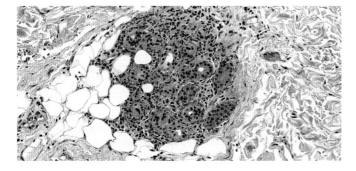

    A. A nutritional deficiency
    B. A storage disorder
    C. Chemotherapy
    D. An internal malignancy
    E. A genodermatosis

15. The drug most frequently associated with the histo-pathologic reaction shown above is:
    A. IVIg
    B. Rituximab
    C. Vemurafenib
    D. Imatinib
    E. Cytarabine

16. Eruptive keratoacanthomas may be a side effect of:
    A. Rituximab
    B. Vemurafenib
    C. Imatinib
    D. Cytarabine
    E. IVIg

17. Histopathologic distinguishing features of a lichenoid drug eruption of utility in differentiating it from lichen planus include:
    A. Satellite cell necrosis and histiocytes
    B. Parakeratosis and eosinophils
    C. Density of infiltrate and plasma cells
    D. Caspary-Joseph spaces
    E. Civatte bodies

18. A 38-year-old male with no prior significant medical history presents with erythematous iris-shaped papules and plaques involving the palms and soles. The best-fit diagnosis is:

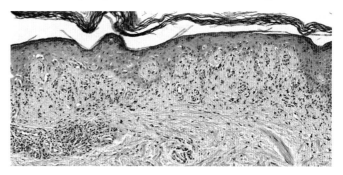

    A. Secondary syphilis
    B. Lichen planus
    C. Erythema multiforme
    D. Toxic epidermal necrolysis
    E. Graft-versus-host disease

19. Biopsy of a sudden-onset blistering rash involving muco-cutaneous surfaces. The most likely diagnosis is:

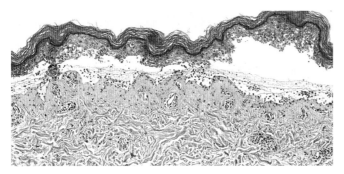

    A. Toxic epidermal necrolysis
    B. Erythema multiforme
    C. Bullous pemphigoid
    D. Lichen planus
    E. Primary syphilis

20. The most likely diagnosis is:

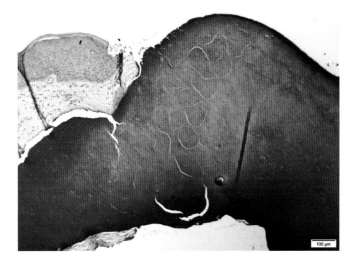

    A. Osteoma cutis
    B. Pilomatricoma
    C. Chondroma
    D. Gouty tophus
    E. Calcinosis cutis

21. The most likely diagnosis is:

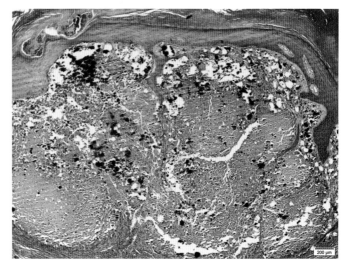

    A. Tumoral calcinosis
    B. Osteoma cutis
    C. Gouty tophus
    D. Subepidermal calcified nodule
    E. Scrotal calcinosis

22. This may be associated with:

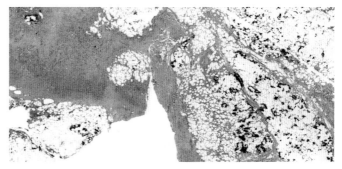

    A. Childhood onset
    B. Hyperthyroidism
    C. End-stage renal disease
    D. Hypercholesterolemia
    E. Dystrophic calcification

23. The most likely diagnosis is:

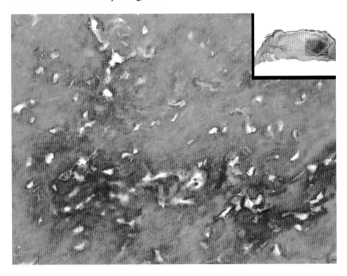

A. Pilomatricoma
B. Osteoma cutis
C. Chondroma
D. Gouty tophus
E. Calcinosis cutis

24. Metabolic disturbances that may be associated with the familial variant of the entity shown above involve:
A. Calcium
B. Sodium
C. Potassium
D. Insulin
E. Adrenaline

25. The most likely diagnosis is:

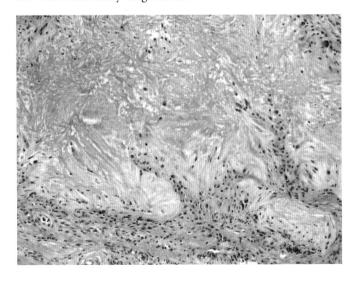

A. Tumoral calcinosis
B. Osteoma cutis
C. Gouty tophus

D. Nodular amyloidosis
E. Scrotal calcinosis

26. The deposits shown in the image above are composed of:
A. Calcium pyrophosphate
B. Monosodium urate
C. Calcium bisphosphonate
D. β_2-microglobulin
E. Phenylalanine

27. The most likely diagnosis is:

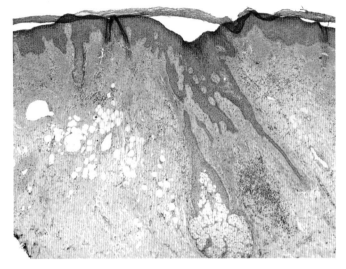

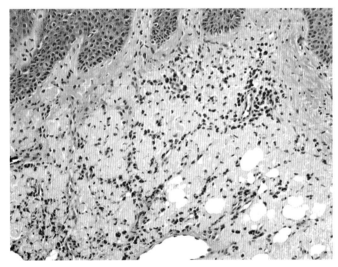

A. Colloid milium
B. Lipoid proteinosis
C. Lichen amyloidosus
D. Macular amyloidosis
E. Nodular amyloidosis

28. Immunohistochemical stains of diagnostic utility (based on the image shown above) include:
    A. CK5/6
    B. CK903
    C. CK7/20
    D. κ/λ
    E. CD45RO

29. The most likely diagnosis is:

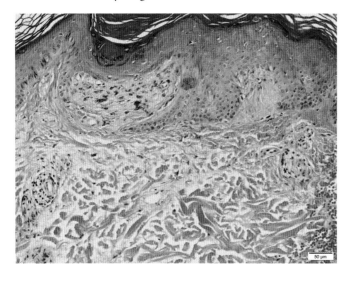

    A. Colloid milium
    B. Lipoid proteinosis
    C. Lichen amyloidosus
    D. Subepidermal calcified nodule
    E. Nodular amyloidosis

30. Immunohistochemical stains of diagnostic utility (based on the image shown above) include:
    A. CD138
    B. CK903
    C. CK7/20
    D. κ/λ
    E. CD45RO

31. The most likely diagnosis is:

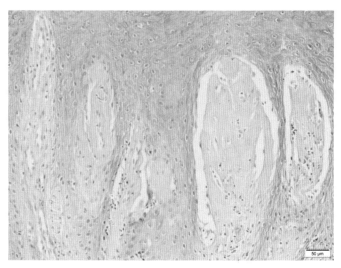

    A. Colloid milium
    B. Lipoid proteinosis
    C. Lichen amyloidosus
    D. Macular amyloidosis
    E. Nodular amyloidosis

32. The most likely diagnosis is:

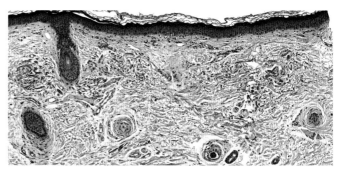

    A. Lipofuscin
    B. Gouty tophus
    C. Argyria
    D. Myospherulosis
    E. Ochronosis

33. The endogenous form of this (based on the image shown above) is due to deficiency of:
    A. Phenylalanine hydroxylase
    B. Glucose-6-phosphatase
    C. Hypoxanthine-guanine phosphoribosyl transferase
    D. Homogentisic acid oxidase
    E. Phosphoribosyl pyrophosphate synthetase

34. The most likely diagnosis is:

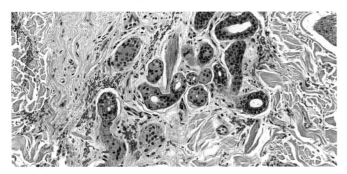

    A. Tattoo
    B. Hemochromatosis
    C. Chrysiasis
    D. Argyria
    E. Ochronosis

35. The most likely diagnosis is:

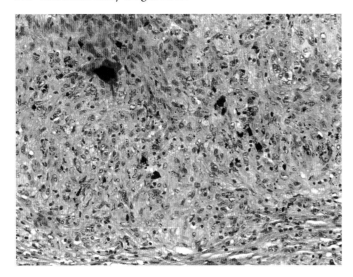

    A. Hemochromatosis
    B. Chrysiasis
    C. Tattoo
    D. Argyria
    E. Ochronosis

36. The most likely causative agent is:

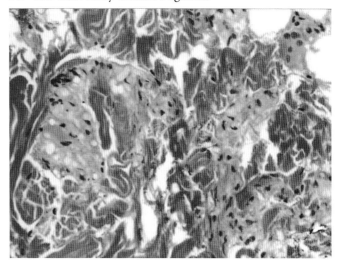

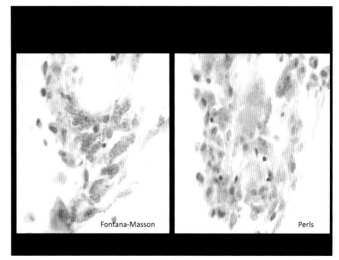

    A. Cadmium
    B. Silver
    C. Minocycline
    D. Silicone
    E. Restylane

37. The most likely causative agent is:

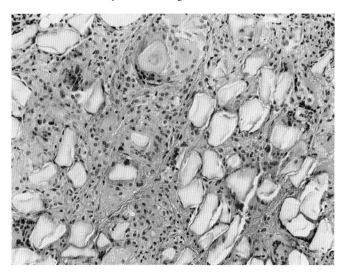

A. Cadmium
B. Restylane
C. Minocycline
D. Silicone
E. Urate

38. The most likely diagnosis is:

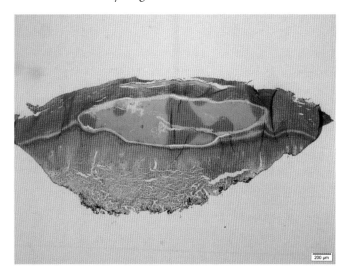

A. Talon noir
B. Subcorneal pustular dermatosis
C. Decubitus ulcer
D. Hemochromatosis
E. Actinic reticuloid

39. The most likely diagnosis is:

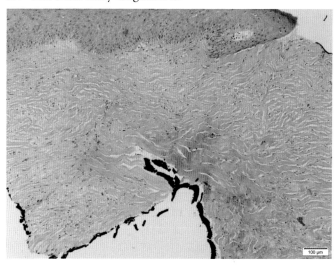

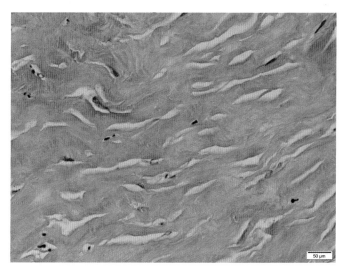

A. Dermatitis artefacta
B. Phototoxic dermatitis
C. Localized scleroderma
D. Lichen sclerosus
E. Radiation dermatitis

40. Photosensitive genodermatoses include all of the following EXCEPT:
A. Xeroderma pigmentosum
B. Cockayne's syndrome
C. Hartnup disease
D. Brooke-Spiegler syndrome
E. Bloom's syndrome

41. The most likely diagnosis is:

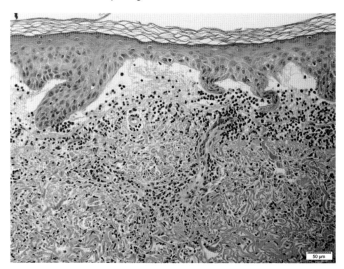

A. Pityriasis lichenoides acuta
B. Sweet's syndrome
C. Polymorphic light eruption
D. Actinic reticuloid
E. Hydroa vacciniforme

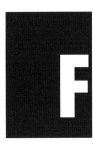

Depositional Diseases and Cutaneous Manifestations of Systemic Disease Answers

Table F1 Cutaneous manifestations related to abnormal vitamin intake

Vitamin	Abnormality	Clinical manifestations	Diagnostic histopathology
A	Deficiency	Night blindness	Absent
	Hypervitaminosis	Vomiting, diarrhea, dry skin, alopecia	Absent
B12	Deficiency	Poikilodermatous pigmentation	Absent
C	Deficiency	Scurvy, follicular hyperkeratosis with "corkscrew" hairs, bleeding gums, spontaneous hemarthrosis	Perifollicular extravasated erythrocytes
D	Deficiency	Rickets, osteomalacia	Absent
K	Deficiency	Bleeding disorders	Vasculopathy
Niacin	Deficiency	Pellagra, diarrhea, dementia, dermatitis, death	Hyperkeratosis, parakeratosis, superficial epidermal pallor, sebaceous gland hyperplasia

Table F2 Select[1] storage disorders

Entity	Gene/enzyme affected	Cutaneous manifestations	Relevant cutaneous histopathology	Distinctive ultrastructural findings
Gaucher's disease	Glucocerebrosidase	None specific	None (skin biopsies consistently negative)	Intracytoplasmic, membrane-bound lysosomal inclusions
G_M1-gangliosidoses	β-galactosidase	Excessive dermal melanocytosis	Vacuolation of fibroblasts, endothelial cells, eccrine glands, elongate melanocytes with fine melanin pigment	Vacuolation of fibroblasts, endothelial cells, smooth muscle cells and eccrine glands
Fabry's disease	α-galactosidase	Angiokeratoma corporis diffusum	Angiokeratoma	Lamellar intracytoplasmic inclusions
Farber's disease	Acid ceramidase	Subcutaneous or periarticular nodules	Fibrotic reticular dermis and subcutis	Curvilinear "Farber" bodies
Krabbe's disease	Galactosylceramidase	None	None	Tubular and crystalline inclusions in Schwann cells
Niemann-Pick disease	Sphingomyelinase	Hyperpigmentation, facial papules, juvenile xanthogranulomas	Dermal "foamy" pale-brown, histiocytic infiltrate	Membrane-bound myelin-like inclusions

[1] Selected based on cutaneous relevance

Table F3 Histopathologic clues to filler reactions

Filler	Trade name	Histopathologic clues
Bovine collagen[1]	Zyderm, Zyplast	Two patterns: First – Non-specific inflammation Second – Dermal palisaded granuloma containing central homogeneous acellular, eosinophilic material (thicker than human collagen) Weakly birefringent
Human-derived collagen[1]	Autologen, Cosmoderm, Cosmoplast, Cymetra	None reported Non-birefringent
Hyaluronic acid[1]	Hylaform, Restylane, Juvederm, Perlane, Macrolane	Dermal FBGCR to extracellular, basophilic, amorphous material, fibrosis Hyaluronic acid positive for Alcian blue at pH 2.7 Non-birefringent
Hyaluronic acid positive dextranomer microparticles[1]	Matridex, Reviderm	Extracellular deposits of filamentous bluish-gray material and dark blue spherical microparticles
Poly-L-lactic acid[1]	Sculptra, New-Fill	FBGCR to translucent, variably sized fusiform/oval/spiky birefringent particles Birefringent
Calcium hydroxylapatite[1]	Radiance, Radiesse	Basophilic microspheres composed of calcium hydroxylapatite, FBGCR, fibrosis Non-birefringent
Paraffin[2]		Replacement of normal dermis and subcutis by variably sized empty pseudocystic spaces Lobular panniculitis, subcutaneous fat has a "swiss cheese" appearance Non-birefringent
Silicone[2]		Variably sized, angulated translucent particles between collagen bundles or within macrophages, asteroid bodies, pseudocystic spaces ("swiss cheese" appearance) *FBGCR typically away from injected site because of migration of filler* Birefringent
Polyvinylpyrrolidone silicone suspension[2]	Bioplastique	Irregular, cystic spaces containing variably sized translucent, jagged, "popcorn" particles in sclerotic stroma FBGCR have characteristic "arabesque" projection into the lumen Non-birefringent
Polymethyl-methacrylate microspheres and bovine collagen[2]	Artecoll, Arteplast, Artefil	Rounded vacuoles of similar size and shape (mimicking normal adipocytes) that correspond to implanted microspheres Non-birefringent
Hydroxyethylmethacrylate and hyaluronic acid[2]	Dermalive, Dermadeep	Pseudocystic spaces containing variably sized, non-birefringent, polygonal, pink, translucent bodies of different shapes and sizes with FBGCR Non-birefringent
Polyacrylamide hydrogel[2]	Aquamid, Interfall, Royamid	Basophilic multi/micro-vacuolated foreign body material corresponding to hydrogel Non-birefringent

[1] Biodegradable;
[2] Non-biodegradable; FBGCR = Foreign body giant cell reaction

Table F4 Cutaneous deposits – an overview

Deposit	Types
Calcium salts	See Table F5
Cartilage	Chondroma
Bone	Osteoma cutis
Hyaline	Gout, amyloid, immunoglobulins, porphyria, lipoid proteinosis, colloid milium
Pigments	Ochronosis, hemosiderin, hemochromatosis, tattoos
Heavy metals	Silver, mercury, gold, arsenic, lead, aluminum, bismuth, titanium, silica, beryllium, zirconium, zinc
Drugs	Antimalarials, phenothiazine, tetracycline, amiodarone, clofazamine, chemotherapeutic agents
Cutaneous implants	See Table F3
Other	Oxalate crystals, myospherulosis, PVP storage disease

Table F5 Calcinosis cutis – classification

Type	Associations	Examples
Dystrophic calcinosis[1]	Inflammatory disease	CREST, dermatomyositis, SLE, PCT
	Neoplastic	Pilomatricoma, trichilemmal cyst, basal cell carcinoma, desmoplastic trichoepithelioma
	Infections	Protozoal, herpes
	Traumatic	Burns, scars, keloid, venous ulcers, radiation sites, auricular calcinosis
	Panniculitis	Pancreatic, lupus profundus
	Genodermatoses	PXE, Werner syndrome, Ehlers-Danlos syndrome
Metastatic calcinosis[2]	Hypervitaminosis D	
	Milk alkali syndrome	
	Hyperparathyroidism	
	Neoplastic	Multiple myeloma, leukemia, lymphoma
Calciphylaxis	Chronic renal failure	
Iatrogenic calcinosis	Intravenous/medication	
Idiopathic	Subepidermal calcified nodule	
	Tumoral calcinosis	
	Scrotal calcinosis	
	Milia-like calcinosis	

[1] Deposition of calcium in dystrophic tissue;
[2] Elevated serum calcium and/or phosphate
CREST = Calcinosis, Raynaud phenomenon, esophageal dysmotility, sclerodactyly, telangiectasia; PCT = Porphyria cutanea tarda; PXE = Pseudoxanthoma elasticum; SLE = Systemic lupus erythematosus

1. **C. Perifollicular extravasated erythrocytes**, shown in the image, are a histopathologic hallmark of vitamin C deficiency (scurvy).

   Typical histopathologic features of scurvy include a non-inflammatory perivascular and perifollicular extravasation of red cells and deposition of hemosiderin near hair follicles with intrafollicular keratotic plugs and coiled hair/s.

   Scurvy is a state of dietary deficiency of vitamin C (ascorbic acid). The human body lacks the ability to synthesize and make vitamin C and therefore depends on exogenous dietary sources such as fruits and vegetables or diets fortified with vitamin C. Vitamin C is functionally *most relevant for the triple-helix formation of collagen*; therefore, vitamin C deficiency results in impaired collagen synthesis. The typical manifestations of vitamin C deficiency, including poor wound healing, are noted in collagen-containing tissues and in organs and tissues such as skin, cartilage, dentine, osteoid, and capillary blood vessels. Pathologic changes in affected children and adults are a function of the rate of growth of the affected tissues; hence, the bone changes are often observed only in infants during periods of rapid bone growth. Defective collagen synthesis leads to defective dentine formation, hemorrhaging into the gums, and loss of teeth.

Hemorrhaging is a hallmark feature of scurvy and can occur in any organ. Hair follicles are one of the common sites of cutaneous bleeding. The bony changes occur at the junction between the end of the diaphysis and growth cartilage. Osteoblasts fail to form osteoid (bone matrix), resulting in cessation of endochondral bone formation. Calcification of the growth cartilage at the end of the long bones continues, leading to the thickening of the growth plate. The typical invasion of the growth cartilage by the capillaries does not occur. Symptoms and signs of scurvy may be remembered by the 4 Hs:

- *Hemorrhage*
- *Hyperkeratosis*
- *Hypochondriasis*
- *Hematologic abnormalities*

Also see Table F1.

2. **A.** Gaucher's disease is due to mutations in glucocerebrosidase.

   Gaucher's disease, the most common of the lysosomal storage diseases, is a form of sphingolipidosis (a subgroup of lysosomal storage diseases) that involves dysfunctional metabolism of sphingolipids. In this disease, glucosylceramide accumulates in cells and certain organs. The disorder is characterized by bruising, fatigue, anemia, low blood platelet count and enlargement of the liver and spleen, and is caused by a hereditary deficiency of the enzyme glucocerebrosidase (also known as glucosylceramidase), which acts on glucocerebroside. When the enzyme is defective, glucocerebroside accumulates, particularly in white blood cells and especially in macrophages (mononuclear leukocytes). Cutaneous manifestations are typically minimal. Extracutaneous manifestations may include enlarged spleen and liver, liver malfunction, skeletal disorders or bone lesions that may be painful, severe neurological complications, swelling of lymph nodes and (occasionally) adjacent joints, distended abdomen, a brownish tint to the skin, anemia, low blood platelet count, and yellow fatty deposits on the white of the eye (sclera).
   Also see Table F2.

3. **D.** Nieman-Pick disease is due to deficiency of sphingomyelinase.

   Niemann-Pick is a group of inherited, severe metabolic disorders in which sphingomyelin accumulates in lysosomes in cells. Mutations in the *SMPD1* gene cause Niemann-Pick disease (types A and B). They produce a deficiency in the activity of the lysosomal enzyme acid sphingomyelinase, which breaks down the lipid sphingomyelin. Cutaneous manifestations include hyperpigmentation, facial papules and juvenile xanthogranulomas.

4. **C.** The best-fit diagnosis for the image shown is acrodermatitis enteropathica (AE).

   Acrodermatitis enteropathica is a rare inherited form of zinc deficiency, clinically characterized by periorificial and acral dermatitis, alopecia, and diarrhea. Histopathologic findings are characteristic, but not specific. *Histopathologic findings vary with the age of the lesion.*

   Early lesions: Show confluent parakeratosis associated with a reduced granular layer. Often, exocytosis of neutrophils into the epidermis is noted, which may be acanthotic and exhibit slight spongiosis. The intracellular edema eventuates into pallor of the upper third of the epidermis. Subsequently, subcorneal and intraepidermal clefts may develop as a result of massive ballooning and reticular degeneration, with necrosis of the keratinocytes.

   Late lesions: Psoriasiform hyperplasia of the epidermis and less epidermal pallor than in early lesions.

5. **C.** Acrodermatitis enteropathica (AE) is due to defects in *ZIP4*.

   AE is an autosomal recessive disorder postulated to occur as a result of mutations in the *SLC39A4* gene that encodes a transmembrane protein that is part of the zinc/iron-regulated transporter-like protein (ZIP) family required for zinc uptake. This protein is highly expressed in the enterocytes in the duodenum and jejunum and, therefore, affected individuals have a decreased ability to absorb zinc from dietary sources. Absence of a binding ligand needed to transport zinc further contributes to zinc malabsorption.

6. **B.** Necrolytic migratory erythema (NME) is a feature of glucagonoma syndrome.

   Glucagonoma syndrome, an uncommon clinicopathologic entity, is characterized by a glucagon-secreting tumor associated with hyperglucagonemia, necrolytic migratory erythema (NME), diabetes mellitus, hypoaminoacidemia, cheilosis, a normochromic, normocytic anemia, venous thrombosis, weight loss, and neuropsychiatric features. The finding of NME was once considered pathognomonic for glucagonoma syndrome. However, several reports indicate that neither glucagonoma nor hyperglucagonemia is necessary for NME. Pseudoglucagonoma syndrome refers to NME in the absence of a glucagon-secreting tumor. NME can be found anywhere on the body, although it has a predilection for the perineum, buttocks, groin, lower abdomen, and lower extremities, areas subject to greater pressure and friction. The lesions wax and wane in a cycle of about 10 days, beginning with an erythematous patch that blisters centrally, erodes, and then crusts over and heals with hyperpigmentation. The lesions are typically annular or polycyclic and may demonstrate confluence in severely affected areas. The histopathologic findings of NME correlate with the clinical state of evolution of the lesion. It is important to take *more than one biopsy*, as early lesions may easily be mistaken for spongiotic dermatitis.

Early lesions: A mild perivascular dermal lymphocytic infiltrate and epidermal spongiosis.

Older lesions: The epidermis classically shows hyperparakeratosis, acanthosis, an absent granular layer, and pallor of keratinocytes in the upper layers of the epidermis. Vacuolar degeneration and necrosis in the superficial layers result in a characteristic cleft-like detachment from the deeper epidermis. The infiltrate may also include neutrophils and eosinophils.

7. E. Reduced activity of UPG decarboxylase leads to porphyria cutanea tarda.

   Reduced activity of UPG decarboxylase leads to porphyria cutanea tarda and hepatoerythropoietic porphyria (step 5, see below).

   Biosynthesis of heme consists of the following steps:

   Step 1: Glycine + succinyl COA catalyzed by aminolevulinic acid (ALA) synthetase gets converted to ALA

   Step 2: ALA to porphobilinogen catalyzed by ALA dehydratase

   Step 3: Porphobilinogen (PBG) to hydroxymethylbilane catalyzed by PBG deaminase (reduced activity leads to acute intermittent porphyria)

   Step 4: Hydroxymethylbilane to uroporphyrinogen (UPG) III catalyzed by UPG III cosynthase (reduced activity leads to congenital erythropoietic porphyria)

   Step 5: UPG III to coproporphyrinogen (CPG) III catalyzed by UPG decarboxylase (reduced activity leads to porphyria cutanea tarda and hepatoerythropoietic porphyria)

   Step 6: CPG III to protoporphyrinogen (PPG) IX catalyzed by CPG oxidase (reduced activity leads to hereditary coproporphyria)

   Step 7: PPG IX to protoporphyrin IX catalyzed by PPG oxidase (reduced activity leads to variegate porphyria)

   Step 8: Protoporphyrin IX to heme catalyzed by ferrochelatase (reduced activity leads to erythropoietic protoporphyria)

   Porphyria cutanea tarda comprises three major forms: *familial, sporadic* and *toxic*. The unifying feature of all types is *the reduction in activity of uroporphyrinogen decarboxylase* leading to overproduction of hepatic porphyrins. The *familial form* is inherited in an autosomal dominant manner and tends to present earlier than the others. The *sporadic form* typically has its onset in mid-life and has a very strong association with

hepatitis C. The *toxic form* results from exposure to polychlorinated aromatic hydrocarbons. Cutaneous changes occur predominantly on sun-exposed sites such as the face, arms and dorsal aspect of arms.

8. C. "Caterpillar bodies" in porphyria cutanea tarda (PCT) contain collagen IV.

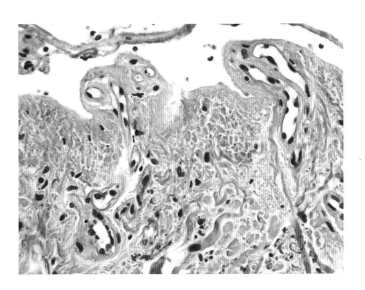

   Histopathologic features of PCT include a pauci-inflammatory subepidermal blister with festooning and the presence of "caterpillar bodies." "Caterpillar bodies" in porphyria cutanea tarda represent basement membrane material and colloid bodies, have a high specificity for PCT and are PAS positive and contain collagen IV.

9. C. Ultrastructural features of PCT include prominent reduplication of the basal laminae with concentric encasement of vessels.

   Regarding the other associations listed:
   - Oval/round juxtanuclear inclusions are seen in Lafora disease
   - Farber bodies are seen in Farber's disease
   - Vacuolation of fibroblasts and endothelial cells is seen in gangliosidosis
   - Zebra bodies are seen in Fabry's disease

10. B. Image shown is that of an accessory tragus.

    The accessory tragus is a relatively common benign congenital anomaly. It may be a sign of other syndromes, such as oculoauricular vertebral dysplasia (Goldenhar syndrome), in which it is a constant feature. Histopathologic features include polypoid architecture with numerous irregularly spaced vellus hair follicles. Eccrine glands are usually present. The stroma includes aggregates of mature adipose tissue, and a central plate of elastic cartilage is seen in most specimens. Small amounts of skeletal muscle may occur in select lesions.

11. A. Image shown is that of an accessory nipple.

Histopathologic features of a supernumerary nipple are identical to that of the regular nipple and include:
- Hyperpigmentation
- Slight hyperkeratosis with acanthosis
- Presence of pilosebaceous structure of Montgomery areolar tubercles
- Presence of smooth muscle bundles typical of the areola
- And possible mammary glands and intradermal straight ducts

A significant increase in the number of clear cells of Toker has been found in supernumerary nipple tissue in select studies.

12. E. Image shown is that of relapsing polychondritis.

Histopathologic features of relapsing polychondritis include chondrolysis, chondritis, and perichondritis. The cartilage loses its basophilia (probably by release of sulfated proteoglycans from the matrix), and the chondrocytes are decreased in number and may appear pyknotic. Early relapsing polychondritis is characterized by a mixed inflammatory infiltrate of lymphocytes, neutrophils, and plasma cells in the perichondrium. As the cartilage degenerates, mononuclear cells and macrophages infiltrate the matrix. The cartilage matrix is eventually destroyed and replaced by fibrous connective tissue. *Despite the presence of clinical erythema, the overlying dermis and epidermis are normal.* Clinically, relapsing polychondritis (RP) is a severe, episodic, and progressive inflammatory condition involving cartilaginous structures, predominantly those of the ears, nose, and laryngotracheobronchial tree. Other affected structures may include the eyes, cardiovascular system, peripheral joints, skin, middle and inner ear, and central nervous system. No laboratory findings are specific for relapsing polychondritis. Anemia, if present, is typically normochromic and normocytic and is associated with a poor prognosis. Non-specific indicators of inflammation (e.g., elevated erythrocyte sedimentation rate, elevated levels of C-reactive protein) are often present. Mild leukocytosis may be detected.

13. D. Image shown fits best for acanthosis nigricans which may represent a cutaneous manifestation of an internal malignancy.

Histopathologic findings of acanthosis nigricans are non-specific and include papillomatosis and mild acanthosis with prominent intervening "valleys" and hyperpigmentation. The dermal papillae project upward as finger-like projections, with occasional thinning of the adjacent epidermis. Pseudohorn cysts may be present. Acanthosis nigricans has been reported with many kinds of cancer, but, by far *the most common underlying malignancy is an adenocarcinoma of gastrointestinal origin, usually a gastric adenocarcinoma.* In 25–50% of cases of malignant acanthosis nigricans, the oral cavity is involved. The tongue and the lips most commonly are affected, with elongation of the filiform papillae on the dorsal and lateral surfaces of the tongue and multiple papillary lesions appearing on the commissures of the lips. Oral lesions of acanthosis nigricans seldom are pigmented. Clinically, acanthosis nigricans is characterized by symmetrical, hyperpigmented, velvety plaques that may occur in almost any location but most commonly appear on the intertriginous areas of the axilla, groin, and posterior neck. The posterior neck is the most commonly affected site in children. An increase in size and number of seborrheic keratoses is known as the Leser-Trélat sign. This sign of multiple eruptive seborrheic keratoses is typically associated with an internal malignancy and represents a paraneoplastic syndrome. Most commonly, the sign is observed with adenocarcinoma, especially of the gastrointestinal tract; however, an eruption of seborrheic keratoses may develop after an inflammatory dermatosis (e.g., eczema, severe sunburn). In this latter case, no associated malignancy is expected. The sign of Leser-Trélat often occurs with malignant acanthosis nigricans, a more accepted sign of internal cancer.

14. C. Image shown is that of neutrophilic eccrine hidradenitis which typically occurs secondary to chemotherapy.

Neutrophilic eccrine hidradenitis (NEH), a self-limited process, was initially described in acute myelogenous leukemia (AML) patients undergoing chemotherapy. Patients with this uncommon, self-limited condition usually present with fever and non-specific cutaneous lesions. More than 70% of oncology patients who develop NEH do so after their first course of chemotherapy. NEH does not appear to portend a worse prognosis for the underlying malignancy when occurring in that setting. The cutaneous manifestations of NEH are highly variable and include lesions that may be solitary or multiple, erythematous or purpuric macules, papules, nodules, or plaques with the trunk or limbs most commonly involved. The cause of NEH is unknown and a direct toxic effect of chemotherapy and a paraneoplastic mechanism have both been proposed to explain NEH in the context of malignancy. Histopathologic findings include a dense neutrophilic infiltrate within and around eccrine glands, with necrosis of eccrine epithelial cells. Some severely neutropenic patients may have a paucity or absence of neutrophils, but necrosis of eccrine glands is evident in all.

15. E. Cytarabine is most frequently associated with neutrophilic eccrine hidradenitis (NEH).

NEH was first described in a patient with acute myeloid leukaemia who had received cytarabine as chemotherapy. Other cytotoxic drugs associated with NEH include chlorambucil, cyclophosphamide, doxorubicin, lomustine, mitoxantrone, topotecan, and vincristine.

16. B. Eruptive keratoacanthomas are frequently associated with vemurafenib.

Approximately 60% of human melanomas harbor mutations in the *BRAF* gene, of which 90% have a substitution of glutamic acid for valine at amino acid 600 (V600E). Given the high prevalence of V600E mutations, therapeutic agents such as vemurafenib, a potent inhibitor of *V600E BRAF*, have been designed and shown to demonstrate complete or partial metastatic melanoma regression in a larger proportion (>80%) of phase 1 study patients and, more recently, a 63% reduction in risk of death and a 74% improvement in progression-free survival in patients with metastatic melanoma. However, cutaneous adverse effects are a common finding with these novel inhibitors with the most frequent being the development of keratoacanthoma-like lesions in approximately 20% of patients on this drug.

17. B. The presence of parakeratosis and eosinophils in a lichenoid drug eruption are helpful features in distinguishing it from lichen planus.

Other features of utility and favoring a lichenoid drug eruption include the presence of plasma cells, and a deeper perivascular and periadnexal infiltrate. Clinically, lichenoid drug eruptions resemble lichen planus, having violaceous papular, often polygonal, pruritic lesions. However, lichenoid drug eruptions tend to have more confluent areas with a slightly more eczematous nature and less (if any) mucosal involvement. The eruption often appears weeks or months following exposure to the responsible agent and may take the same length of time to disappear following withdrawal of the drug, often leaving post-inflammatory hyperpigmentation, particularly in dark-complexioned individuals.

18. C. In conjunction with the clinical presentation, the best-fit diagnosis for the image shown is erythema multiforme.

Erythema multiforme (EM) is an acute, self-limited, and sometimes recurring skin condition that is considered to be a type IV hypersensitivity reaction associated with certain infections, medications, and other various triggers. Erythema multiforme may be present within a wide spectrum of severity. Erythema multiforme minor represents a localized eruption of the skin with minimal or no mucosal involvement. The papules evolve into pathognomonic target or iris lesions that appear within a 72-hour period and begin on the extremities (see the image). Lesions remain in a fixed location for at least 7 days and then begin to heal. Precipitating factors include herpes simplex virus, Epstein-Barr virus, and histoplasmosis. Because this condition may be related to a persistent antigenic stimulus, *recurrence is the rule* rather than the exception, with most affected individuals experiencing 1–2 recurrences per year.

In established lesions of EM, the histopathologic reaction pattern is that of an interface dermatitis with scattered individually necrotic dyskeratotic keratinocytes within or just above the basal layer of the epidermis and an accompanying dermal infiltrate of varied densities composed predominantly of lymphocytes (although occasional eosinophils have been noted in scattered reports). *Typically there are no changes in the horn which is usually basket-weave.*

19. A. In conjunction with the clinical presentation, the best-fit diagnosis for the image shown is toxic epidermal necrolysis.

Toxic epidermal necrolysis (TEN) is a potentially life-threatening dermatologic disorder characterized by widespread erythema, necrosis, and bullous detachment of the epidermis and mucous membranes, resulting in exfoliation and possible sepsis and/or death. Mucous membrane involvement can result in gastrointestinal hemorrhage, respiratory failure, ocular abnormalities, and genitourinary complications. Mucous membrane erosions (seen in 90% of cases) generally *precede the skin lesions* by 1–3 days. The most frequently affected mucosal membrane is the oropharynx, followed by the eyes and genitalia. Most cases of TEN are drug induced, typically occurring within 1–3 weeks of therapy initiation and rarely occurring after more than 8 weeks. The most commonly implicated agents include the following:

- Sulfonamide antibiotics
- Antiepileptic drugs
- Oxicam non-steroidal anti-inflammatory drugs
- Allopurinol

TEN is a clinical diagnosis, confirmed by histopathologic analysis of lesional skin. Skin biopsy, harvested at the earliest possible stage, is important in establishing an accurate diagnosis and directing specific therapeutic modalities. Necrotic keratinocytes with full-thickness epithelial necrosis and detachment and a minimal inflammatory infiltrate is consistent with the diagnosis of TEN.

20. E. Image shown is that of calcinosis cutis.

Calcinosis cutis is a term used to describe a group of disorders in which calcium deposits form in the skin.

Calcinosis cutis is classified into 4 major types based on the etiopathogenesis:
- Dystrophic
- Metastatic
- Iatrogenic
- Idiopathic

The clinical presentation of calcinosis cutis can vary according to the diagnosis and underlying process. In general, multiple, firm, whitish dermal papules, plaques, nodules, or subcutaneous nodules are found in a distribution characteristic for the specific disorder. At times, these lesions may be studded with a yellow-white, gritty substance. Specifics relating to the different types are as follows:

Dystrophic calcinosis cutis: Calcification is usually localized to a specific area of tissue damage, though it may be generalized in some disorders.

Metastatic calcinosis cutis: Calcium deposition frequently is widespread. Large deposits are frequently found around large joints, such as knees, elbows, and shoulders, in a symmetrical distribution. Visceral organ deposition of calcium in the lung, kidneys, blood vessels, and stomach actually occurs more frequently than deposition within the skin or muscle.

Idiopathic calcinosis cutis: Calcification most commonly is localized to one general area.

Iatrogenic calcinosis cutis: Calcification generally is located at the site of an invasive procedure, though diffuse deposition may occur.

Histopathologic findings include variably sized basophilic deposits within the dermis, with or without a surrounding foreign-body giant cell reaction. Calcium deposition may be confirmed on Von Kossa and alizarin red stains.

Also see Table F5.

21. D. The most likely diagnosis for the image shown is subepidermal calcified nodule.

These lesions usually develop in early childhood and are typically solitary, though multiple lesions can also be present. The nodules most commonly occur on the face, though they may occur anywhere. The pathogenesis is unknown, but the lesions may be due to calcification of adnexal structures. In terms of histopathology, the calcium deposits are typically small, globular and superficial.

22. C. Image shown is that of calciphylaxis which may be associated with end-stage renal disease.

Calciphylaxis (calcific uremic arteriolopathy) is a life-threatening variant of metastatic calcification that occurs almost exclusively in the setting of end-stage renal insufficiency. Its prevalence in patients in hemodialysis is

almost 4%. Clinically, it presents with hard, tender, erythematous but cold necrotic plaques with subsequent eschar formation, usually on the lower extremities or abdomen. Most cases progress acutely, although more protracted, subacute presentation may also occur. In terms of histopathologic features, the *sine qua non* of calciphylaxis is calcification of subcutaneous vessel walls. There is usually epidermal ulceration. *Peri-eccrine calcification, albeit noted rarely, is believed to be highly specific for calciphylaxis.* Variable findings include pandermal ischemic necrosis with secondary subepidermal clefting, sparse neutrophils, and vascular thrombosis. Laboratory findings include elevated serum calcium and phosphate levels. Elevated parathyroid hormone levels are also expected. Exceptional cases in patients without renal insufficiency have been associated with metastatic breast cancer or Crohn's disease.

23. B. Image shown is that of osteoma cutis.

Osteoma cutis refers to the presence of bone within the skin in the absence of a pre-existing or associated lesion. There are four clinical types: isolated, widespread, multiple miliary facial, and plate-like osteomas. Hence, they may present as single or multiple hard nodules, miliary tumors, or plaques. The face, scalp, extremities, digits, and subungual areas are most commonly affected. A familial occurrence of Albright hereditary osteodystrophy may be present. Other relevant syndromic associations include Gardner syndrome (colonic polyposis, retinal hyperplasia, and other osseous and soft tissue growths). Histopathologic findings include small spicules to large masses of mature bone deposited in the dermis or subcutaneous tissue. Spicules of bone may enclose areas of mature fat, recapitulating a medullary cavity, but hematopoietic elements are seldom observed.

24. A. Metabolic alterations in calcium may be associated with familial osteoma cutis.

Serum calcium, phosphorus, and parathyroid hormone (PTH) levels help to define Albright hereditary osteodystrophy.

25. C. Image shown is that of gouty tophus.

In regular H&E stained sections, chronic tophaceous gouty deposits frequently show large pale pink acellular areas, which represent dissolved urate crystals, surrounded by histiocytes and multinucleate giant cells. Pseudogout also demonstrates pale pink areas that may be surrounded by histiocytes and multinucleate giant cells. On higher-power views, however, the crystals are purple and rhomboid and therefore can be distinguished from gout on routine H&E stained sections. Clinically, the spontaneous onset of excruciating pain, edema, and inflammation in the metatarsal-phalangeal joint of the great toe (podagra) is highly suggestive of acute crystal-induced arthritis and is the initial joint manifestation in 50% of gout cases.

26. **B.** The deposits in gout are composed of monosodium urate monohydrate crystals.

Gout and pseudogout are the 2 most common crystal-induced arthropathies. Pseudogout is caused by calcium pyrophosphate crystals and is more accurately termed calcium pyrophosphate disease. Elevated serum uric acid levels are the principal risk factor for developing gout. Although gout is associated with hyperuricemia, gout attacks are triggered not by a particular level of uric acid but typically by acute changes in the level of uric acid. Genetic disorders associated with overproduction of uric acid include:
- Hypoxanthine-guanine phosphoribosyl transferase deficiency (Lesch-Nyhan syndrome)
- Glucose-6-phosphatase deficiency (von Gierke disease)
- Fructose 1-phosphate aldolase deficiency
- Superactivity of phosphoribosyl pyrophosphate synthetase (PRPP)

27. **E.** The most likely diagnosis for the image shown is nodular amyloidosis.

Histopathologic findings characteristic of nodular amyloidosis are that of an eosinophilic amorphous deposit. The amyloid deposits are not limited to the papillary dermis but involve the entire dermis and may extend to subcutaneous fat. Amyloid deposition may be particularly prominent in walls of small blood vessels and surrounding individual adipocytes. An accompanying inflammatory infiltrate composed of varying numbers of plasma cells is typically present. When stained with Congo red and viewed with polarized light, deposits exhibit a characteristic apple-green birefringence. Pagoda red is even more specific for amyloid, and staining with thioflavin T is very sensitive.

Nodular amyloidosis, initially reported by Gottron in 1950, is typically benign and limited to the skin. However, lesions are more often persistent. Reported rates of progression to systemic disease are derived from case series with small numbers of patients; these rates vary from 7% to nearly 50%. The clinical presentation is that of brownish pink/red, firm nodules that can present at any cutaneous site including the face, scalp, extremities, trunk and genitalia, although acral areas are preferentially involved.

28. **D.** Immunohistochemical stains of diagnostic utility in nodular amyloidosis are κ/λ.

Also called amyloidosis cutis nodularis atrophicans or tumefactive amyloid, the amyloid in nodular amyloidosis is

believed to derive from local plasma cells, in contrast to lichenoid and macular amyloidosis, which have keratinocyte-derived amyloid. Plasma cells produce immunoglobulin light chains that are precursors to the amyloid fibril protein(s) termed amyloid L. Reports differ regarding the clonality of this population of plasma cells. In some instances, plasma cells have been monoclonal, suggesting that nodular amyloidosis is a neoplastic disorder.

29. **C.** The most likely diagnosis for the image shown is lichen amyloidosus.

Diagnostic histopathologic findings in lichen amyloidosus include the presence of amorphous, eosinophilic deposits in the papillary dermis, usually at the tips of the dermal papillae. *Identical histopathologic findings are present in macular amyloidosis.* Differences between these two entities are based on clinical presentation.

Lichen amyloidosus – Presents as intensely pruritic, red-brown hyperkeratotic papules most commonly seen on the pretibial surfaces (although it can also occur on the feet and the thighs). Lichen amyloidosus has been reported in association with select syndromes such as multiple endocrine neoplasia type 2A (MEN 2A), also known as Sipple syndrome (cardinal triad of this autosomal dominant syndrome is medullary thyroid carcinoma, pheochromocytoma, and hyperparathyroidism).

Macular amyloidosis – Presents as poorly defined hyperpigmented and rippled patches on the trunk. There appears to be a predilection for the interscapular region of adult females.

30. **B.** Antibodies to CK903, a high molecular weight cytokeratin, are of diagnostic utility in lichen amyloidosus.

Amyloid deposits in localized cutaneous amyloidosis (LCA, macular amyloidosis and lichen amyloidosus) bind to antikeratin antibodies as they are believed to be derived from epidermal keratinocytes. These deposits contain sulfhydryl groups, pointing to altered keratin as a source for these deposits. *There are no differences in staining characteristics of cytokeratins between deposits of macular amyloidosis and lichen amyloidosus.* The cytokeratins detected in amyloid deposits of LCA are believed to be of the basic type (type II). This may be because, in amyloidogenesis, acidic cytokeratins such as cytokeratin 14 are degraded faster than basic types.

31. **A.** The most likely diagnosis for the image shown is colloid milium.

Histopathologic findings diagnostic for colloid milium include fissured dermal eosinophilic deposits. Colloid cannot be distinguished from amyloid under light microscopy alone and because colloid, like amyloid, stains positively for periodic acid-Schiff stain, it can be difficult to distinguish it from amyloid. *However, colloid is usually negative for the amyloid stain methyl (crystal) violet.* Colloid may also sometimes yield weakly positive results and may show green birefringence with Congo red stain.

Colloid milium, a degenerative condition linked to excessive sun exposure and possibly exposure to petroleum products and hydroquinone, is a relatively uncommon condition characterized by the presence of multiple, dome-shaped, amber- or flesh-colored papules developing on light-exposed skin and the observance of dermal deposits of colloid under light microscopy. There are 4 distinct variants: (1) an adult-onset type, (2) a nodular form (nodular colloid degeneration), (3) a juvenile form that is inherited, and (4) a pigmented form, thought to be due to excess hydroquinone use for skin bleaching. The origin of the colloid deposition in the dermis is not certain, but it is thought to be due to degeneration of elastic fibers in the adult form and due to degeneration of UV-transformed keratinocytes in the juvenile form. The clinical presentation is that of crops of amber, waxy, partially translucent, firm papules on light-exposed skin, with the cheeks, periorbital area, nose, ears, and neck most frequently involved, ranging from 1–5 mm in diameter. Gelatinous material can be expressed. In the pigmented form, the papules are gray-black and confluent or clustered.

32. E. The most likely diagnosis for the image shown is ochronosis.

    Histopathologic examination shows yellow-brown, banana-shaped fibers in the papillary dermis. Early histopathologic findings include basophilia of the collagen fibers in the upper dermis, homogenization and swelling of the collagen bundles, and altered texture and arrangement of elastic fibers in the dermis resembling solar elastosis. Exogenous ochronosis, in which bluish black pigmentation of skin and cartilage is noted iatrogenically by exogenous agents, has been seen after exposure to antimalarials and noxious substances including phenol, trinitrophenol, benzene, hydroquinone, mercury, resorcinol, and picric acid. Exogenous ochronosis-like pigmentation may also occur after the topical application of hydroquinone, limited to sites of application. The hyperpigmentation may fade slightly after discontinuing the agent, but the discoloration is usually permanent. Hyperpigmentation typically appears after 6 months continual product use. The highest reported incidence of this syndrome occurs in South African Blacks. The mechanism of hyperpigmentation is speculated to involve effects on tyrosinase or alternatively by inhibiting homogentisic acid oxidase locally resulting in deposition.

33. D. Endogenous ochronosis, or alkaptonuria, is an autosomal recessive disease, which is caused by deficiency of homogentisic acid oxidase.

    In contrast to exogenous ochronosis, endogenous ochronosis, or alkaptonuria, is an autosomal recessive disease, which is caused by deficiency of homogentisic acid oxidase and results in tissue accumulation of homogentisic acid, which is an insoluble pigment that binds collagen and may induce a blue-black hyperpigmentation called ochronosis. There is marked similarity in the histopathologic findings of endogenous and exogenous ochronosis. Alkaptonuria is distinguished clinically in as much as patients exhibit a multitude of systemic symptoms that are absent in the exogenous form. These features include arthritis, scleral pigmentation, cartilaginous pigmentation, black ear wax, renal calculi/failure, urine that turns dark on standing (oxidized product) and calcification and stenosis of heart valves.

34. D. The most likely diagnosis for the image shown is argyria.

    Histopathologic findings diagnostic for argyria include the presence of small, round, brown-black fine granules singly or in clusters evident with routine staining. They appear in greatest numbers in the basement membrane zone surrounding sweat glands. These silver granules also favor the connective-tissue sheaths around pilosebaceous structures and nerves. They have a predilection for elastic fibers and are best visualized as strikingly refractile with dark-field illumination. An increase in the amount of melanin in exposed skin also appears to occur.

    Argyria results from prolonged contact with or ingestion of silver salts. Argyria is characterized by gray to gray-black staining of the skin and mucous membranes produced by silver deposition. Silver may be deposited in the skin either from industrial exposure or as a result of medications containing silver salts. Clinically, a permanent and irreversible metallic tinge occurs in the skin of patients with argyria. Early on, a gray-brown staining of the gums develops, later progressing to involve the skin diffusely. The cutaneous pigmentation usually is a slate-gray, metallic, or blue-gray color and may be clinically apparent after a few months, but the characteristic clinical appearance usually takes many years and depends on the degree of exposure. The hyperpigmentation is most apparent in the sun-exposed areas of skin, especially the forehead, nose, and hands. In some patients, the entire skin acquires a slate blue-gray color and the sclerae, nail beds, and mucous membranes may also become hyperpigmented.

35. C. The most likely diagnosis for the image shown is tattoo deposits.

    A tattoo is the result of the deposition of exogenous pigment into the skin. This may be purposeful or accidental. Accidental tattoos may occur after abrasion injuries introducing asphalt, graphite, or carbon into the injured skin. Rarely, medically induced tattoos have developed after the use of ferrous subsulfate solution (Monsel's solution) for coagulation purposes. While traumatic tattoos are not rare, decorative tattoos are more common.

Histopathologic reaction patterns associated with tattoo deposits are diverse and include a spongiotic reaction pattern, lichenoid dermatitis, granulomatous reaction, and even a morphea-like reaction. The composition of tattoo pigment colors is as follows:

Black – Carbon (India ink), iron oxide, logwood

Blue – Cobalt aluminate

Brown – Ferric oxide, silica

Green – Chromic oxide, lead chromate, phthalocyanine dyes, malachite

Purple – Manganese, aluminum

Red – Mercuric sulfide (cinnabar), sienna (ferric hydrate), sandalwood, brazilwood, organic pigments (aromatic azo compounds), cadmium red

White – Titanium oxide, zinc oxide, lead white

Yellow – Cadmium sulfide

Several cutaneous disorders show a predilection for tattooed skin. These include lichen planus, psoriasis, sarcoidosis, and lupus erythematosus. Whether disease localized to the tattoo represents the Köebner phenomenon or results from a locus minoris resistentiae that predisposes the area to disease is unclear. Although rare, eruptive keratoacanthomas have been commonly reported in both red and multicolored tattoos.

36. **C.** The most likely diagnosis for the image shown is minocyclin-induced reaction.

Histopathologically, the pigment is evident in macrophages, in dermal dendrocytes and in eccrine myoepithelial cells. The pigment may also be deposited on elastic tissue fibers or lie free within the dermis. The pigment is positive with Perls's as well as Fontana-Masson but is PAS negative. Clinically, there are distinct types of minocycline-induced hyperpigmentation:

Type 1 – Blue-gray coloration on the face in areas of inflammation

Type 2 – Blue-gray coloration on normal skin on the skin of the shins and forearms

Type 3 – The least common, characterized by diffuse muddy brown or blue-gray discoloration in sun-exposed areas

Type 4 – Blue-gray pigmentation in scars

Of note, the more recent view is that a combination of these types can be seen in the same patient.

Regarding other drug-induced pigmentary disorders:

Amiodarone pigmentation – Results in a photodistributed lipofuscinosis with accumulation of lysosomal laminated bodies within macrophages; these granules within macrophages stain positively with periodic acid-Schiff stain

Phenothiazine pigmentation – Accumulation of pigment-laden macrophages around superficial blood vessels; these macrophages stain with Fontana-Masson stain, but not Perls's stain

Chemotherapeutic agent–induced pigmentation – Interface dermatitis and pigment incontinence

Antimalarial pigmentation – Pigment granules are noted both extracellularly and within dermal macrophages and stain for hemosiderin and/or melanin

37. **B.** The best-fit diagnosis for the image shown is Restylane deposits.

Restylane is a biodegradable filler. Histopathologic clues to Restylane deposits are the presence of extracellular, basophilic, amorphous material composed of hyaluronic acid that is positive for Alcian blue at pH 2.7 and negative for polariscopy (also see Table F3).

38. **A.** The most likely diagnosis for the image shown is talon noir.

Histopathologic clues to the diagnosis of talon noir are pools of hemorrhage in the stratum corneum. Clinically presenting typically as bilateral, roughly symmetrical pigmentation on the heels, talon noir or calcaneal petechiae are usually traumatic in nature.

39. **E.** The most likely diagnosis for the image shown is radiation dermatitis.

Histopathologic features of radiation-related change vary with stage.

Acute radiation dermatitis (occurring within 90 days of initiating treatment): Findings include apoptotic keratinocytes, vacuolization of the basal layer, and epidermal edema. Depending upon the radiation dose, epidermal necrosis with blister formation and sloughing of the epidermis may be seen. These changes manifest clinically as "moist desquamation." Hyperkeratosis is seen with dry desquamation. Dermal changes include dermal and endothelial cell edema, vasodilation, erythrocyte extravasation, and fibrin thrombi in vessels. An inflammatory infiltrate is noted throughout the dermis

Late-stage or chronic radiation dermatitis (occurring months to years after radiation exposure): This is characterized by dermal fibrosis and poikilodermatous skin changes, including hyperpigmentation and hypopigmentation, atrophy, and telangiectasias, eosinophilic homogenized sclerosis of dermal collagen, scattered, large, atypical fibroblasts, absence of pilosebaceous units, and vascular changes. The deep vessels show fibrous thickening, sometimes with luminal obliteration and recanalization, whereas telangiectases are prominent in the upper dermis.

Radiation dermatitis is one of the most common side effects of radiotherapy for cancer, affecting approximately 95% of patients receiving radiotherapy. The skin changes depend upon the radiation dose and include erythema, edema, pigment changes, hair loss, and dry or moist desquamation.

40. **D.** Brooke-Spiegler syndrome is NOT a photosensitive genodermatosis.

Features of Brooke-Spiegler syndrome, a rare autosomal dominant disorder, include various adnexal tumors including multiple cylindromas, trichoepitheliomas and spiradenomas. Photosensitive genodermatoses include:

- Xeroderma pigmentosum
- Cockayne's syndrome
- Bloom's syndrome
- Hartnup disease
- Rothmund-Thompson syndrome
- Smith-Lemli-Opitz syndrome
- Kindler's syndrome

41. **C.** The most likely diagnosis for the image shown is polymorphic light eruption (PMLE).

The most striking histopathologic feature in PMLE is edema in the superficial dermis. A tight, perivascular lymphocytic infiltrate may also be observed in the upper and mid dermis. When clinically eczematous, spongiosis, edema, dyskeratosis, and basal cell vacuolization may be observed. Occasionally, neutrophils and eosinophils may be present in the infiltrate. Polymorphic light eruption is an acquired disease and is the most common of the idiopathic photodermatoses. PMLE is characterized by recurrent, abnormal, delayed reactions to sunlight, ranging from erythematous papules, papulovesicles, and plaques to erythema multiforme-like lesions on sunlight-exposed surfaces. Despite the diverse clinical presentations, *within any one patient, only one clinical form is consistently manifested*. PMLE tends to manifest in the spring and is a recurrent condition. Sunlight is clearly the primary etiologic factor for PMLE. The onset of the disease is sudden. The accompanying rash is pruritic and, in some instances, painful. Thirty minutes to several hours of exposure are required to trigger the eruption. Sun-exposed sites are primarily affected, but auto sensitization may lead to a generalized involvement.

1. Spindle cell pseudotumors are typically associated with:
   A. Atypical mycobacteria
   B. Visceral leishmaniasis
   C. Subcutaneous phaeohyphomycosis
   D. Pityrosporum folliculitis
   E. Ecthyma gangrenosum

2. Bullous impetigo is *most commonly* caused by:
   A. *Pseudomonas*
   B. *Yersinia*
   C. *Streptococcus*
   D. *Staphylococcus*
   E. *Listeria*

3. Staphylococci are:
   A. Catalase negative
   B. Gram-negative
   C. Coagulase positive

4. Common pathogenic species of staphylococci include all of the following EXCEPT:
   A. *Staphylococcus aureus*
   B. *Staphylococcus epidermidis*
   C. *Staphylococcus saprophyticus*
   D. *Staphylococcus caseolyticus*

5. Sexually transmitted chlamydia produces all of the following EXCEPT:
   A. Condyloma lata
   B. Lymphogranuloma venereum
   C. Pelvic inflammatory disease
   D. Acute epididymitis
   E. Reiter's syndrome

6. Body lice are the principal vectors of transmission of the causative organism in:
   A. Bubonic plague
   B. Q fever
   C. Scrub typhus
   D. Epidemic typhus
   E. Babesiosis

7. Bacterial endotoxin-mediated disease includes all of the following EXCEPT:
   A. Diphtheria
   B. Staphylococcal scalded skin syndrome
   C. Botulism
   D. Tetanus
   E. Legionnaire's disease

8. Which is the following is NOT caused by streptococci:
   A. Impetigo
   B. Erysipelas
   C. Erythema nodosum
   D. Scarlet fever
   E. Carbuncle

9. Which of the following may be caused by staphylococci:
   A. Impetigo
   B. Erysipelas
   B. Thrush
   C. Erythema nodosum
   D. Scarlet fever

10. Cutaneous manifestations of an overabundance of cory-neforms include:
    A. Thrush
    B. Erthyrasma
    C. Erysipelas
    D. Keratoderma
    E. Erysipeloid

11. Erysipeloid is associated with:
    A. *Pseudomonas aeruginosa*
    B. *Streptococcus pyogenes*
    C. *Staphylococcus aureus*
    D. *Corynebacterium diphtheriae*
    E. *Erysipelothrix rhusiopathiae*

12. *Corynebacterium minutissimum:*
    A. Is a Gram-negative diplococcus
    B. Is normal skin flora
    C. Has a predilection for the scalp
    D. Is negative on Wood's lamp examination

13. Lupus vulgaris is a form of:
    A. Lupus erythematosus
    B. Metastatic tuberculosis
    C. Reinfection tuberculosis
    D. Orofacial tuberculosis
    E. Disseminated tuberculosis

14. Scrofuloderma is best described as:
    A. Cutaneous involvement secondary to direct extension
    B. Cutaneous involvement secondary to disseminated tuberculosis
    C. Cutaneous involvement secondary to erythema induratum
    D. Cutaneous involvement secondary to orofacial tuberculosis
    E. Cutaneous involvement secondary to lupus vulgaris

15. The causative organism in Buruli ulcer is:
    A. *Mycobacterium marinum*
    B. *Mycobacterium kansasi*
    C. *Mycobacterium simiae*
    D. *Mycobacterium scrofulaceum*
    E. *Mycobacterium ulcerans*

16. Which of the following is NOT a Group I mycobacterium:
    A. *Mycobacterium marinum*
    B. *Mycobacterium kansasi*
    C. *Mycobacterium simiae*
    D. *Mycobacterium scrofulaceum*

17. Mycobacteria classified as "rapid growers" include:
    A. *Mycobacterium marinum*
    B. *Mycobacterium kansasi*
    C. *Mycobacterium simiae*
    D. *Mycobacterium scrofulaceum*
    E. *Mycobacterium chelonae*

18. Entities classified under "tuberculids" include:
    A. Lichen scrofulosorum
    B. Tuberculoid leprosy
    C. Borderline leprosy
    D. Sarcoidosis
    E. Lepromatous leprosy

19. The causative organism in swimming pool granuloma:
    A. Is a Group IV mycobacterium
    B. Is a rapid grower
    C. Is a photochromogen
    D. Will grow at 37 °C

20. Tuberculoid leprosy:
    A. Is common in western USA
    B. Is paucibacillary
    C. Is unstable clinically
    D. Expresses T_{H2} cytokines

21. Lucio's phenomenon is associated with:
    A. Tuberculoid leprosy
    B. Necrotizing vasculitis
    C. Erythema nodosum
    D. Lepra (type I) reaction
    E. Indeterminate leprosy

22. The primary hosts in anthrax are:
    A. Cats
    B. Herbivores
    C. Humans
    D. Birds
    E. Bats

23. The causative organism in granuloma inguinale is:
    A. *Haemophilus ducreyi*
    B. *Yersinia pseudotuberculosis*
    C. *Brucella abortus*
    D. *Klebsiella granulomatis*
    E. *Bacillus anthracis*

24. Which of the following is NOT caused by *Bartonella*:
    A. Malakoplakia
    B. Cat scratch disease
    C. Bacillary angiomatosis
    D. Verruca peruana
    E. Trench fever

25. This is an example of a:

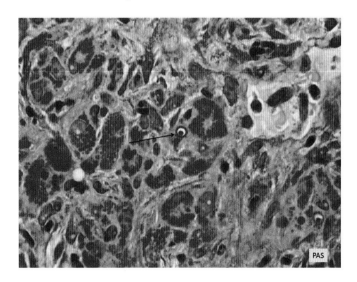

    A. Schaumann body
    B. Michaelis-Gutmann body
    C. Asteroid body
    D. Dutcher body
    E. Russell body

26. This (based on the above image) is associated with:
    A. Sarcoidosis
    B. Listeriosis
    C. Malakoplakia
    D. Tularemia
    E. Rhinoscleroma

27. This is an example of:

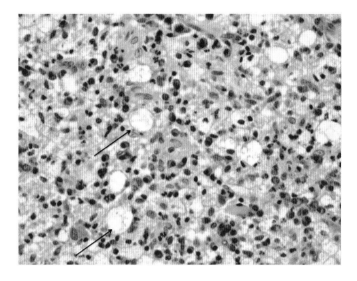

    A. Dutcher cell
    B. Michaelis-Gutmann body
    C. Asteroid body
    D. Russell body
    E. Mikulicz cell

28. This (based on the above image) is associated with:
    A. Sarcoidosis
    B. Listeriosis
    C. Malakoplakia
    D. Tularemia
    E. Rhinoscleroma

29. Tick-transmitted rickettsial infections include:
    A. Epidemic typhus
    B. Murine typhus
    C. Q fever
    D. Rickettsialpox
    E. Rocky mountain spotted fever

30. Mite-transmitted rickettsial infections include:
    A. Epidemic typhus
    B. Murine typhus
    C. Q fever
    D. Rickettsialpox
    E. Rocky mountain spotted fever

31. Penile ulcerations occur in the acute form of all of the following EXCEPT:
    A. Syphilis
    B. Gonorrhea
    C. Chancroid
    D. Granuloma inguinale
    E. Genital herpes

32. Which of the following is INCORRECT regarding Lyme disease:
    A. Tick transmitted
    B. Caused by *Rickettsia*
    C. Caused by spirochetes
    D. Deer are the preferred hosts
    E. Small mammals can serve as hosts

33. "Strawberry mucosa" is associated with:
    A. Psittacosis
    B. Listeriosis
    C. Corynebacteria
    D. Malakoplakia
    E. Trichomoniasis

34. All of the following are correct regarding *Neisseria gonorrhoeae* EXCEPT:
    A. Causes urethritis in affected males
    B. Is a facultative intracellular pathogen
    C. Makes proteases capable of lysing IgA
    D. Produces exotoxins
    E. Capsular polysaccharides contribute to virulence

35. The causative organism in lymphogranuloma venereum is:
    A. *Haemophilus ducreyi*
    B. *Yersinia pseudotuberculosis*
    C. *Chlamydia trachomatis*
    D. *Klebsiella granulomatis*
    E. *Neisseria gonorrhoeae*

36. Which of the following is a feature of primary syphilis:
    A. Chancre
    B. Chancroid
    C. Gumma
    D. Hutchinson's teeth
    E. Tabes dorsalis

37. Which of the following is associated with secondary syphilis:
    A. Chancre
    B. Charcot's joints
    C. Mucocutaneous eruption
    D. Gumma
    E. Tabes dorsalis

38. Hutchinson's triad includes:
   A. Interstitial keratitis, 8th nerve deafness, notched incisors
   B. Stomatitis, 7th nerve palsy, iridocyclitis
   C. Mucositis, 5th nerve palsy, iridocyclitis
   D. Arthritis, uveitis, stomatitis
   E. Arthritis, deafness, urethritis

39. Hutchinson's triad is associated with:
   A. Primary syphilis
   B. Secondary syphilis
   C. Tertiary syphilis
   D. Latent syphilis
   E. Congenital syphilis

40. Which of the following is NOT associated with tertiary syphilis:
   A. Gumma
   B. Chancre
   C. Tabes dorsalis
   D. Charcot's joints
   E. Obliterative endarteritis

41. The causative organism in yaws is:
   A. *Borrelia burgdorferi*
   B. *Neisseria gonorrhoeae*
   C. *Treponema pallidum*
   D. *Klebsiella granulomatis*
   E. *Francisella tularensis*

42. Which of the following is the most common cause of dermatophyte infection worldwide:
   A. *Trichophyton rubrum*
   B. *Trichophyton violaceum*
   C. *Trichophyton mentogrophytes*
   D. *Trichophyton tonsurans*
   E. *Microsporum canis*

43. Favus (tinea capitis favosa) is most characteristic of infection by:
   A. *Trichophyton rubrum*
   B. *Trichophyton violaceum*
   C. *Trichophyton mentogrophytes*
   D. *Trichophyton schoenleinii*
   E. *Trichophyton tonsurans*

44. Common causative organisms of tinea barbae, tinea corporis and tinea cruris are:
   A. *Trichophyton rubrum, Trichophyton violaceum, Trichophyton mentogrophytes*
   B. *Trichophyton rubrum, Trichophyton mentogrophytes, Microsporum canis*
   C. *Trichophyton mentogrophytes, Microsporum canis, Trichophyton tonsurans*

   D. *Trichophyton rubrum, Trichophyton mentogrophytes, Epidermophyton floccosum*
   E. *Trichophyton mentogrophytes, Trichophyton violaceum, Epidermophyton floccosum*

45. Pseudohyphae are characteristic of:
   A. Onychomycosis
   B. Candidiasis
   C. Phaeohyphomycosis
   D. Alternariosis
   E. Chromomycosis

46. The most likely causative organism is:

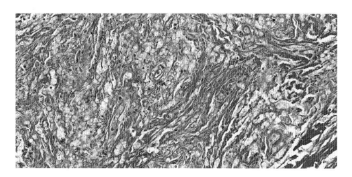

   A. *Cryptococcus neoformans*
   B. *Blastomyces dermatitidis*
   C. *Coccidioides immitis*
   D. *Histoplasma capsulatum*
   E. *Leishmania donovani*

47. The most likely diagnosis is:

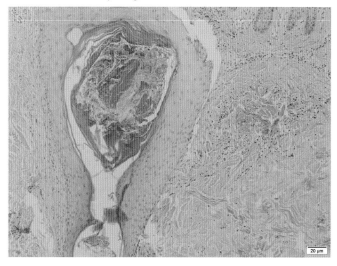

A. Majocchi's granuloma
B. Pityrosporum folliculitis
C. Inflamed cyst
D. Tinea pedis
E. Pityriasis versicolor

48. The causative organism (based on the above image) is:
    A. *Tinea capitis*
    B. *Tinea faciei*
    C. *Malassezia furfur*
    D. *Pityriasis versicolor*
    E. *Candida albicans*

49. The causative organism most likely is:

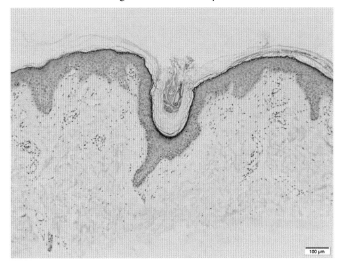

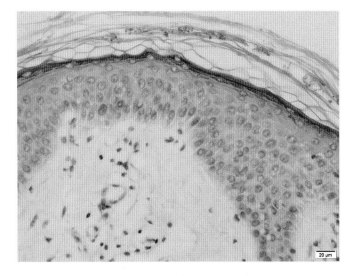

A. *Tinea capitis*
B. *Tinea faciei*
C. *Fonsecaea pedrosoi*
D. *Pityrosporum ovale*
E. *Candida albicans*

50. Which of the following is NOT a dematiaceous fungus:
    A. *Fonsecaea pedrosoi*
    B. *Cladosporium carrioni*
    C. *Phialophora compacta*
    D. *Blastomyces dermatitidis*
    E. *Exophiala jeanselmei*

51. The best-fit diagnosis is:

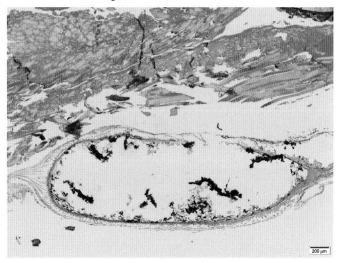

A. Sporotrichosis
B. Phaeohyphomycosis
C. Chromomycosis
D. Coccidiomycosis
E. Paracoccidiomycosis

52. This is associated with:

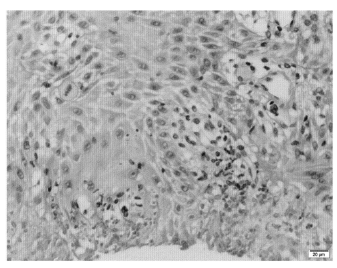

A. Sporotrichosis
B. Phaeohyphomycosis
C. Chromomycosis

D. Coccidiomycosis

E. Paracoccidiomycosis

53. The best-fit diagnosis is:

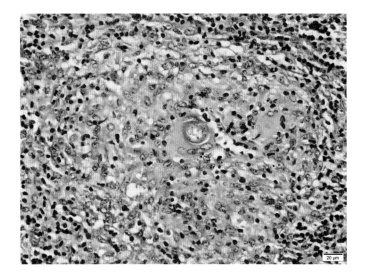

A. Sporotrichosis

B. Phaeohyphomycosis

C. Chromomycosis

D. Coccidiomycosis

E. Paracoccidiomycosis

54. This (based on the above image) is endemic in:
A. Mississippi
B. Africa
C. India
D. Mexico

55. The best-fit diagnosis is:

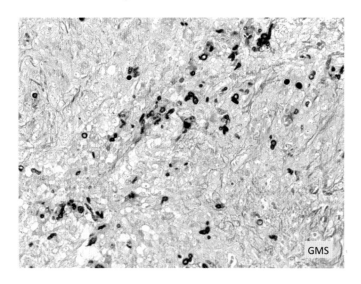

A. Sporotrichosis

B. Phaeohyphomycosis

C. Chromomycosis

D. Coccidiomycosis

E. Paracoccidiomycosis

56. Broad-based buds, lack of endospores and lack of a capsule are typical of:
A. Sporotrichosis
B. Phaeohyphomycosis
C. Blastomycosis
D. Coccidiomycosis
E. Paracoccidiomycosis

57. The best-fit diagnosis is:

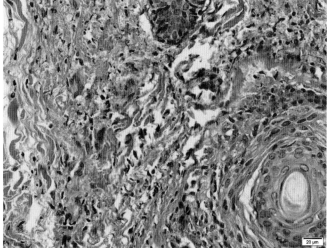

A. Sporotrichosis

B. Histoplasmosis

C. Chromomycosis

D. Coccidiomycosis

E. Paracoccidiomycosis

58. This organism (based on the above image) is endemic in:
A. Latin America
B. Northeastern USA
C. Northwestern USA
D. Southeastern USA
E. Southwestern USA

59. The best-fit diagnosis is:

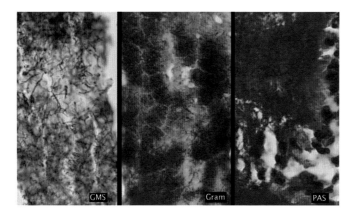

    A. Mycetoma
    B. Phaeohyphomycosis
    C. Necrobiosis lipoidica
    D. Scrofuloderma
    E. Necrotizing fasciitis

60. *Nocardia* is a:
    A. Gram-negative, acid-fast coccus
    B. Gram-negative, acid-fast bacillus
    C. Gram-positive, acid-fast coccus
    D. Gram-positive, acid-fast bacillus

61. The best-fit diagnosis is:

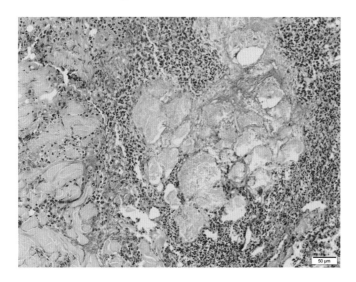

    A. Nocardiosis
    B. Actinomycosis
    C. Mucormycosis
    D. Aspergillosis
    E. Fusariosis

62. The best-fit diagnosis is:

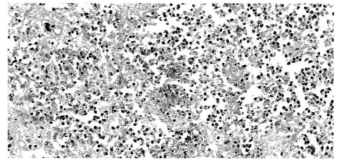

    A. Nocardiosis
    B. Actinomycosis
    C. Mucormycosis
    D. Aspergillosis
    E. Fusariosis

63. The best-fit diagnosis is:

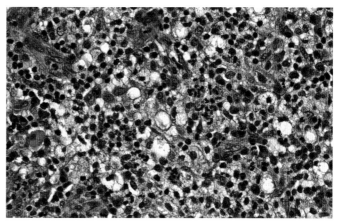

    A. Nocardiosis
    B. Actinomycosis
    C. Mucormycosis
    D. Aspergillosis
    E. Rhinosporidiosis

64. The most likely diagnosis is:

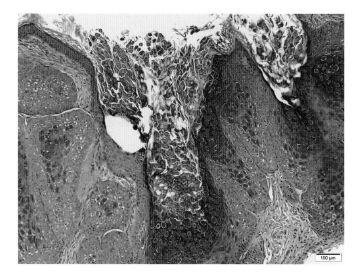

   A. Condyloma acuminatum
   B. Epidermodysplasia verruciformis
   C. Molluscum contagiosum
   D. Bowenoid papulosis
   E. Eczema herpeticum

65. The causative organism of Milker's nodule is:
   A. Poxviridae
   B. Herpesviridae
   C. Papovaviridae
   D. Parvoviridae
   E. Picornaviridae

66. Ecthyma contagiosum is also known as:
   A. Monkeypox
   B. Varicella
   C. Measles
   D. Orf
   E. Vaccinia

67. Which of the following is NOT a member of the Poxviridae family:
   A. Monkeypox
   B. Varicella
   C. Molluscum
   D. Orf
   E. Vaccinia

68. Which of the following statements is correct regarding HSV-1 and HSV-2:
   A. Earliest changes in HSV-1 alone involve epidermal nuclei
   B. Both are biologically and serologically distinct
   C. Ballooning degeneration is only typical of HSV-1
   D. Reticular degeneration is only typical of HSV-2
   E. Eosinophilic viral inclusions are only seen in HSV-2

69. Herpes zoster:
   A. Occurs almost exclusively in children
   B. Is highly infectious
   C. Results from reactivation of latent VZV infection
   D. Typically presents with a non-contiguous dermatomal rash
   E. Causes eczema herpeticum

70. The most likely causative organism is:

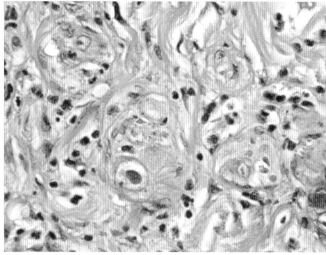

   A. EBV
   B. HHV-6
   C. HHV-8
   D. CMV
   E. HPV-1

71. Epstein–Barr virus belongs to the:
   A. Poxviridae family
   B. Herpesviridae family
   C. Papovaviridae family
   D. Parvoviridae family
   E. Picornaviridae family

72. Which of the following is NOT EBV associated:
   A. Infectious mononucleosis
   B. Burkitt's lymphoma
   C. Nasopharyngeal carcinoma
   D. Post-transplant lymphoproliferative disorder
   E. Cervical cancer

73. Plantar warts are associated with:
   A. HPV-1
   B. HPV-5
   C. HPV-6
   D. HPV-13
   E. HPV-32

74. The best-fit diagnosis is:

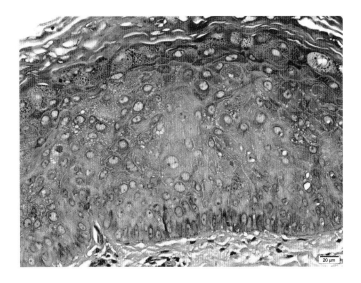

A. Verruca vulgaris
B. Verruca plana
C. Epidermodysplasia verruciformis
D. Condyloma acuminatum
E. Bowenoid papulosis

75. The causative organism (based on the above image) is associated with all of the following EXCEPT:
A. HPV-1
B. HPV-3
C. HPV-5
D. HPV-6
E. HPV-8

76. The HPV strain most commonly implicated in bowenoid papulosis is:
A. HPV-1
B. HPV-3
C. HPV-5
D. HPV-10
E. HPV-16

77. Measles belongs to the:
A. Poxviridae family
B. Paramyxoviridae family
C. Papovaviridae family
D. Parvoviridae family
E. Picornaviridae family

78. The causative organism of fifth disease is a:
A. Pox virus
B. Papova virus
C. Parvo virus
D. Picorna virus
E. Toga virus

79. Hand, foot and mouth disease is caused by:
A. Coxsackie virus
B. Parvo virus
C. HTLV-1
D. Hepatitis B virus
E. CMV

80. Giannoti-Crosti syndrome is characterized by:
A. Follicular and mucous membrane lesions and cicatricial alopecia
B. Sebaceous neoplasms and internal malignancies
C. Relapsing rash, meningitis and an ascending polyneuropathy
D. Non-relapsing rash, hepatitis and lymphadenopathy
E. Arthritis, hepatitis and meningitis

81. The best-fit diagnosis is:

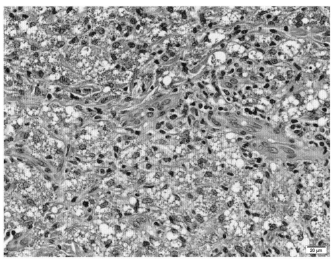

A. Chromomycosis
B. Histoplasmosis
C. Cryptococcosis
D. Leishmaniasis
E. Botryomycosis

82. Mucocutaneous leishmaniasis is caused by:
A. *Leishmania tropica*
B. *Leishmania mexicana*
C. *Leishmania braziliensis*
D. *Leishmania donovani*

83. The causative organism in kala-azar is:
A. *Leishmania tropica*
B. *Leishmania mexicana*
C. *Leishmania braziliensis*
D. *Leishmania donovani*

84. Larva migrans is associated with:
    A. *Taenia solium*
    B. *Schistosoma hematobium*
    C. *Dirofilaria repens*
    D. *Ancylostoma braziliense*
    E. *Onchocerca volvulus*

85. This is an image of a/an:

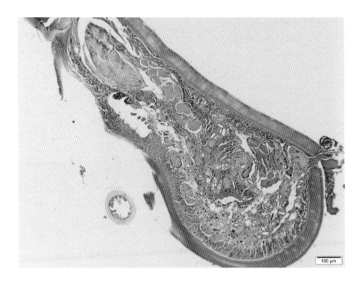

    A. Sarcoptes mite
    B. Intact tick
    C. Demodex mite
    D. Crab louse
    E. Sand flea

86. Cercarial dermatitis is associated with:
    A. Schistosomiasis
    B. Cysticercosis
    C. Echinococcosis
    D. Gnathostomiasis
    E. Dirofilariasis

87. This is an image of a/an:

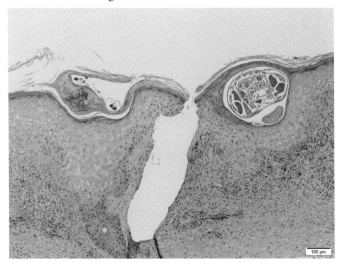

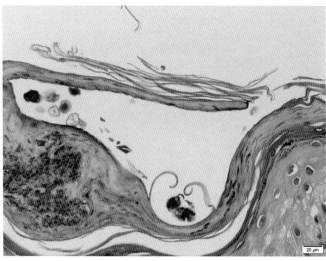

    A. Sand flea
    B. Intact tick
    C. Demodex mite
    D. Crab louse
    E. Sarcoptes mite

88. This is an image of a/an:

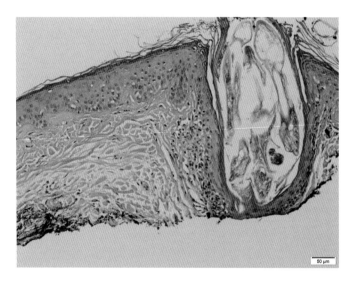

    A. Sarcoptes mite
    B. Intact tick
    C. Demodex mite
    D. Crab louse
    E. Sand flea

89. The best-fit diagnosis is:

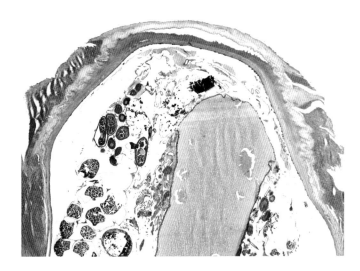

    A. Scabies
    B. Pediculosis
    C. Demodicosis
    D. Tungiasis
    E. Amoebiasis

90. Pitted keratolysis is associated with:
    A. Psittacosis
    B. Listeriosis
    C. Corynebacteria
    D. Malakoplakia
    E. Clostridia

Infections

Answers

Table G1 Clues to infections and infestations – histopathologic reaction pattern based and inflammatory infiltrate based

Reaction pattern		Entities to commonly consider
Granulomatous	Palisaded	Phaeohyphomycosis, mycobacterial, treponemal, sporotrichosis, cryptococcosis, cat scratch disease, lymphogranuloma venerum, schistosomiasis, coccidiomycosis
	Tuberculoid	Tuberculosis, tuberculids, tuberculoid leprosy, secondary/tertiary syphilis, Majocchi's granuloma, cryptococcosis, histoplasmosis, leishmaniasis
	Suppurative	Atypical mycobacteria, lymphogranuloma venereum, actinomycosis, nocardiosis, mycetoma, cryptococcosis, aspergillosis
	Histiocyte rich	Atypical mycobacteria, lepromatous leprosy, leishmaniasis, malakoplakia
Inflammatory cell type based	Histiocyte and plasma-cell rich	Rhinoscleroma, syphilis, yaws, granuloma inguinale
	Plasma-cell rich	Syphilis, yaws, lymphogranuloma venereum, chancroid, leishmaniasis, trypanosomiasis
	Eosinophil rich	Arthropod bite, helminthiasis, subcutaneous phycomycosis
	Neutrophil rich	Impetigo, ecthyma, cellulitis, erysipelas, granuloma inguinale, chancroid, erythema nodosum leprosum, Lucio's phenomenon, yaws, actinomycosis, nocardiosis, mycetoma, phaeohyphomycosis, aspergillosis, mucormycosis

Parasitized inflammatory cells	Parasitized macrophages	Rhinoscleroma, granuloma inguinale, lepromatous leprosy, histoplasmosis, leishmaniasis, toxoplasmosis
	Parasitized MNGCs	Prototothecosis, schistosomiasis, demodeciosis
Psoriasiform		Candidiasis, tinea imbrecata
Spongiotic		Dermatophytoses, candidiasis, cercarial dermatitis, arthropod bite
Intraepidermal vesiculation		Herpes, orf, Milker's nodule, erysipeloid, dermatophytoses, candidiasis
Folliculitis		Dermatophytoses, pityrosporum folliculitis, herpes, demodex infestation, larva migrans
Vasculitis		Erythema nodosum leprosum, Lucio's phenomenon, necrotizing fasciitis, meningococcal/gonnococccal septicemia, cytomegalovirus infection, rickettsial infection, spider bite, recurrent herpes
Spindle cell pseudotumors		Atypical mycobacteria, histioid leprosy, acrodermatitis chronica atrophicans
Invisible dermatosis		Erythrasma, pityriasis versicolor, dermatophytoses, pitted keratolysis

MNGCs = Multinucleate giant cells

Table G2 Rickettsial infections

Transmitting vector	Organism	Disease
Tick	*Rickettsia rickettsiae*	Rocky mountain spotted fever
	Rickettsia conorii	Boutonneuse fever
	Rickettsia africae	African tick bite fever
	Rickettsia sibirica	Siberian tick typhus
	Rickettsia australis	Queensland tick typhus

Table G2 Rickettsial infections (*cont.*)

Transmitting vector	Organism	Disease
Mite	*Rickettsia akari* *Orientia tsutsugamushi*	Rickettsialpox Scrub typhus
Louse	*Rickettsia prowazekii*	Epidemic typhus
Flea	*Rickettsia mooseri*	Murine typhus
Aerosol	*Coxiella burnettii*	Q fever

Table G3 Classification of mycobacteria other than *Mycobacterium tuberculosis* (MOTT)

Group	Classification	Species
I	Photochromogens	*M*[*]*. marinum* *M. kansasi* *M. simiae*
II	Scotochromogens	*M. scrofulaceum* *M. flavescens* *M. szulgai*
III	Nonchromogens	*M. ulcerans* *M. avium-intracellulare* complex *M. gastrii* *M. terrae* *M. xenopi* *M. hemophilum* *M. novum* *M. nonchromogenicum*
IV	Rapid growers	*M. fortuitum* complex: *M. fortuitum* *M. chelonae* *M. abscessus* *M. phlei* *M. vaccae* *M. smegmatis* *M. diernhoferi*

[*] *M. = Mycobacterium*

Table G4 Mycetomas – granule color-based working classification

Category	Granule color	Causative organism/s
Eumycetomas	Black	*Madurella mycetomatis, M. grisea* *Leptosphaeria senegalensis* *Exophilia jeanselmei* *Curvularia lunata*
	Pale	*Phialophora verrucosa, P. parasitica* *Cladophialophora bantiana* *Pyrenchaeta romeroi* *Petriellidium boydii* *Aspergillus nidulans, A. flavus* *Fusarium* spp. *Acremonium* spp. *Neotestudina rosatii* Dermatophytes
	Brown	*Neoscytalidium dimidiatum*
Actinomycetomas	Red Yellow Pale	*Actinomadura pelletieri* *Streptomyces somaliensis* *Nocardia brasiliensis, N. cavae, N. asteroides* *Actinomadura madurae*

Table G5 HPV associations – a "cheat sheet"

Disease	Associated HPVs
Plantar wart	HPV-1, -2, - 60, -63, -65, -66
Common wart	HPV-2, -3
Common warts in the immunosuppressed	HPV-75, -76, -77
Plane wart	HPV-3
Epidermodysplasia verruciformis	HPV-3, -5, -6, -8, -9, -10, -12, -14, -17, -19, -22, -24
Anogenital wart	HPV-6
Warts in meat/fish handlers	HPV-7
Heck's disease	HPV-13, -32
Bowenoid papulosis	HPV-16

Table G6 Classification of leishmaniasis – a short guide

Clinical disease	Causative organism/s
Cutaneous/oriental leishmaniasis	*L*[*]*. tropica* (Africa) *L. mexicana* (Central and South America)
Mucocutaneous/American leishmaniasis	*L. braziliensis*
Visceral leishmaniasis (kala-azar)	*L. donovani*

[*] *L. = Leishmania*

Table G7 Fungal infections – "at a glance"

Disease	Causative organism/s	Key histopathologic clues	Image
Majocchi's granuloma	*Trichophyton rubrum, Microsporum canis, Trichophyton violaceum, Trichophyton tonsurans, Trichophyton mentogrophytes*	Perifollicular granulomas	
Superficial candidiasis	*Candida albicans*	Pseudohyphae	
Cryptococcosis	*Cryptococcus neoformans*	Yeast-like with refractile walls Mucinous capsule	

Table G7 Fungal infections – "at a glance" (*cont.*)

Disease	Causative organism/s	Key histopathologic clues	Image
Pityrosporum folliculitis	*Malassezia furfur*	Ruptured folliculitis Basophilic debris spilling into adjacent dermis Single as well as aggregates of spores within the follicle	
Blastomycosis	*Blastomyces dermatitidis*	Yeast-like with broad-based buds Doubly refractile thick walls Multiple nuclei	
Coccidiomycosis	*Coccidioides immitis*	Thick-walled spherules/ sporangia Multiple endospores/ sporangiospores within sporangia	

Table G7 Fungal infections – "at a glance" (cont.)

Disease	Causative organism/s	Key histopathologic clues	Image
Histoplasmosis	*Histoplasma capsulatum*	Yeast-like organisms with a surrounding clear halo	
Chromomycosis	*Fonsecaea pedrosoi, Fonsecaea compacta, Phialophora verrucosa, Cladosporium carrionii, Aureobasidium pullulans*	Round, thick-walled, golden brown cells/ sclerotic bodies/ medlar bodies/ muriform cells	
Phaeohyphomycosis	*Exophiala jeanselmei, Wangiella dermatidis*	Circumscribed cyst with/ without central wood splinter Brown filamentous hyphae/yeast-like structures in wall	

Table G7 Fungal infections – "at a glance" (*cont.*)

Disease	Causative organism/s	Key histopathologic clues	Image
Sporotrichosis	*Sporothrix schenckii*	Cigar bodies Blastospore surrounded by rays of eosinophilic material/ sporothrix asteroid	
Mycetoma	See Table G4	Grains surrounded by eosinophilic fringe	
Nocardiosis	*Nocardia asteroides, Nocardia brasiliensis, Nocardia caviae*	Gram-positive Weakly acid-fast Finely branched filaments	

Table G7 Fungal infections – "at a glance" (*cont.*)

Disease	Causative organism/s	Key histopathologic clues	Image
Mucormycosis	*Rhizopus, Mucor, Absidia*	Broad, non-septate hyphae Branch at right angles	
Fusariosis	*Fusarium* spp.	Hyaline, septate hyphae Branching at acute or right angles *Resembles aspergillosis*	
Aspergillosis	*Aspergillus flavus*	Septate hyphae Dichotomous branching at acute or right angles	

Table G7 Fungal infections – "at a glance" (*cont.*)

Disease	Causative organism/s	Key histopathologic clues	Image
Rhinosporidiosis	*Rhinosporidium seeberi*	Large spherical spherules/ sporangia Multiple endospores/ sporangiospores within sporangia	

Table G8 Artistic rendition of cutaneous infections

What you see	Description	Interpretation
	"Sulfur granules" Delicate (<1 μm) filaments Gram-positive, non-acid fast	**Actinomycosis**
	White/red/yellow granules Narrow (0.5–1 μm), intertwined filaments	**Actinomycotic mycetoma**
	White/yellow/brown/black granules Hyphae (2–6 μm) Numerous chlamydospores Swollen cells at periphery	**Eumycotic mycetoma**

Table G8 Artistic rendition of cutaneous infections (*cont.*)

What you see	Description	Interpretation
	Narrow, delicate (0.5–1 μm) filaments Branching at right angles Beaded/granular Partially acid-fast	**Nocardiosis**
	Broad hyphae (12 μm average) Almost non-septate Non-dichotomous, irregular branching (sometimes at 90°)	**Zygomycosis**
	Septate hyphae (3–12 μm) Dichotomous branching at 45° angles Radial growth pattern	**Aspergillosis**
	Septate hyphae (2–6 μm) Two types of conidiation: Unbranched/branched with canoe-shaped macroconidia Long/short small 1–2-celled conidia singly/clusters	**Fusariosis**
	Colorless, branched, septate hyphae Hyphae often in chains of arthroconidia	**Dermatophytosis**
	Brown-pigmented, septate hyphae (2–6 μm) Dark, budding, yeast-like forms also may be present	**Phaeohyphomycosis**
	Sclerotic bodies (brown, thick-walled with horizontal and vertical septae, 5–12 μm) Occasionally brown septate hyphal forms present	**Chromoblastomycosis**
	Yeast-like cells Variably shaped (2–6 μm) Characteristic, elongate "cigar bodies"	**Sporotrichosis**

Table G8 Artistic rendition of cutaneous infections (*cont.*)

What you see	Description	Interpretation
	Yeast-like cells Small (2–4 μm) Ovoid, budding on a narrow base Characteristically within macrophages Clustered when extracellular	**Histoplasmosis**
	Yeast-like cells Round to oval (8–15 μm) Broad-based budding Thick walled	**Blastomycosis**
	Yeast-like cells Round to oval, large (3–30 μm) Multiple budding (buds attached to parent cell by narrow budding)	**Paracoccidiomycosis**
	Round to oval, budding yeast cells (3–6 μm) Branching septate hyphae and pseudohyphae Chains of budding cells	**Candidiasis**
	Yeast-like Mostly round (2–20 μm) Encapsulated Thin, dark walls Narrow-based budding	**Cryptococcosis**
	Round, oval sporangia (2–25 μm) Polyhedral endospores in sporangia No budding	**Prototothecosis**
	Spherules (10–100 μm) Thin-walled mature spherules Round endospores within spherules No budding	**Coccidiomycosis**
	Large, round sporangia (100–350 μm) Thick-walled sporangia Variably sized endospores Zonally arranged endospores No budding	**Rhinosporidiosis**

1. **A.** Spindle cell tumors are typically associated with infections by atypical mycobacteria.

   Mycobacterial spindle cell pseudotumor is a rare entity, probably representing an unusually pronounced histiocytic response to mycobacterial infection that can mimic a mesenchymal neoplasm. Most reported cases have occurred in immunocompromised patients, particularly in patients with HIV/AIDS and organ transplant recipients. More recently, a similar reaction pattern has been reported in association with TNF-alpha blockade. Mycobacterial spindle cell pseudotumor has been reported with various species of mycobacteria (see Table G1). Most commonly reported is the *Mycobacterium avium-intracellulare* complex, likely due to the high prevalence of infection with this organism, especially during the AIDS epidemic. *Mycobacterium tuberculosis* has been associated with spindle cell pseudotumor in which no visible organisms were seen on special stains (infection was detected by polymerase chain reaction). Reports of mycobacterial pseudotumor due to *Mycobacterium bovis* have been reported in the lymph nodes of neonates who were infected with attenuated strains in the bacille Calmette-Guérin (BCG) vaccination. Other mycobacterial species reported in spindle cell pseudotumor include *M. haemophilum* and *M. simiae*. Most mycobacterial spindle cell pseudotumors reported typically demonstrate many mycobacteria within the spindle cells. Other entities that may show a similar histopathologic reaction pattern include histioid leprosy and acrodermatitis chronica atrophicans.

2. **D.** Bullous impetigo is most commonly caused by staphylococcus.

   Bullous impetigo, caused almost exclusively by *Staphylococcus aureus*, is commonly due to exfoliative toxins of *S. aureus* termed exfoliatins A and B. These exotoxins cause a loss of cell adhesion in the superficial dermis, which, in turn, causes blisters and skin sloughing by cleaving of the granular cell layer of the epidermis.

   Both *S. aureus* and group A beta hemolytic streptococci (GABHS) cause non-bullous impetigo; *S. aureus* accounts for approximately 80% of cases, GABHS accounts for 10% of cases, and both organisms are recovered in 10% of cases. *S. aureus* produces bacteriotoxins toxic to streptococci. These bacteriotoxins may be the reason that only *S. aureus* is isolated in lesions that are caused predominantly by streptococci. While in the past, GABHS and *S. aureus* were equally frequent causative agents for non-bullous impetigo, currently *S. aureus* accounts for 50–60% of cases. In developing nations and warm climates, however, GABHS is still the more common cause.

3. **C.** Staphylococci are coagulase positive.

   The microscopic appearance of *Staphylococcus aureus* is round and resembles that of a sphere (cocci). Because of the way the bacteria divide and multiply, it will appear in clusters or tetrads. In Greek, staphylococcus means "clusters of grapes." The use of a common bacteriological stain, the Gram stain, helps to identify *S. aureus*. The organism will appear purple using this staining technique ("*Gram positive*"). When grown on bacteriological media, *Staphylococcus aureus* appears as a large white to golden colony. The majority of the time the colony of *Staphylococcus aureus* produces a zone of hemolysis surrounding the colony. Staph is not very fastidious and grows well, either aerobically or under anaerobic conditions, and produces good growth within 24 hours. *All staphylococci produce the enzyme catalase* when introduced to hydrogen peroxide. This test easily differentiates the staphylococci from the streptococci. *It also produces the enzyme coagulase* which allows the organism to produce a clot in rabbit plasma. *This is a key test to differentiate S. aureus from other staphylococci.*

4. **D.** *Staphylococcus caseolyticus* is NOT a common pathogenic species of staphylococcus.

   Regarding other species mentioned:
   - *S. aureus* is associated with pyogenic infections, toxin-induced diseases (such as gastroenteritis, toxic shock syndrome and scalded skin syndrome)
   - *S. epidermidis*, the most frequent coagulase-negative staph species to be isolated from the skin, is associated with infections secondary to implanted prosthetic devices
   - *S. saprophyticus*, also coagulase negative, is associated with 15–30% of urinary tract infections in sexually active women

5. **A.** Condyloma lata are NOT produced by chlamydia.
   Condyloma lata are characteristic papular lesions found on the penis or vulva in secondary syphilis and are caused by *Treponema pallidum*.
   Chlamydia trachomatis, an obligate intracellular pathogen, is a common cause of sexually transmitted urethritis and cervicitis. It is associated with pelvic inflammatory disease in females and with non-gonorrheal urethritis and acute epididymitis in males. Reiter's syndrome (genital infection plus conjunctivitis plus polyarthritis) is also a result of infection by *C. trachomatis*, as is lymphogranuloma venereum.

6. **D.** Body lice are the principal vectors of transmission of the causative organism in epidemic typhus.

   The causative organism, *Rickettsia prowazekii*, is a small bacteria-like obligate intracellular parasite that infects endothelial cells. Scrub typhus and Q fever are also rickettsial diseases causing vasculitis, but they are transmitted by mite and droplets respectively (also see Table G2). Bubonic plague is caused by *Yersinia pestis* and babesiosis by the malaria-like protozoan, *Babesia microti* (this organism is transmitted by the same deer tick that carries Lyme disease).

7. **E.** The pathogenicity of Legionnaire's disease, caused by Gram-negative *Legionella pneumophilia*, is NOT related to exotoxin production.

Ubiquitous in aquatic environments, the Gram-negative *Legionella* organism is a facultative, intracellular parasite of protozoa. The pathogenesis of legionellosis is largely due to the ability of *Legionella pneumophilia* to invade and grow within alveolar macrophages. *L. pneumophila* causes 2 distinct disease entities. Legionnaire's disease (LD) is characterized by pneumonia. Pontiac fever is a short-term, milder illness than LD and is not characterized by pneumonia, instead manifesting as fever and myalgias that resolve without treatment.

All of the other entities are the result of exotoxin production by the causative organisms.

8. **E.** Carbuncle is NOT caused by streptococci.

Carbuncles are deep-seated suppurative lesions of the skin and subcutaneous tissues that spread laterally beneath the fascia and then erupt on the skin surface with multiple adjacent sinuses. They are commonly caused by *Staphylococcus aureus*.

Impetigo is caused by either gr A streptococci (90%) or staphylococci (10%).

Erysipelas is caused by group A β-hemolytic streptococci.

Erythema nodosum is associated with γ-hemolytic streptococci as well as other infections.

Scarlet fever is caused by streptococcal infection and mediated by a phage-encoded pyrogenic exotoxin.

9. **A.** Impetigo may be caused by staphylococci.

Impetigo is caused by either group A streptococci (90%) or staphylococci (10%).

All the other entities are associated with infection by streptococci (see above).

Thrush is caused by *Candida albicans*.

10. **B.** Erythrasma is a cutaneous manifestation of an overabundance of coryneforms.

Erythrasma is caused by *Corynebacterium minutissimum* and presents as a well-defined, red-to-brown, scaling patch with a predilection for skin folds. The biopsy often appears normal.

The other two conditions associated with an overabundance of coryneforms include trichomycosis and pitted keratolysis.

11. **E.** Erysipeloid is associated with *Erysipelothrix rhusiopathiae*.

Erysipeloid is an acute bacterial infection of traumatized skin and other organs. Erysipeloid is caused by the microorganism *Erysipelothrix rhusiopathiae* (insidiosa),

which has long been known to cause animal and human infections. Direct contact between meats infected with *E. rhusiopathiae* and traumatized human skin results in erysipeloid. Humans acquire erysipeloid after direct contact with infected animals. Erysipeloid is more common among farmers, butchers, cooks, homemakers, and anglers. The infection is more likely to occur during the summer or early fall. Cutaneous forms of erysipeloid usually are self-limited even without treatment; therefore, skin-limited erysipeloid has a fairly good prognosis with no long-term sequelae.

12. **B.** *Corynebacterium minutissimum* is normal skin flora.

Erythrasma is caused by *Corynebacterium minutissimum*, a component of the normal skin flora. *C. minutissimum* is a Gram-positive, non-spore-forming, aerobic or facultative bacillus. Under conditions of moisture and occlusion, *C. minutissimum* proliferates in the upper levels of the stratum corneum. Erythrasma *most commonly involves the toe webs, followed by the groin and axilla*. A Wood's lamp examination depicting coral-red fluorescence confirms the diagnosis of erythrasma. This fluorescence is due to the production of porphyrins by *C. minutissimum*. The organism is difficult to detect on hematoxylin and eosin stained slides and thus presents as an invisible dermatosis; visualization may be enhanced by use of special stains such as periodic acid-Schiff and Giemsa.

13. **C.** Lupus vulgaris is the most common form of reinfection tuberculosis.

Lupus vulgaris (also known as tuberculosis luposa) are painful cutaneous tuberculosis skin lesions with a nodular appearance, most often on the face around the nose, eyelids, lips, cheeks, ear and neck. The lesions may ultimately develop into disfiguring skin ulcers if left untreated. Lupus vulgaris often develops due to inadequately treated pre-existing tuberculosis. It may also develop at the site of BCG vaccination. Rarely, it has been shown to be associated with tattoo marks and also with long-term bindi use, so-called "bindi tuberculosis." On diascopy, it shows characteristic "apple-jelly" color. Biopsy typically reveals paucibacillary tuberculoid granulomas.

14. **A.** Scrofuloderma is best described as cutaneous involvement secondary to direct extension.

Scrofuloderma also known as "tuberculosis cutis colliquativa" occurs when the skin becomes involved by direct extension from an underlying tuberculous infection (usually lymphadenitis). Although uncommon, scrofuloderma should be considered in cases of persistent lymphadenitis, particularly when there is cutaneous extension in patients from countries where tuberculosis is endemic.

15. **E.** *Mycobacterium ulcerans* is the causative organism in Buruli ulcer.

    Buruli ulcer, caused by *Mycobacterium ulcerans*, is a chronic, debilitating, necrotizing disease of the skin and soft tissue. Buruli ulcer is an emerging infectious disease and *is the third most common mycobacterial disease of the immunocompetent host*, after tuberculosis and leprosy. Although it has been reported in over 33 countries around the world, the greatest burden of disease is in the tropical regions of West and Central Africa, Australia, and Japan. It primarily affects children aged 5–15 years. Buruli ulcers generally begin as a painless dermal papule or subcutaneous edematous nodule, which, over a period of weeks to months, breaks down to form an extensive necrotic ulcer with undermined edges. The destructive effects are due to production of a soluble polyketide exotoxin called mycolactone, which can diffuse extensively in the subcutaneous tissue. Because mycolactone has both immunosuppressive and cytotoxic properties, dramatic tissue destruction occurs without inducing inflammation or systemic symptoms, such as fever, malaise, or adenopathy.

16. **D.** *Mycobacterium scrofulaceum* is NOT a Group I mycobacterium.

    Mycobacterium scrofulaceum is a scotochromogen or Group II mycobacterium. Other members in this group include *M. flavescens* and *M. szulgai* (also see Table G3).

17. **E.** Of the mycobacteria listed, *Mycobacterium chelonae* is the only one that is a rapid grower.

    Other members in this category (Group IV) include:

    M. fortuitum complex (*M. fortuitum, M. chelonae, M. abscessus*)
    M. phlei
    M. vaccae
    M. smegmatis
    M. diernhoferi

    Also see Table G3.

18. **A.** Lichen scrofulosorum is a tuberculid.

    Overall, tuberculids are heterogeneous groups of cutaneous lesions that occur in association with tuberculosis elsewhere. They typically occur in patients who have a heightened sensitivity or allergy to the organism. Papulonecrotic tuberculids (PNTs) and lichen scrofulosorum are still widely accepted as true tuberculids. Lichen scrofulosorum (also known as "tuberculosis cutis lichenoides") is a rare tuberculid that presents as a lichenoid eruption of minute papules in children and adolescents with tuberculosis. The lesions are usually asymptomatic, closely grouped, skin-colored to reddish-brown papules, often perifollicular and are

mainly found on the abdomen, chest, back, and proximal parts of the limbs. The eruption is usually associated with a strongly positive tuberculin reaction.

19. **C.** *Mycobacterium marinum*, the causative organism in swimming pool granuloma, is a photochromogen.

    Other characteristics of Group I mycobacteria include slow grower and lack of growth at 37 °C. A swimming pool granuloma occurs when water containing *Mycobacterium marinum* bacteria enters a break in the skin. Signs of a skin infection appear about 2 to 3 weeks later. Also see Table G3.

20. **B.** Tuberculoid leprosy is paucibacillary.

    The clinical manifestations of leprosy depend on the nature of the host's immune response to infection with *Mycobacterium leprae* and range from lepromatous leprosy (uncontrolled replication with nerve damage from high-titer infection) to tuberculoid leprosy (nerve and organ damage predominantly from the host granulomatous immune response). Tuberculoid leprosy is relatively stable clinically and the most common type in India and Africa. The lepromin test is positive. T_{HI} cytokines (particularly IL-2 and IFN-γ) are more strongly expressed in tuberculoid leprosy than in the other subtypes.

21. **B.** Lucio's phenomenon is associated with necrotizing vasculitis.

    Lucio's phenomenon is an acute lepra reaction in diffuse lepromatous leprosy characterized by cutaneous infarctions secondary to a necrotizing vasculitis. Lucio's phenomenon is seen almost exclusively in patients from the Caribbean and Mexico with diffuse, lepromatous leprosy, especially in untreated cases. It is characterized by recurrent crops of large, sharply demarcated, ulcerative lesions, affecting mainly the lower extremities, but may generalize and become fatal as a result of secondary bacterial infection and sepsis. The mechanism of pathogenesis is thought to be immune-complex mediated.

22. **B.** Herbivores are the primary host for anthrax.

    Anthrax is a zoonosis that primarily affects herbivorous animals. It is an occupational hazard of those handling hair/wool/hide/carcasses of infected animals. The causative organism is *Bacillus anthracis*, a rod-shaped, Gram-positive, aerobic bacterium. The lethality of the anthrax disease is due to the bacterium's two principal virulence factors: the poly-D-glutamic acid capsule, which protects the bacterium from phagocytosis by host neutrophils, and the tripartite protein toxin, called anthrax toxin. Anthrax toxin is a mixture of three protein components: protective antigen (PA), edema factor (EF), and lethal factor (LF). PA plus LF produces lethal toxin, and PA plus EF produces edema toxin. These toxins cause death and tissue swelling (edema), respectively. Clinically, eschar formation is characteristic and the "swab extraction tube system" has demonstrated good recovery of viable *B. anthracis* in culture. Humans are the incidental and not the primary host for anthrax.

23. **D.** The causative organism in granuloma inguinale is *Klebsiella granulomatosis*.

    The intracellular organism responsible for granuloma inguinale was initially described by Donovan over a century ago and, subsequently, the bacterium was classified in 1913 as *Calymmatobacterium granulomatis*. The molecular structure of the causative organism was similar to that of *Klebsiella* species and thus it was reclassified as the Gram-negative pleomorphic bacillus *Klebsiella granulomatis*. The mode of transmission of granuloma inguinale primarily occurs through sexual contact. Although the exact incubation period for granuloma inguinale is unknown, it ranges from a day to a year, with the median time being 50 days. The easiest method to visualize the organism is *via* smears from the base of the ulcer. The organisms are seen within the cytoplasm of histiocytes. Characteristically, they exhibit bipolar staining, which has been likened to a safety-pin appearance ("Donovan bodies").

24. **A.** Malakoplakia is NOT caused by *Bartonella*.

    Bartonella is a genus of Gram-negative bacteria. It is the only genus in the family Bartonellaceae. Facultative intracellular parasites, *Bartonella* species can infect healthy people, but are considered especially important as opportunistic pathogens. *Bartonella* species are transmitted by vectors such as ticks, fleas, sand flies, and mosquitoes. At least eight *Bartonella* species or subspecies are known to infect humans.

    The best known ones are the following:

    B. bacilliformis – Carrion's fever (Oroya fever, verruca peruana)
    B. quintana – Trench fever, bacillary angiomatosis, endocarditis
    B. clarridgeiae – Cat scratch disease
    B. henselae – Cat scratch disease, bacillary angiomatosis, peliosis hepatitis, endocarditis, bacteremia with fever, neuroretinitis

25. **B.** Image shown is that of a Michaelis-Gutmann body (M-G body).

    Michaelis-Gutmann bodies (M-G bodies) are concentrically layered basophilic inclusions found in the urinary tract. They are 2–10 μm in diameter, and are thought to represent remnants of phagosomes mineralized by iron and calcium deposits.

26. **C.** Michaelis-Gutmann bodies (M-G bodies) are associated with malakoplakia.

    M-G bodies are a pathognomonic feature of malakoplakia, an inflammatory condition that affects the genitourinary system. They were discovered in 1902 by Leonor Michaelis and Carl Gutmann. Malakoplakia is a rare granulomatous disease of infectious etiology. The name is derived from the Greek *malakos* (soft) and *plakos* (plaque), describing its usual clinical presentation as friable yellow soft plaques.

27. **E.** Arrows highlight the Mickulicz cell.

    The arrows highlight the Mikulicz cell – a large macrophage with clear cytoplasm that contains the bacilli; *this cell is specific to the lesions in rhinoscleroma*. Histopathologic findings correspond to clinical stages:
    - In the catarrhal (or atrophic) stage, squamous metaplasia and a non-specific subepithelial infiltrate of polymorphonuclear leukocytes with granulation tissue are observed.
    - In the granulomatous stage, the diagnostic features include chronic inflammatory cells, Russell bodies, pseudoepitheliomatous hyperplasia, and groups of large vacuolated histiocytes that contain *Klebsiella rhinoscleromatis* organisms (Mikulicz cells). However, the groups, clusters, or sheets of large (100 to 200 μm) vacuolated histiocytes (i.e. Mikulicz cells) that contain the causative agent are most striking. Although the organisms are occasionally visible on standard hematoxylin and eosin stains, they are more readily demonstrated by using silver impregnation Warthin-Starry stains. Electron microscopy reveals large phagosomes filled with bacilli and surrounded by a finely granular or fibrillar material that is arranged in a radial pattern. This finding represents the accumulation of antibodies on the bacterial surface (type A granules), as well as the aggregation of bacterial mucopolysaccharides surrounded by antibodies (type B granules).

28. **E.** The Mickulicz cell is specific to rhinoscleroma.

    Mickulicz cells are seen in rhinoscleroma, a chronic granulomatous condition of the nose and other structures of the upper respiratory tract. Rhinoscleroma is a result of infection by the bacterium *Klebsiella rhinoscleromatis*.

29. **E.** Rocky mountain spotted fever is a tick-transmitted rickettsial infection.

    Other tick-transmitted rickettsial infections include Boutonneuse fever, African tick bite fever, Siberian tick typhus and Queensland tick typhus. Also see Table G2.

30. **D.** Rickettsialpox is mite transmitted.

    The causative organism of Rickettsialpox is *Rickettsia akari*. The only other mite-transmitted rickettsial disease is Scrub typhus, although the causative organism is different (*Orientia tsutsugamushi*). Also see Table G2.

31. **B.** Gonorrhea does NOT produce a penile ulcer.

    In males, gonococcal infection produces a mucopurulent discharge and meatal inflammation but no ulceration. Infection may extend retrograde into the posterior urethra, epididymis, prostate and seminal vesicles. Urethral strictures and sterility are the result of chronic infection in untreated males. All of the other entities listed (syphilis, chancroid, granuloma inguinale and genital herpes) can cause a penile ulcer.

32. **B.** Lyme disease is NOT caused by rickettsia.

    Lyme disease is caused by the spirochete *Borrelia burgdorferi*. Lyme disease is classified as a zoonosis, as it is transmitted to humans from a natural reservoir among small mammals and birds by ticks that feed on both sets of hosts. Hard-bodied ticks of the genus *Ixodes* are the main vectors of Lyme disease (also the vector for *Babesia*). Most infections are caused by ticks in the nymphal stage, because they are very small and thus may feed for long periods of time undetected. Larval ticks are very rarely infected. Although deer are the preferred hosts of the adult stage of deer ticks, and tick populations are much lower in the absence of deer, ticks generally do not acquire Lyme disease spirochetes from deer. Rather, deer ticks acquire *Borrelia* microbes from infected small mammals and occasionally birds, including the white-footed mouse, *Peromyscus leucopus*.

33. **E.** "Strawberry mucosa" is associated with trichomoniasis.

    Trichomoniasis is a common sexually transmitted parasitic infection caused by the flagellate *Trichomonas vaginalis*.

34. **D.** *Neisseria gonorrhoeae* does NOT produce exotoxins.

    N. gonorrhoeae is a facultative intracellular pathogen that causes pelvic inflammatory disease in females and urethritis in males. Capsular polysaccharides contribute to the virulence of the organism by inhibiting phagocytosis in the absence of anti-gonococcal antibodies. *Neisseria* make proteases that are capable of lysing IgA.

35. **C.** The causative organism of lymphogranuloma venereum is *C. trachomatis*.

    Regarding other organisms listed:

    Haemophilus ducreyi causes chancroid
    Yersinia pseudotuberculosis causes Far East scarlet-like fever
    Klebsiella granulomatosis causes granuloma inguinale
    Neisseria gonorrhoeae causes gonorrhea

36. **A.** Chancre is a feature of primary syphilis.

    The incubation period for primary syphilis is 14 to 21 days. Symptoms of primary syphilis are a small, painless open sore or ulcer (called a chancre) on the genitals, mouth, skin, or rectum that heals by itself in 3 to 6 weeks as well as enlarged lymph nodes in the area of the sore.

37. **C.** A mucocutaneous eruption is associated with secondary syphilis.

    The symptoms of secondary syphilis start 4 to 8 weeks after the primary syphilis. The symptoms may include a skin rash (usually on the palms of the hands and soles of the feet), sores called mucous patches (in or around the mouth, vagina, or penis), moist, warty patches (called condylomata lata) in the genitals or skin folds, fever, malaise, loss of appetite, arthralgias, enlarged lymph nodes, changes in vision and even hair loss.

38. **A.** Hutchinson's triad consists of interstitial keratitis, malformed teeth (Hutchinson incisors and mulberry molars), and eighth nerve deafness.

    Hutchinson's triad is named after Sir Jonathan Hutchinson (1828–1913). It is a common pattern of presentation for congenital syphilis.

39. **E.** Hutchinson's triad is associated with congenital syphilis.

    Congenital syphilis is caused by transplacental transmission of spirochetes; the transmission rate approaches 90% if the mother has untreated primary or secondary syphilis. Fetal infection can develop at any time during gestation. Manifestations are defined as *early* if they appear in the first 2 years of life and *late* if they develop after age 2 years.

    About 60% of infants born with congenital syphilis are asymptomatic at birth. Symptoms develop within the first 2 months of life. In symptomatic infants, the most common physical finding, reported in almost 100% of cases, is hepatomegaly; biochemical evidence of liver dysfunction is usually observed. The other common findings are skeletal abnormalities, rash, and generalized lymphadenopathy. Radiographic abnormalities, periostitis or osteitis, involve multiple bones and are seen in the vast majority of symptomatic infants, but they also can be found in one-fifth of infants with no symptoms or relevant findings on physical examination. Sometimes, the lesion is painful and an infant will favor an extremity (pseudopalsy). The rash is maculopapular and may involve palms and soles. In contrast to acquired syphilis, a vesicular rash and bullae may develop. These lesions are also highly contagious. Mucosal involvement may present as rhinitis ("snuffles"). Nasal secretions are highly contagious. Hematological abnormalities include anemia and thrombocytopenia. Some have leukocytosis.

Abnormal CSF examination is seen in half of symptomatic infants but also can be found in 10% of those who are asymptomatic.

Manifestations of late-onset congenital syphilis (diagnosed >2 years) include neurosyphilis, bone involvement (saber shins, saddle nose), teeth involvement (notched, peg-shaped incisors, Hutchinson teeth), pigmentary involvement (linear scars, rhagades, at the corners of the mouth), interstitial keratitis (typically presents in the first or second decade of life), sensory-neural hearing loss (eighth cranial nerve deafness, presents between age 10 and 40 years) and the classic Hutchinson triad.

40. **B.** Chancre is NOT associated with tertiary syphilis.

Tertiary neurosyphilis presents with symptoms of meningitis or with focal deficits consistent with stroke. The mnemonic device PARESIS is an aid to recall the following symptoms and signs: *Personality, Affect, Reflexes* (e.g., hyperactive), *Eye* (e.g., Argyll Robertson pupils), *Sensorium* (e.g., illusions, delusions, hallucinations), *Intellect* (e.g., decreased recent memory, orientation, judgment, insight) and *Speech* abnormalities. Gumma, a localized destructive lesion, can appear in virtually any tissue in tertiary syphilis. Other lesions present only in tertiary syphilis include tabes dorsalis and Charcot's joints. Obliterative endarteritis, the histopathologic hallmark of syphilis, can occur in any stage of syphilis including tertiary syphilis.

41. **C.** *Treponema pallidum* is the causative organism of yaws.

Yaws is the most prevalent infectious, non-venereal treponemal disease and is caused by *Treponema pallidum pertenue*. Yaws, endemic syphilis (bejel), and pinta collectively constitute the endemic treponematoses. Yaws is transmitted by direct skin contact and primarily affects children younger than 15 years, with a peak incidence in those aged 6–10 years. Similar to syphilis, yaws can persist for years as a chronic, relapsing disease.

42. **A.** *Trichophyton rubrum* is the most common cause of dermatophyte infection worldwide.

Trichophyton rubrum is the most common causative agent of dermatophytosis worldwide, mainly occupying the human feet, skin, and between fingernails. *T. rubrum* is known to be one of the most prominent anthrophilic species of dermatophytes, a fungus commonly causing skin diseases, appearing in various shades of white, yellow, brown, and red. It may also be found in various textures, being waxy, cottony, or smooth. Even though it is commonly observed, *T. rubrum* infections are incredibly hard to diagnose, and difficult to differentiate from other dermatophytes. The fungal pathogen's ability to produce and secrete proteolytic enzymes is a major virulence factor.

43. **D.** Favus is most characteristic of infection by *Trichophyton schonleinii*.

Rarely, favus is caused by *Trichophyton violaceum*, *Trichophyton mentagrophytes* var *quinckeanum*, or *Microsporum gypseum*. Favus typically affects scalp hair but also may infect glabrous skin and nails.

44. **D.** *Trichophyton rubrum, T. mentogrophytes, Epidermophyton floccosum* are common causative organisms of tinea barbae, tinea corporis and tinea cruris.

45. **B.** Pseudohyphae are characteristic of *Candida albicans*.

While both hyphae and pseudohyphae are filaments that are composed of fungal cells arranged next to each other as a chain, they can be found in polymorphic fungi and in some dimorphic fungi, and components help to bear reproductive structures, differences between them are as follows:

- Hyphae may or may not contain septa, whereas pseudohyphae always contain septa
- There is no constriction at the location of septa found in hyphae, whereas a constriction is found in pseudohyphae
- Hyphae can be coenocytic (single celled, multinuclear) or multicellular, but pseudohyphae are always multicellular
- Hyphae do not show budding whereas pseudohyphae do show budding through which they grow continuously
- Hyphae are always stationary, whereas pseudohyphae are used to invade cells by growing faster by budding, showing some kind of mobility

Also see Table G7 and Table G8.

46. **A.** Image shown is that of *Cryptococcus neoformans*.

C. neoformans is the most common species in the USA and other temperate climates throughout the world and is found in aged pigeon droppings. Worldwide, *C. neoformans* serotype A causes most cryptococcal infections in immunocompromised patients, including patients infected with HIV. *C. gattii* rarely infects persons with HIV infection and other immunosuppressed patients. Patients infected with *C. gattii* are usually immunocompetent, respond slowly to treatment, and are at risk for developing intracerebral mass lesions (e.g., cryptococcomas). *C. neoformans* reproduces by budding and forms round yeast-like cells that are 3–6 μm in diameter. Within the host and in certain culture media, a large polysaccharide capsule surrounds each cell. The principal site or sites of infection (i.e., pulmonary, CNS, disseminated disease) dictate the medical history of patients with symptomatic cryptococcal disease. Factors that are especially important include the presence of coexisting conditions associated with immunosuppression (e.g., steroid use, malignant disease, transplantation) or HIV infection.

India ink, which outlines the organisms by negative contrast, helps to identify the yeast cells in fluids or macerated tissue samples. In fixed tissue, the capsule of *C. neoformans* may also be stained with mucicarmine, which preferentially stains mucopolysaccharides. Tissue sections can be stained with the Fontana-Masson stain to detect melanin precursors in the yeast cell wall. The presence of melanin or melanin precursors is useful in differentiating *C. neoformans* from other yeasts. Also see Table G7 and Table G8.

47. **B.** Image shown is that of pityrosporum folliculitis.

The diagnosis of pityrosporum folliculitis is based on clinical suspicion of the classic presentation of pruritic papulopustules found in a follicular pattern on the back, chest, upper arms, and occasionally the neck of young to middle-aged adults. They are rarely present on the face. An improvement in the lesions with empiric antimycotic therapy supports a clinical diagnosis of pityrosporum folliculitis.

The basic lesion observed is that of folliculitis. The ostium of the hair follicles is dilated, partially disrupted with keratin plugging, cellular debris, and an inflammatory infiltrate including lymphocytes, histiocytes, and neutrophils. Some follicles may be cystic and ruptured. Single as well as aggregates of spores are noted within the follicle. A useful aid to the diagnosis is the presence of basophilic debris adjacent to a partially disrupted follicle. Also see Table G7.

48. **C.** The causative organism of pityrosporum folliculitis is *Malassezia furfur*.

Yeasts, specifically *Malassezia furfur*, are the pathogenic agents in pityrosporum folliculitis. *M. furfur* has been linked to several skin diseases, including seborrheic dermatitis, folliculitis, confluent and reticulated papillomatosis, and pityriasis versicolor. In 1874, Malassez first described round and oval budding yeasts from scales of patients with seborrheic dermatitis. He coined the phrases "bottle bacillus of Unna" to describe the small oval cells in the scale and "spore of Malassez" to name the bud that is observed in association with the yeast. Saborouraud proposed the *Pityrosporum* genus in 1904 to describe the budding yeast cells without hyphal elements from normal skin. Later, in the 1900s, *Pityrosporum ovale* and *Pityrosporum orbiculare* were isolated. Pityrosporum folliculitis is caused by *Malassezia* species that *are part of the cutaneous microflora* and not by exogenous species.

49. **D.** The most likely causative organism is *Pityrosporum ovale*.

Pityrosporum ovale (also known as *P. orbicularis* and *Malassezia furfur*) is a dimorphic lipophilic yeast that normally resides in the skin. It is an opportunistic infection and causes pityriasis versicolor, a chronic asymptomatic scaling dermatosis associated with overgrowth of the hyphal form of *P. ovale*. Clinically, it is characterized by well-demarcated scaling patches with variable pigmentation occurring most commonly on the trunk. *Pityrosporum* infections, although not contagious and secondary to an overgrowth of resident cutaneous flora under certain favorable conditions, are chronic and recurrent. Image shows numerous round budding yeasts (blastoconidia) and short septate hyphae (pseudomycelium) giving the so called "*spaghetti and meatballs*" appearance.

50. **D.** *Blastomyces dermatitidis* is NOT a dematiaceous fungus.

Subcutaneous dematiaceous fungal infections, which include chromoblastomycosis and phaeohyphomycosis, are a heterogeneous group of clinical entities caused by dematiaceous or pigmented fungi that are found in soil. These infections have a wide spectrum of clinical presentations that depend largely on the specific causative organism and on the integrity of the host's immune response. Chromoblastomycosis and phaeohyphomycosis are both caused by pigmented fungi and share a number of clinical features and causative organisms, yet are considered two distinct clinical entities. Phaeohyphomycosis designates fungal infections caused by pheoid or melanized fungi and characterized histopathologically by the presence of septate hyphae, pseudohyphae, and yeasts. Etiologic agents of phaeohyphomycosis include *Exophiala, Phoma, Bipolaris, Phialophora, Colletotrichum, Curvularia, Alternaria, Exserohilum*, and *Phialemonium* spp. Etiologic agents of chromomycosis include *Fonsecaea pedrosoi, Phialophora compacta, Phialophora verrucosa, Cladosporium carrioni, Aureobasidium pullalans* and *Rhinocladiella aquapersa*. Other species implicated include *Exophiala jeanselmei* and *Wangiella dermatitidis*. Other dematiaceous fungi include the dimorphic fungus *Sporothrix schenkii, Tinea nigra* and *Alternaria*.

51. **B.** Image shown is that of phaeohyphomycosis.

The clinical presentation of phaeohyphomycosis depends on the immune status of the host: superficial (tinea nigra and black piedra); cutaneous (scytalidiosis) and corneal; subcutaneous (mycotic cyst); and systemic phaeohyphomycosis in the immunocompromised host.

The mycotic cyst is a localized form, characterized by subcutaneous asymptomatic nodular lesions that develop after traumatic implantation of fungi, especially on the extremities. The average size of the cysts is 2.5 cm. KOH examination reveals pigmented yeasts, pseudohyphae, and hyphae. In terms of histopathology, the characteristic lesion, as evidenced in the figure, is a circumscribed cyst or chronic abscess in the deep dermis or subcutis. The wall of this is typically composed of compressed fibrous tissue with an adjacent granulomatous tissue reaction. A wood splinter or foreign body may be seen in the central cystic portion and brown filamentous hyphae may be seen in the wall, in the giant cells or even in the debris. Also see Table G7 and Table G8.

52. **C.** Image shown is that of chromomycosis.

The diagnosis of chromoblastomycosis rests on identification of thick-walled, multiseptate, brown, sclerotic cells termed *medlar bodies, copper pennies*, or *muriform cells* (shown in the image). These pathognomonic features can be observed in tissue biopsy specimens or by direct microscopic examination of a scraping of black dots from the surface of the nodule with 10% potassium hydroxide. Identification of the causative fungal species can be achieved by tissue culture but is not reliably positive. Chromoblastomycosis is a subcutaneous infection with highest prevalence in the tropics; it is typically seen in immunocompetent hosts and results from traumatic inoculation of skin by pigmented fungi. The principal causative agents are fungi of the genera *Fonsecaea* (tropical forests), *Cladophialophora* (dry climates), and *Phialophora*. *Fonsecaea* is most commonly isolated except in Australia where *Cladosporium carrioni* is typically responsible. The disease is most commonly observed in agriculturists on the lower legs, which likely explains the observed propensity for men of lower socioeconomic status. Chromoblastomycosis typically presents with an asymptomatic papule or nodule that develops slowly over years into a localized verrucous plaque that expands and leaves behind a central sclerotic or keloidal scar. The lesion may have characteristic black dots on the surface, which represent the host's attempt at transepidermal elimination of fungal elements. The disease most often remains localized, but satellite lesions from autoinoculation and lymphatic spread have been documented. Also see Table G7 and Table G8.

53. **D.** Image shown is that of coccidiomycosis.

Infection is typically transmitted by inhalation of airborne spores of *Coccidioides immitis* or *C. posadasii*. The vast majority of coccidioidal infections result from airborne transmission. Pulmonary infection can result from inhalation of a single spore in humans, but high inoculum exposures are more likely to result in symptomatic disease. Inhaled *C. immitis* or *C. posadasii* arthroconidia (i.e., spores) are deposited into the terminal bronchiole.

The arthroconidia enlarge to form spherules, which are round double-walled structures measuring approximately 20–100 μm in diameter. The spherules undergo internal division within 48–72 hours and become filled with hundreds to thousands of offspring (i.e., endospores).

Rupture of the spherules leads to the release of endospores, which mature to form more spherules. As an arthroconidium transforms into a spherule, the resulting inflammation results in a local pulmonary lesion. Extracts of *C. immitis* organisms react with complement, leading to the release of mediators of chemotaxis for neutrophils. Some of the endospores are engulfed by macrophages, initiating the acute inflammation phase. If the infection is not cleared during this process, a new set of lymphocytes and histiocytes descend on the infection site, leading to granuloma formation with the presence of giant cells. This is the chronic inflammation phase. People with severe disease may have both acute and chronic forms of inflammation. Also see Table G7 and Table G8.

54. **D.** Coccidiomycosis is endemic in Mexico.

Coccidiomycosis is caused by *Coccidioides immitis*, a soil fungus native to the San Joaquin Valley of California, and by *C. posadasii*, which is endemic to certain arid-to-semiarid areas of the southwestern USA, northern portions of Mexico, and scattered areas in Central America and South America. Although genetically distinct, the 2 species are morphologically identical.

55. **A.** Image shown is that of sporotrichosis.

Sporotrichosis is characterized histopathologically by granulomatous inflammation with occasional asteroid bodies. The sporothrix may be present in the tissue as yeast-like forms, as elongate cells ("cigar bodies") or, albeit rarely, as hyphae. The "sporothrix asteroid" is the pathognomonic finding and is characterized by a blastospore surrounded by radiating strands of intensely basophilic, hyaline material.

Sporotrichosis is a subacute or chronic infection caused by the saprophytic dimorphic fungus *Sporothrix schenckii*. The characteristic infection involves suppurating subcutaneous nodules that progress proximally along lymphatic channels (lymphocutaneous sporotrichosis).

In lymphocutaneous sporotrichosis, the primary lesion develops at the site of cutaneous inoculation, typically in the distal upper extremities. After several weeks, new lesions appear along the lymphatic tracts. Patients with this form are typically afebrile and not systemically ill. The lesions usually cause minimal pain. The fixed cutaneous form is characterized by a painless violaceous or erythematous plaque that may ulcerate or become verrucous. This presentation should be considered when a wound fails to heal. There are no satellite lesions. The disseminated cutaneous form is usually seen in immunosuppressed individuals. This form of the disease can be the initial presentation of HIV infection or may develop as part of an immune reconstitution syndrome. Also see Table G7 and Table G8.

56. **C.** Blastomycosis is characterized by broad-based buds and lack of an endospore and capsule.

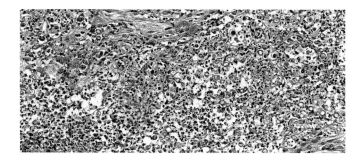

Microscopically, yeasts 8–20 μm in size, with single, broad-based buds, double refractile walls, and multiple nuclei, are extremely characteristic of *Blastomyces dermatitidis*. *B. dermatitidis* mold has a distinctive "lollipop" appearance with oval conidia, 2–4 μm in diameter, at the tips of thin conidiophores. They also have thin septate hyphae, 1–2 μm in diameter. Blastomycosis is a fungal infection caused by inhalation of aerosolized conidia (spores) of *Blastomyces dermatitidis*. Clinical presentations occur across a wide spectrum, ranging from an asymptomatic, self-limited pulmonary infection to widely disseminated life-threatening disease. Blastomycosis is endemic to the USA and Canada and most cases are clustered around the Mississippi and Ohio River Valley states and Canadian provinces around the Great Lakes. Within the USA, the most commonly affected states are Arkansas, Illinois, Kentucky, Louisiana, Mississippi, North Carolina, Tennessee, and Wisconsin. Exposure to soil is the common factor associated with contracting this disease. Blastomycosis is recognized increasingly in immunocompromised hosts, particularly in patients with acquired immune deficiency syndrome (AIDS). Also see Table G7 and Table G8.

57. **B.** The best-fit diagnosis for the image shown is histoplasmosis.

Tissue biopsy results may reveal the presence of yeast forms in tissue through hematoxylin and eosin staining. Using the Grocott-Gomori methenamine-silver procedure, yeast may be detected in areas of caseation necrosis. Typically, numerous parasitized macrophages containing small ovoid, yeast-like organisms with a clear surrounding halo are evident. *Histoplasma capsulatum* is a dimorphic fungus that remains in a mycelial form at ambient temperatures and grows as yeast at body temperature in mammals. Infection causes histoplasmosis. Most individuals with histoplasmosis are asymptomatic. Those who develop clinical manifestations are usually immunocompromised or are exposed to a high quantity of inoculum. *Histoplasma* species may remain latent in healed granulomas and recur, resulting in cell-mediated immunity impairment.

Clinical presentations include asymptomatic pulmonary histoplasmosis, symptomatic pulmonary histoplasmosis, acute diffuse pulmonary histoplasmosis, chronic pulmonary histoplasmosis, acute respiratory distress syndrome, disseminated histoplasmosis, broncholithiasis, mediastinal granuloma, fibrosing mediastinitis, endobronchial histoplasmosis, and lung nodules. Also see Table G7 and Table G8.

58. **D.** Histoplasmosis is endemic in southeastern parts of USA.

Although the fungus that causes histoplasmosis can be found in temperate climates throughout the world, it is endemic to the Ohio, Missouri, and Mississippi River valleys in the USA. Internationally, the fungus is predominantly found in river valleys in North and Central America, eastern and southern Europe, and parts of Africa, eastern Asia, and Australia.

The soil in areas endemic for histoplasmosis provides an acidic damp environment with high organic content that is good for mycelial growth. Highly infectious soil is found near areas inhabited by bats and birds, such as caves and chicken coops. Decaying trees and riverbanks also make good habitats for incubations. Birds cannot be infected by the fungus and do not transmit the disease; however, bird excretions contaminate the soil, thereby enriching the growth medium for the mycelium. In contrast, bats can become infected and they transmit histoplasmosis through droppings. Contaminated soil can be potentially infectious for years. Outbreaks of histoplasmosis have been associated with construction and renovation activities that disrupt contaminated soil. In addition, travelers to endemic areas are at risk for histoplasmosis because airborne spores can travel hundreds of feet.

59. **A.** The best-fit diagnosis for the image shown is mycetoma.

Mycetoma is a chronic infection of skin and subcutaneous tissue. The condition was first described in the mid-1800s and was initially named Madura foot, after the region of Madura in India where the disease was first identified. Mycetoma infection can be caused by fungi or bacteria (see Table G4). When caused by fungi, it is referred to as mycotic mycetoma or eumycetoma. When it is caused by bacteria, it usually involves infection by the actinomycetes group; such cases are called actinomycotic mycetoma or actinomycetoma. Involvement of the lower extremities is common, and the disease presentation, whether caused by fungi or bacteria, is quite similar. Mycetoma occurs most often in farmers, shepherds, Bedouins, nomads, and people living in rural areas. Frequent exposure to penetrating wounds by thorns or splinters is a risk factor, especially in combination with contaminated soil material.

Actinomycetoma can be caused by the following:

Nocardia species
Actinomadura madurae
Actinomadura pelletieri
Streptomyces somaliensis

Eumycetoma is mainly caused by the following:

Petriellidium boydii (*Scedosporium apiospermum*)
Madurella mycetomatis or *M. grisea*

The color of the grains is sometimes helpful in pinpointing the exact etiologic agent. For example, the grains of *M. mycetomatis* or *M. grisea* are typically black, while those of *Petriellidium boydii* and several actinomycetes are usually faint yellowish or white.

60. **D.** *Nocardia* is a Gram-positive, acid-fast bacillus.

Nocardia organisms are branching, beaded, filamentous, Gram-positive bacteria with a characteristic morphology (also see Table G8). *Nocardia* are typically weakly acid-fast after traditional staining and positive on modified acid-fast staining. *N. brasiliensis* is the most common cause of progressive cutaneous and lymphocutaneous (sporotrichoid) disease.

Nocardial species can cause mycetoma, a chronic, swollen, purulence-draining, subcutaneous infection of the extremities, typically encountered in tropical areas of the world, but also reported from the southern USA, Central and South Americas, and Australia. It is usually ascribed to *N. brasiliensis*.

61. **C.** The best-fit diagnosis for the image shown is mucormycosis.

Stains of fixed tissues with hematoxylin and eosin (H&E) or specialized fungal stains, such as Grocott methenamine-silver or periodic acid-Schiff (PAS) stains, show pathognomonic changes of mucormycosis of broad-based (typically 10–20 μm diameter), irregular, ribbon-like, non-septate hyphae with irregular branching that may occur at right angles. Vascular invasion and necrosis are the characteristic consequences of the infective process. Also see Table G7 and Table G8.

Mucormycosis refers to several different diseases caused by infection with fungi in the order of Mucorales. *Rhizopus* species are the most common causative organisms. In descending order, the other genera with mucormycosis-causing species include *Mucor, Cunninghamella, Apophysomyces, Absidia, Saksenaea, Rhizomucor,* and other species. Most mucormycosis infections are life threatening, and risk factors, such as diabetic ketoacidosis and neutropenia, are present in most cases. Severe infection of the facial sinuses, which may extend into the brain, is the most common presentation. Based on

anatomic localization, mucormycosis can be classified as 1 of 6 forms: (1) rhinocerebral, (2) pulmonary, (3) cutaneous, (4) gastrointestinal, (5) disseminated, and (6) uncommon presentations.

62. **D.** The best-fit diagnosis for the image shown is aspergillosis.

Aspergillus hyphae are histologically distinct from other fungi in that the hyphae have frequent septae, which branch at 45° angles (also see Table G7 and Table G8). The hyphae are best visualized in tissue with silver stains. Although many species of *Aspergillus* have been isolated in nature, *A. fumigatus* is the most common cause of infection in humans. *Aspergillus* species are ubiquitous molds found in organic matter. Although more than 100 species have been identified, the majority of human illness is caused by *Aspergillus fumigatus* and *Aspergillus niger* and, less frequently, by *Aspergillus flavus* and *Aspergillus clavatus*. The transmission of fungal spores to the human host is *via* inhalation. The four most common manifestations of *Aspergillus* are as follows: lung disease (i.e., allergic bronchopulmonary aspergillosis), aspergilloma, chronic necrotizing pulmonary aspergillosis, and invasive aspergillosis.

63. **E.** The best-fit diagnosis for the image shown is rhinosporidiosis.

Rhinosporidiosis is a chronic granulomatous infection of the mucous membranes that usually manifests as vascular friable polyps that arise from the nasal mucosa or external structures of the eye. Rhinosporidiosis is endemic in India, Sri Lanka, South America, and Africa. The etiologic agent of rhinosporidiosis, *Rhinosporidium seeberi,* has traditionally been considered a fungus. Recent 18S ribosomal ribonucleic acid (rRNA) gene analysis has placed *R. seeberi* into a novel group of aquatic parasites of the class Mesomycetozoea, some of which cause similar diseases in amphibians and fish. The life cycle begins with a round endospore that is 6–10 μm in diameter. The endospore grows to become a thick-walled sporangium 100–350 μm in diameter that contains up to several thousand endospores. These structures are similar to the smaller endospores (2–5 μm in diameter) and spherules (30–60 μm in diameter) of *Coccidioides immitis.*

The sporangia of *R. seeberi* are observed under the normal epithelium. They are associated with immune cells, including neutrophils, lymphocytes, plasma cells, and multinucleated giant cells, often in scattered granulomas. Also see Table G7 and Table G8.

64. **C.** Image shown is that of molluscum bodies.

The striking feature of molluscum infection is the presence of intracytoplasmic, eosinophilic, granular inclusions within the keratinocytes of the basal, spinous, and granular layers of the epidermis. These inclusions, the *Henderson-Paterson bodies*, can measure 35 μm in diameter. Ultrastructural studies have shown that these bodies are membrane-bound sacs that contain numerous molluscum contagiosum virions. The viral particles increase in size as they progress up toward the granular layer, causing compression of the nucleus to the periphery of the infected keratinocytes.

Molluscum contagiosum is a viral disease caused by a DNA poxvirus and is largely (if not exclusively) a disease of humans. It is an unclassified member of the Poxviridae family (i.e., poxviruses). Clinically, it causes characteristic skin lesions consisting of single or, more often, multiple, rounded, dome-shaped, pink, waxy papules that are usually 2–5 mm (rarely up to 1.5 cm in the case of a giant molluscus) in diameter. The papules are umbilicated and typically contain a caseous plug. The poxviruses are a large group of viruses with a high molecular weight. They are the largest animal viruses, only slightly smaller than the smallest bacteria, and are just visible using light microscopy. They are complex DNA viruses that replicate in the cytoplasm and are especially adapted to epidermal cells. They cannot be grown in tissue culture or eggs. Humans are the host for the following 3 types of molluscum contagiosum virus:

Orthopoxvirus – This resembles variola (smallpox) and vaccinia, which are ovoid

Parapoxvirus – These are orf and Milker's nodule viruses, which are cylindrical

Unclassified (with features that are intermediate between those of the orthopox and parapox groups) – These are intermediate in structure and include molluscum contagiosum virus and tanapox

65. **A.** The causative organism of Milker's nodule is parapoxvirus belonging to the Poxviridae family.

The etiologic organism is the Milker's nodule virus, also called paravaccinia virus. The Milker's nodule virus is a 140 nm × 310 nm, double-stranded DNA poxvirus, a member of the cylindrical subgroup (see above). The disease is a zoonosis, endemic to and common in cattle worldwide. Infections in cattle are also known as bovine papular stomatitis. Human disease is contracted through direct transmission (i.e., handling of infected cow teats, calf muzzles, or other sites of active bovine infection) or through indirect transmission (i.e., handling of virally contaminated objects). The course of Milker's nodule is usually self-limited, running from 14–72 days, with infrequent systemic symptoms and little or no scarring.

The histopathologic appearance of Milker's nodule varies with the stage of the disease and is similar to orf. Early lesions show ballooning of keratinocytes, spongiform appearance of vacuolated cells with wispy eosinophilic cytoplasm, vesicle formation, prominent cell membranes, and pyknotic nuclei. There may be eosinophilic intracytoplasmic viral inclusions and rarely intranuclear inclusions. Later in the course of disease, Milker's nodules demonstrate irregular acanthosis with pronounced deep extensions of thin rete ridges. Epidermal necrosis is variable.

66. **D.** Ecthyma contagiosum is also known as orf.

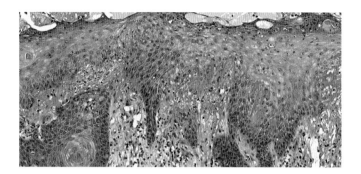

Orf occurs in humans with an occupational or household exposure to the virus. The incubation period is 3–7 days, and then orf usually appears as a small papule; 95% of cases occur on the hands. Orf generally manifests as a solitary lesion. Dermoscopic examination demonstrates a well-defined nodule with a central crust, white structureless areas, and white shiny streaks, surrounded by dotted vessels, hairpin vessels, and a fine peripheral scale.

In terms of histopathologic findings, the epidermis usually shows marked pseudoepitheliomatous hyperplasia. Necrosis of the epidermis with ulceration occurs in the center of the lesion. The orf viral infection causes intranuclear and intracytoplasmic inclusion bodies with vacuolization and disaggregation of keratinocytes. Pyknosis of individual keratinocytes occurs as does a dense inflammatory infiltrate of plasma cells, macrophages, histiocytes, and lymphocytes.

67. **B.** Varicella does NOT belong to the Poxviridae family.

Members of the Poxviridae family include cowpox, vaccinia, variola, monkeypox, molluscum contagiosum, Milker's nodule and orf.

Varicella belongs to the Herpesviridae family. Other members of this include HSV, HZV, CMV and EBV.

68. **B.** HSV-1 and HSV-2 are biologically and serologically distinct.

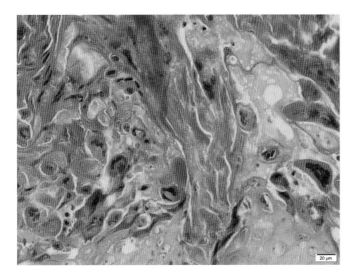

Histopathologic changes shown above are common *to both* HSV-1 and HSV-2. Briefly, these include ballooning degeneration, reticular degeneration, acantholysis and the distinctive viral cytopathic changes of *m*argination of chromatin, *m*ultinucleation and *m*olding evident in keratinocytes. HSV belongs to the alpha herpesvirus group. It is a non-enveloped virus that is approximately 160 nm in diameter with a linear, double-stranded DNA genome. The overall sequence homology between HSV-1 and HSV-2 is about 50%. HSV-1 has tropism for oral epithelium, while HSV-2 has tropism for genital epithelium. HSV infection is mediated through attachment *via* ubiquitous receptors to cells, including sensory neurons, leading to establishment of latency.

HSV-1 and HSV-2 are characterized by the following unique biological properties:

- *Neurovirulence* (the capacity to invade and replicate in the nervous system)
- *Latency* (the establishment and maintenance of latent infection in nerve cell ganglia proximal to the site of infection): In orofacial HSV infections, the trigeminal ganglia are most commonly involved, while, in genital HSV infection, the sacral nerve root ganglia (S2-S5) are involved
- *Reactivation*: The reactivation and replication of latent HSV, always in the area supplied by the ganglia in which latency was established, can be induced by various stimuli (e.g., fever, trauma, emotional stress, sunlight, menstruation), resulting in overt or covert recurrent infection and shedding of HSV. In immunocompetent persons who are at an equal risk of acquiring HSV-1 and HSV-2 both orally and genitally, HSV-1 reactivates more frequently in the oral rather than the genital region. On the other hand, HSV-2 reactivates 8–10 times more commonly in the genital region than in the orolabial

regions. Reactivation is more common and severe in immunocompromised individuals.

69. **C.** Herpes zoster results from reactivation of latent VZV infection.

Reactivation of varicella-zoster virus (VZV) that has remained dormant within dorsal root ganglia, often for decades after the patient's initial exposure to the virus in the form of varicella (chickenpox), results in herpes zoster (shingles). Although it is usually a self-limited dermatomal rash with pain, herpes zoster can be far more serious; in addition, acute cases often lead to post-herpetic neuralgia (PHN) and are responsible for a significant economic burden.

Herpes zoster typically occurs in the elderly, is not infectious, and a contiguous dermatomal distribution is typical. Eczema herpeticum is caused by HSV not zoster.

70. **D.** The best-fit diagnosis for the image shown is cytomegalovirus (CMV).

CMV is a lytic virus that causes a cytopathic effect *in vitro* and *in vivo*. The pathologic hallmark of CMV infection is an enlarged cell with viral inclusion bodies. The microscopic description given to these cells is most commonly an "owl's eye," depicted in the image. CMV is a double-stranded DNA virus and is a member of the Herpesviridae family. CMV shares many attributes with other herpes viruses, including genome, virion structure, and the ability to cause latent and persistent infections. CMV has the largest genome of the herpes viruses. At least 60% of the US population has been exposed to CMV, with a prevalence of more than 90% in high-risk groups (e.g., unborn babies whose mothers become infected with CMV during pregnancy or people with HIV).

CMV has been detected *via* culture (human fibroblast), serologies, antigen assays, PCR, and cytopathology. The IgM level is elevated in patients with recent CMV infection, or there is a 4-fold increase in IgG titers. False-positive CMV IgM results may be seen in patients with EBV or HHV-6 infections, as well as in patients with increased rheumatoid factor levels. Antigenemia is defined as the detection of the CMV pp65 antigen in leukocytes.

71. **B.** EBV belongs to the Herpesviridae family.

The other family members include, CMV, herpes simplex virus type 1 (HSV-1 or HHV-1) and herpes simplex virus type 2 (HSV-2 or HHV-2), varicella zoster virus (VZV), human herpes virus (HHV)-6, HHV-7, and HHV-8.

72. **E.** Cervical cancer is associated with HPV and NOT EBV.

Epstein-Barr virus (EBV), or human herpesvirus 4, is a gamma herpesvirus that infects more than 95% of the world's population. The most common manifestation of primary infection with this organism is *acute infectious mononucleosis*, a self-limited clinical syndrome that most frequently affects adolescents and young adults. Infection with Epstein-Barr virus is also associated with *lymphoproliferative disorders* especially *post-transplant lymphoproliferative disorders* in immunocompromised hosts, as well as *nasopharyngeal carcinoma* and *Burkitt's lymphoma*. Most non-Hodgkin lymphomas are associated with Epstein-Barr virus, and evidence of the Epstein-Barr virus genome is demonstrable in many of these tumors. Epstein-Barr virus is also associated with Hodgkin lymphoma, in which the Epstein-Barr virus genome is present in the Reed-Sternberg cell. The EBNA1 protein interferes with tumor growth factor-beta signaling by downregulating *Smad2*; this interference with tumor-suppressor functions may contribute to tumor formation. In patients with AIDS, Epstein-Barr virus is associated with hairy leukoplakia, leiomyosarcoma, CNS lymphoma, and lymphoid interstitial pneumonitis in children. However, only approximately one half of acquired immunodeficiency syndromes (AIDS)-associated Burkitt lymphomas contain Epstein-Barr virus genomes, which suggests a more complex interaction between chronic human immunodeficiency virus (HIV) infection and immune system defects. Antibodies to Epstein-Barr virus antigens measured for clinical purposes include antibodies to viral capsid antigen (VCA), early antigens (EAs), and EBNA. EAs are expressed early in the lytic cycle, whereas VCA and membrane antigens are structural viral proteins expressed late in the lytic cycle. EBNA is expressed in latently infected cells. Primary acute Epstein-Barr virus infection is associated with VCA-IgM, VCA-IgG, and absent EBNA antibodies. The antibody pattern in recent infection (3–12 months) includes positive findings for VCA-IgG and EBNA antibodies, negative VCA-IgM antibodies, and usually, positive EA antibodies.

After 12 months, the pattern is the same as in recent infection, *except EA antibodies are not present.*

73. **A.** Plantar warts are typically associated with HPV-1.

Other HPVs associated with plantar warts include HPV-2, -60, -63, -65 and -66 (see Table G5).

74. **C.** The best-fit diagnosis for the image shown is epidermodysplasia verruciformis (EDV).

The classic histopathologic manifestation of epidermodysplasia verruciformis, shown in the image, is a verruca plana-like lesion with mild hyperkeratosis and acanthosis, in which the keratinocytes contain perinuclear halos and blue-gray pallor, as is demonstrated in the image. Perinuclear halos are a specific cytopathic effect, that is, clear cells in the granular and spinous layers with occasional enlarged, hyperchromatic, atypical nuclei, are present.

Epidermodysplasia verruciformis is a rare, inherited disorder inherited in an autosomal recessive manner that predisposes patients to widespread human papillomavirus (HPV) infection and cutaneous squamous cell carcinomas. The pathophysiology of epidermodysplasia verruciformis is linked to defective cell-mediated immunity, with elucidation of mutations in *EVER1* and *EVER2* genes (band 17q25). Their gene products are integral membrane proteins localized to the endoplasmic reticulum. Epidermodysplasia verruciformis usually begins in infancy or early childhood, with the development of various types of flat, wartlike lesions and confluent plaques on the skin, especially on dorsal hands, extremities, face, and neck. The diagnosis of epidermodysplasia verruciformis should be suspected in the clinical setting of numerous verrucous lesions or when lesions are resistant to appropriate therapy.

Pertinent physical findings are limited to the skin and rarely occur on the mucosa. Primary skin lesions manifest as 2 types, although they generally are polymorphic. The first type is flat, wart-like lesions resembling verruca plana; they are flat-topped papules with scaly, hyperpigmented or hypopigmented, sometimes confluent, patches or plaques. The second type is verrucous or seborrheic keratosis-like lesions; they are commonly seen on sun-exposed skin, including dorsum of hands.

75. **A.** HPV-1 is NOT associated with epidermodysplasia verruciformis (EDV).

Patients with epidermodysplasia verruciformis are usually infected with multiple types of HPV, including common types that affect individuals without epidermodysplasia verruciformis (e.g., HPV types 3 and 10) and those unique to epidermodysplasia verruciformis, the so called epidermodysplasia verruciformis–associated HPVs (EDV-HPVs).

More than 30 EDV-HPVs, such as types 4, 5a, 5b, 8, 9, 12, 14, 15, 17, 19–25, 36–38, 47, and 50, have been identified in epidermodysplasia verruciformis lesions. HPV-5 and HPV-8 have been isolated in more than 90% of epidermodysplasia verruciformis-associated squamous cell carcinomas. Epidermodysplasia verruciformis-associated HPVs can be divided into 2 groups:

- Group with high oncogenic potential (HPV types 5, 8, 10, and 47): More than 90% of epidermodysplasia verruciformis-associated skin cancers contain these virus types
- Group with low oncogenic potential (HPV types 14, 20, 21, and 25): These types are usually detected in benign skin lesions

Also see Table G5.

76. **E.** HPV-16 is the HPV strain associated with bowenoid papulosis.

Also see Table G5 for other HPV associations.

77. **B.** The causative virus of measles belongs to the Paramyxoviridae family.

A number of important human diseases are caused by paramyxoviruses. These include mumps, measles, and respiratory syncytial virus (RSV), which is the major cause of bronchiolitis and pneumonia in infants and children.

78. **C.** Parvo virus is the causative organism of fifth disease.

Erythema infectiosum (also known as fifth disease) is usually a benign childhood condition characterized by a classic slapped-cheek appearance and a lacy exanthem. It results from infection with human parvovirus (PV) B19, an erythrovirus.

79. **A.** Coxsackie virus is the causative organism of hand, foot and mouth (HFM) disease.

Coxsackieviruses belong to the family Picornaviridae and the genus *Enterovirus*, which also includes poliovirus and echovirus.

Group A coxsackieviruses tend to infect the skin and mucous membranes and cause herpangina, acute hemorrhagic conjunctivitis (AHC), and hand, foot and mouth (HFM) disease; Coxsackie A16 is the causative organism in most cases of HFM disease

Group B coxsackieviruses tend to infect the heart, pleura, pancreas, and liver, causing pleurodynia, myocarditis, pericarditis, and hepatitis

80. **D.** A non-relapsing rash, hepatitis and lymphadenopathy characterize Giannoti-Crosti syndrome.

The cutaneous eruption of Gianotti-Crosti syndrome (papular acrodermatitis of childhood) is characterized by monomorphous pale, pink-to-flesh-colored or erythematous 1–10 mm papules or papulovesicles localized symmetrically and acrally over the extensor surfaces of the extremities, the buttocks, and the face. Other findings include fever, lymphadenopathy, hepatosplenomegaly and pharyngeal erythema, oropharyngeal ulcers or vesicles. The prognosis is excellent. This syndrome is generally a benign, self-limited condition. The eruption usually starts to resolve after 6–8 weeks. While this syndrome is *typically associated with hepatitis B*, many other viruses such as hepatitis A, CMV, HSV-1, HSV-6, EBV, adenovirus, rotavirus, parainfluenza and coxsackievirus have been implicated.

81. **D.** Leishmaniasis is the best-fit diagnosis for the image shown.

For a biopsy confirmation of leishmaniasis, a punch or incisional/excisional biopsy specimen should be obtained and *should include the ulcer or nodule border with both affected and unaffected tissue.* The parasite consists of a nucleus and a kinetoplast surrounded by a cell wall.

Visualization of all 3 features (i.e., nucleus, cell membrane, and an eccentrically located kinetoplast) is required to make a diagnosis based on microscopy findings. Even with visualization of amastigotes – the so-called Leishman-Donovan bodies, which have a sensitivity of 50% to 70% – a species-specific diagnosis cannot be ascertained. An important step in histopathologic analysis is searching for amastigotes within macrophages, *usually best found beneath the epidermis.* Each amastigote measures 2–4 µm in diameter, so tiny as to require high power magnification to visualize, is a dull blue-gray color with hematoxylin and eosin staining, and is found in clusters in the cytoplasm of dermal macrophages. Organisms tend to cluster at the periphery of the macrophages ("marquee sign"). In addition to dermal macrophages, the other cell line capable of harboring *Leishmania* parasites is the epidermal Langerhans cell, which migrates from the epidermis to the site of infection in the dermis. In chronic relapsing cutaneous leishmaniasis, also referred to as leishmania recidivans, infections occur within a scar from a previous primary acute cutaneous leishmanial infection. This produces variable epidermal changes and pseudoepitheliomatous hyperplasia, which may be seen if no grenz zone is present. Giemsa, Brown-Hopps, Gram, or Leishman stains are all used to enhance *Leishmania* organisms on touch preparations, tissue aspiration, or biopsy samples.

82. **C.** *Leishmania braziliensis* is the causative organism of mucocutaneous leishmaniasis.

Mucocutaneous leishmaniasis usually occurs after the apparent resolution of cutaneous infection, although it can coexist with skin involvement. Lesions normally appear within 2 years of cutaneous infection, but may take as many as 30 years. The route of infection spread may be either hematogenous or lymphatic. *L. braziliensis* accounts for most cases of mucocutaneous leishmaniasis, but *L. panamensis, L. guyanensis*, and *L. amazonensis* have also been implicated. Also see Table G6.

83. **D.** *Leishmania donovani* is the causative organism in kala-azar.

Visceral leishmaniasis is also known as kala-azar and often affects the liver, spleen, and bone marrow. Visceral leishmaniasis is caused by *Leishmania donovani, Leishmania infantum*, or *Leishmania chagasi.* Cutaneous leishmaniasis in those with resolved visceral leishmaniasis is referred to as post-kala-azar dermal leishmaniasis.

84. **D.** Larva migrans is associated with *Ancylostoma braziliense.*

Ancylostoma braziliense (hookworm of wild and domestic dogs and cats) is the most common cause of cutaneous larva migrans. It can be found in the central and southern USA, Central America, South America, and the Caribbean.

85. **B.** Image shown is that of an intact tick.

86. **A.** Cercarial dermatitis is associated with schistosomiasis.

    Swimmer's itch is an itchy rash that can occur after swimming or wading outdoors. Also known as cercarial dermatitis, swimmer's itch is most common in freshwater lakes and ponds, but it occasionally occurs in salt water. The rash is a short-term immune reaction occurring in the skin of humans that have been infected by water-borne schistosomatidae. The genera most commonly associated with swimmer's itch in humans are *Trichobilharzia* and *Gigantobilharzia*.

87. **E.** Image shown is that of scabies.

    The histopathologic features of scabies are distinctive enough to suggest the diagnosis, although they are common to a variety of arthropod reactions. If a burrow is excised, mites, larvae, ova, and feces may be identified within the stratum corneum. Typically, the larvae (3 pairs of legs) migrate to the skin surface and burrow into the intact stratum corneum to make short burrows, called molting pouches.

    Human scabies is an intensely pruritic skin infestation caused by the host-specific mite *Sarcoptes scabiei hominis*. Scabies is a great clinical imitator. Its spectrum of cutaneous manifestations and associated symptoms often results in delayed diagnosis. In fact, the term "7-year itch" was first used with reference to persistent, undiagnosed infestations with scabies. The *S. scabiei hominis* mite that infects humans is female and is large enough (0.3–0.4 mm long) to be seen with the naked eye. (The male is about half this size.) The mite has 4 pairs of legs and crawls at a rate of 2.5 cm/min; it is unable to fly or jump. Although its life cycle occurs completely on the host, the mite is able to live on bedding, clothes, or other surfaces at room temperature for 2–3 days, while remaining capable of infestation and burrowing. At temperatures below 20 °C, *S. scabiei* are immobile, although they can survive such temperatures for extended periods.

88. **C.** Image shown is that of the demodex mite.

    This hair follicle mite is the only metazoan organism commonly found in the pilosebaceous components of the eyelid of humans. *Demodex folliculorum* (all stages) is found in small hair follicles and eyelash hair follicles. In all forms, immature and adult, it produces follicular distention and hyperplasia, and increases keratinization leading (in eyelashes) to cuffing, which consists of keratin and lipid moieties. *Demodex brevis* (all stages) is present in the eyelash sebaceous glands, small hair sebaceous glands, and lobules of the meibomian glands. Demodectic mites produce histologically observable tissue and inflammatory changes, epithelial hyperplasia, and follicular plugging.

89. **D.** Image shown is that of tungiasis.

    Tungiasis is an infestation by the burrowing flea *Tunga penetrans* or related species. The flea has many common names, being known in various locations as the chigger flea, sand flea, chigoe, jigger, nigua, pigue, or le bicho de pe. Typical areas of involvement include the plantar surface of the foot, the intertriginous regions of the toes, and the periungual regions. Infestation in its simplest form is manifested by the appearance of a white patch with a black dot.

    Histopathologic examination reveals an intraepidermal cavity lined by an eosinophilic cuticle, which represents the body of the flea. In the cavity are round to oval eggs, hollow ring-like components of the tracheal system, and the digestive tract. A thick band of striated muscle runs from the head to the terminal orifice. Usually, an inflammatory infiltrate is present in the subjacent dermis.

90. **C.** Pitted keratolysis is associated with corynebacteria.

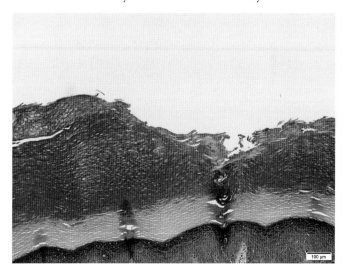

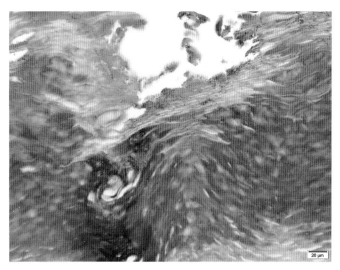

Pitted keratolysis is a skin disorder characterized by crateriform pitting that primarily affects the pressure-bearing aspects of the plantar surface of the feet and, occasionally, the palms of the hand, as collarettes of scale. The manifestations of pitted keratolysis are due to a superficial cutaneous bacterial infection. Pitted keratolysis is caused by a cutaneous infection with *Micrococcus sedentarius* (now renamed *Kytococcus sedentarius*), *Dermatophilus congolensis*, or species of *Corynebacterium*, *Actinomyces, or Streptomyces*. Under appropriate conditions (i.e., prolonged occlusion, hyperhidrosis, increased skin surface pH), these bacteria proliferate and produce proteinases that destroy the stratum corneum, creating pits.

Histopathologic findings are not specific and reveal a crater limited to the stratum corneum. The microorganisms, cocci, and filamentous forms may be seen with H&E staining, but they are detected more easily with Gram stain, periodic acid-Schiff stain, or methenamine-silver stain.

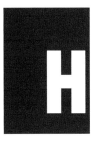

Tumors
Questions

1. The most likely diagnosis is:

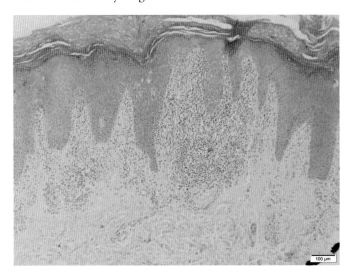

A. Seborrheic keratosis
B. Lichen simplex chronicus
C. Prurigo nodularis
D. Familial dyskeratotic comedones
E. Inflammatory linear verrucous epidermal nevus

2. The most likely diagnosis is:

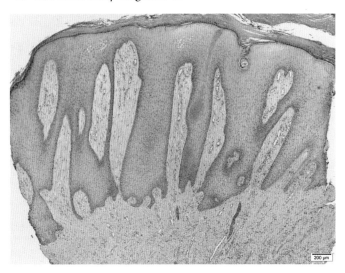

A. Seborrheic keratosis
B. Keratoacanthoma
C. Squamous cell carcinoma
D. Prurigo nodularis
E. Inflammatory linear verrucous epidermal nevus

3. The most likely diagnosis is:

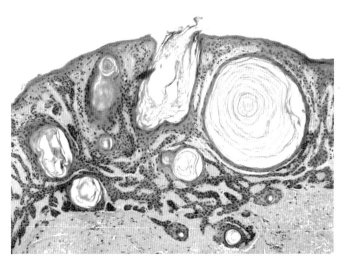

A. Nevus sebaceus
B. Keratoacanthoma
C. Seborrheic keratosis
D. Prurigo nodularis
E. Inflammatory linear verrucous epidermal nevus

4. An increase in size and number of these (based on the image shown above) is known as:
A. Auspitz sign
B. Leser-Trélat sign
C. Nikolsky's sign
D. Ugly duckling sign
E. Buschke-Ollendorf sign

5. The best-fit diagnosis is:

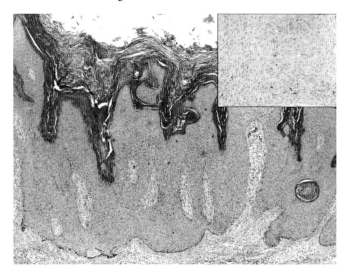

    A. Melanoacanthoma
    D. Clear cell acanthoma
    C. Large cell acanthoma
    D. Epidermolytic acanthoma
    E. Clear cell papulosis

6. The best-fit diagnosis is:

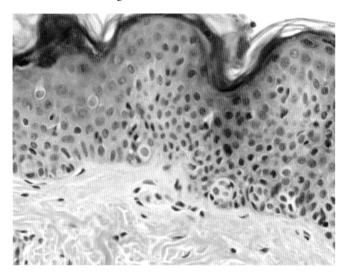

    A. Melanoacanthoma
    D. Clear cell acanthoma
    C. Large cell acanthoma
    D. Epidermolytic acanthoma
    E. Clear cell papulosis

7. The best-fit diagnosis is:

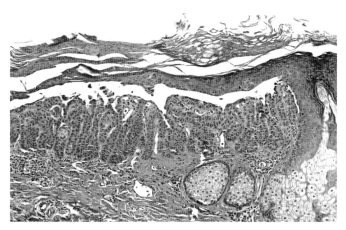

    A. Stucco keratosis
    B. Seborrheic keratosis
    C. Arsenical keratosis
    D. Actinic keratosis
    E. Bowenoid papulosis

8. The best-fit diagnosis is:

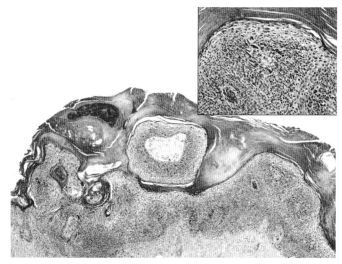

    A. Stucco keratosis
    B. Seborrheic keratosis
    C. Bowen's disease
    D. Actinic keratosis
    E. Arsenical keratosis

9. Biopsy of one of many verrucous papules on the labia. The best-fit diagnosis is:

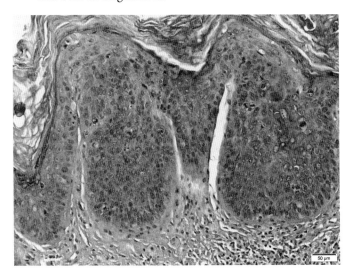

A. Bowen's disease
B. Bowenoid papulosis
C. Condyloma acuminatum
D. Actinic cheilitis
E. Verruca vulgaris

10. The HPV strain most commonly implicated in the above (based on the image shown above) is:
A. HPV-1
B. HPV-3
C. HPV-5
D. HPV-10
E. HPV-16

11. Predisposition to multiple cancers of this type is associated with:

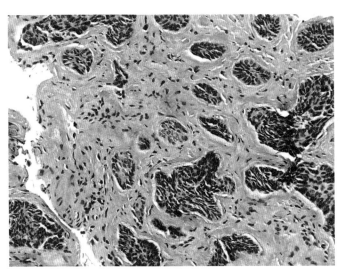

A. Muir-Torre syndrome
B. Birt-Hogg-Dubé syndrome
C. Brooke-Spiegler syndrome
D. Gorlin-Goltz syndrome
E. NAME/LAMB syndrome

12. Mutations in which of the following genes is associated (based on answer to question 11) with this syndrome:
A. *HRAS*
B. *PTEN*
C. *PTCH1*
D. *BAP1*
E. *CDK4*

13. The best-fit diagnosis is:

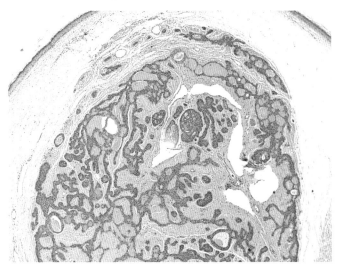

A. Metatypical carcinoma
B. Fibroepithelioma
C. Trichoblastoma
D. Trichoepithelioma
E. Spiradenoma

14. Marjolin's ulcer refers to:
A. Squamous cell carcinoma arising in sites of chronic injury
B. Recurrent basal cell carcinoma
C. Malignant melanoma arising in sites of chronic sun damage
D. Bowen's disease in mucosal sites
E. Prurigo nodularis, impetiginized and traumatized

15. Which of the following would be expected to be positive in this entity:

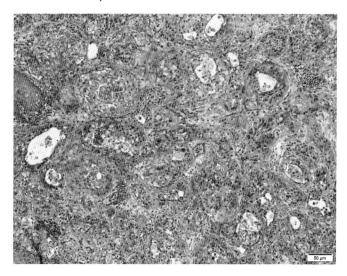

A. CK7, CK20, p16
B. CK15, Bcl-2, CD10
C. CD10, CD34, p21
D. MSH2, MLH1, CK20
E. CK5/6, CK903, p40

16. Which of the following is NOT a high-risk feature for squamous cell carcinoma:
A. Perineural invasion
B. Acantholytic subtype
C. Head and neck location
D. p40 positivity
D. Extension into subcutis

17. A genetic predisposition to cutaneous squamous cell carcinoma may be associated with:
A. Brooke-Spiegler syndrome
B. Muir-Torre syndrome
C. Rothmund-Thomson syndrome
D. NAME syndrome
E. Burt-Hogg-Dubé syndrome

18. The mutation most commonly detected in cutaneous squamous cell carcinoma involves:
A. *MSH2*
B. *KRAS*
C. *TP53*
D. *Rb*
E. *MLH1*

19. The best-fit diagnosis is:

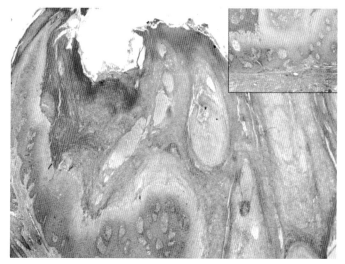

A. Squamous cell carcinoma
B. Verrucous carcinoma
C. Verruca vulgaris
D. Bowen's disease
E. Prurigo nodularis

20. The best-fit diagnosis is:

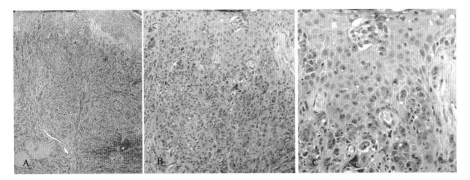

    A. Mucoepidermoid carcinoma
    B. Metaplastic mucocele
    C. Mucinous oncocytoma
    D. Merkel cell carcinoma
    E. Adenomatous eccrine metaplasia

21. The best-fit diagnosis is:

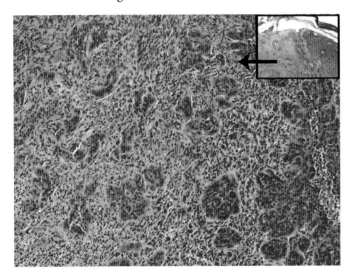

    A. Atypical fibroxanthoma
    B. Metatypical carcinoma
    C. Undifferentiated pleomorphic sarcoma
    D. Spindle cell squamous carcinoma
    E. Metaplastic carcinoma

22. The best-fit diagnosis is:

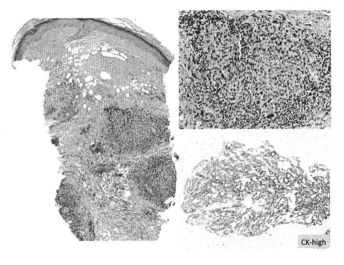

    A. Cutaneous lymphadenoma
    B. Merkel cell carcinoma
    C. Carcinosarcoma
    D. Lymphoepithelioma-like carcinoma
    E. Nasopharyngeal carcinoma

23. The best-fit diagnosis for this biopsy of a yellow nail is:

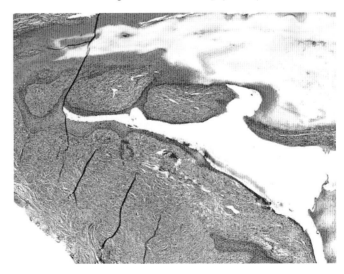

A. Onychomycosis
B. Onychopapilloma
C. Onychomatrixoma
D. Onycholemmal carcinoma
E. Normal nail

24. Which of the following is correct regarding subungual keratoacanthomas:
    A. Typically present as multiple lesions
    B. More destructive than subungual squamous cell carcinoma
    C. Associated with HPV-3 and HPV-5
    D. Characterized by progressive peripheral growth with coincident central healing
    E. Perineural invasion frequent

25. Which of the following is correct regarding kerato-acanthoma centrifugum marginatum:
    A. Characterized by progressive peripheral growth with coincident central healing
    B. Cutaneous marker for Muir-Torre syndrome
    C. Associated with polyoma virus
    D. Perineural invasion frequent

26. Keratoacanthomas associated with Muir-Torre syndrome exhibit which of the following immunoprofiles:
    A. Positive MLH1 and MSH6
    B. Negative TP53 and p40
    C. Negative BAP1, positive BRAFV600E
    D. Positive CK7 and MSH2
    E. Negative MSH2 and MLH1

27. Disorders characterized by hyperpigmentation include all of the following EXCEPT:
    A. Chediak-Higashi syndrome
    B. Dowling-Degos disease
    C. Peutz-Jeghers syndrome
    D. Laugier-Hunziker syndrome
    E. Macules of Albright syndrome

28. These are a feature of all of the following EXCEPT:

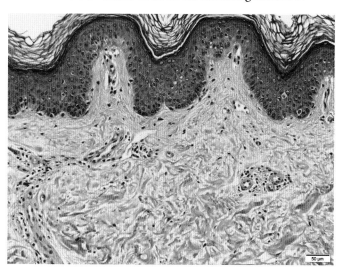

A. McCune-Albright syndrome
B. Laugier-Hunziker syndrome
C. LAMB syndrome
D. Peutz-Jeghers syndrome
E. Chediak-Higashi syndrome

29. The best-fit diagnosis is:

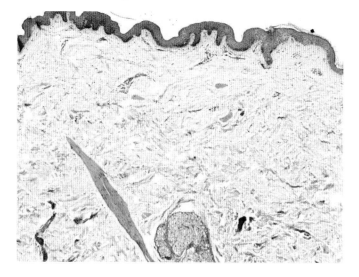

A. Junctional nevus
B. Dysplastic nevus
C. Pigmented seborrheic keratosis
D. Ink-spot lentigo
E. Melanoacanthoma

30. The best-fit diagnosis is:

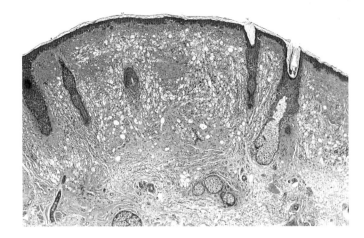

    A. Metastatic renal cell carcinoma
    B. Clear cell syringoma
    C. Balloon cell nevus
    D. Balloon cell melanoma
    E. Clear cell angiofibroma

31. The best-fit diagnosis is:

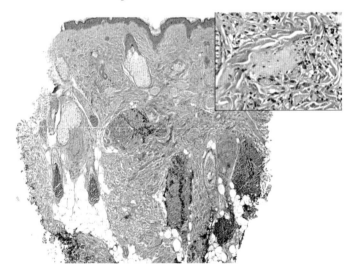

    A. Metastatic melanoma
    B. Deep penetrating nevus
    C. Cellular blue nevus
    D. Neurothekeoma
    E. Dermal melanocytic hamartoma

32. Mutations in which of the following (based on question 31) suggest these are part of the Spitz spectrum:
    A. HRAS
    B. KRAS
    C. GNAQ

    D. BAP1
    E. NF

33. Which of the following is a characteristic of a recurrent nevus:
    A. Follicular extension
    B. Mitotically active dermal component
    C. Pigmented dermal component
    D. Loss of HMB45 gradient
    E. Trizonal pattern

34. Mucosal melanomas express mutations in:
    A. BRAF
    B. HRAS
    C. BAP1
    D. KIT
    E. GNAQ

35. Uveal melanomas express mutations in:
    A. BRAF
    B. HRAS
    C. BAP1
    D. KIT
    E. GNAQ

36. The best-fit diagnosis is:

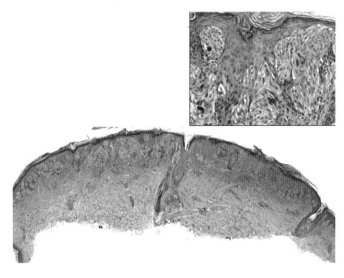

    A. Deep penetrating nevus
    B. Ancient nevus
    C. Dysplastic nevus
    D. Spitz nevus
    E. Malignant melanoma

37. These (based on the image shown above) are typically associated with mutations in:
    A. BRAF
    B. HRAS

C. *BAP1*
D. *KIT*
E. *GNAQ*

38. Which of the following is NOT helpful in differentiating Spitz nevus from spitzoid melanoma:
    A. HRAS status
    B. HMB45 gradient
    C. Ki-67 index
    D. Imaging mass spectrophotometry
    E. S100A6 staining

39. The best-fit diagnosis is:

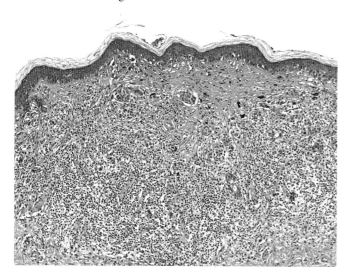

    A. Meyerson's nevus
    B. Traumatized nevus
    C. Spitz nevus
    D. Malignant melanoma
    E. Halo nevus

40. The histopathologic differential diagnosis might include all of the following EXCEPT:

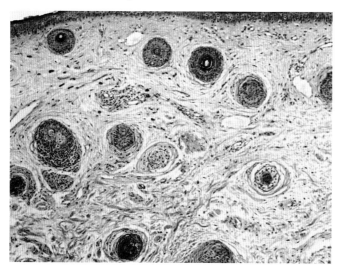

A. Hori's nevus
B. Nevus of Ota
C. Nevus of Ito
D. Cellular blue nevus
E. Sun's nevus

41. A Reed nevus is a variant of which of the following:
    A. Blue nevus
    B. Deep penetrating nevus
    C. Spitz nevus
    D. Meyerson's nevus
    E. Congenital nevus

42. Which of the following is NOT a feature of a dysplastic nevus:
    A. >5.00 mm in diameter
    B. Confluent pagetoid spread
    C. "Shoulder"
    D. Lamellar and concentric fibroplasia
    E. Cytologic atypia

43. High-risk gene mutations in melanoma include:
    A. *CDKN2A*
    B. *MSH6*
    C. *PTCH1*
    D. *SMOH*
    E. *COL1A1*

44. The best-fit diagnosis is:

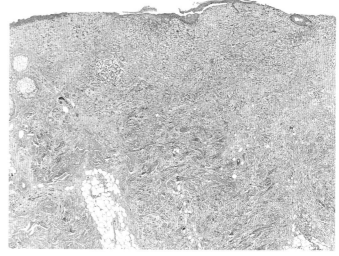

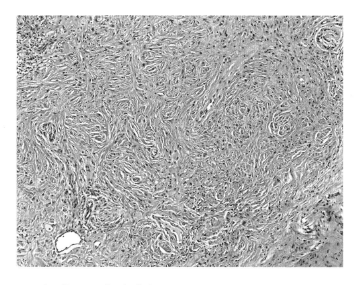

A. Desmoplastic Spitz nevus
B. Deep penetrating nevus
C. BAP-1 inactivated melanocytic tumor
D. Inflamed scar
E. Desmoplastic melanoma

45. These (based on the image shown above) are associated with mutations in:
    A. *BRAF*
    B. *Rb*
    C. *KIT*
    D. *RETp*
    E. *GNAQ*

46. The best-fit diagnosis is:

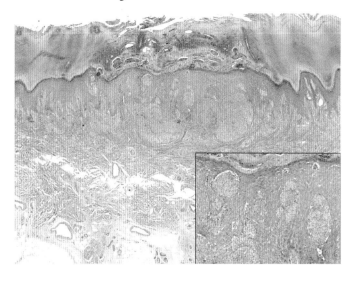

A. Tinea nigra
B. Nevus of special site
C. BAP-1 inactivated melanocytic tumor
D. Acral melanoma
E. Superficial spreading melanoma

47. These (based on the image shown above) are associated with mutations in:
    A. *BRAF*
    B. *Rb*
    C. *KIT*
    D. *RETp*
    E. *GNAQ*

48. The best-fit diagnosis is:

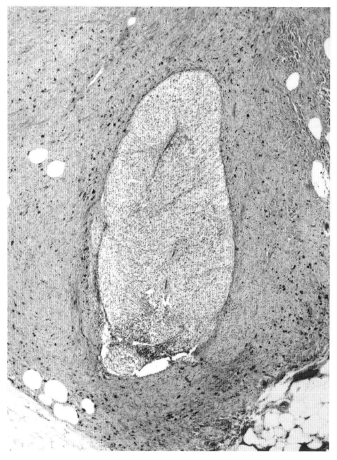

A. Congenital proliferative nodule
B. Cellular blue nevus
C. Deep penetrating nevus
D. Plexiform Spitz nevus
E. Dermal melanocyte hamartoma

49. The best-fit diagnosis is:

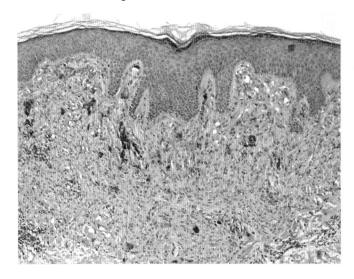

    A. Epithelioid blue nevus
    B. Deep penetrating nevus
    C. Cellular blue nevus
    D. Dermal melanocyte hamartoma
    E. Plexiform Spitz nevus

50. Multiple lesions (based on the image shown above) are associated with:
    A. McCune-Albright syndrome
    B. Laugier-Hunziker syndrome
    C. Carney's complex syndrome
    D. Peutz-Jeghers syndrome
    E. Chediak-Higashi syndrome

51. Biallelic loss of *BAP1* is associated with mutations in:
    A. *BRAF*
    B. *Rb*
    C. *KIT*
    D. *RETp*
    E. *GNAQ*

52. Chromosomes targeted in the FISH melanoma first generation probes included:
    A. 2 and 6
    B. 6 and 11
    C. 7 and 10
    D. 7 and 13
    E. 19 and 22

53. The best-fit diagnosis is:

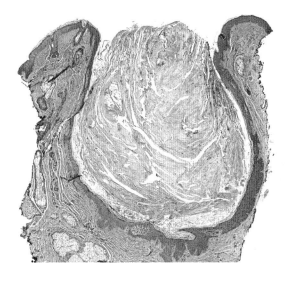

    A. Epidermal inclusion cyst
    B. Keratosis pilaris atrophicans
    C. Dilated pore of Winer
    D. Inverted follicular keratosis
    E. Tumor of the follicular infundibulum

54. The best-fit diagnosis is:

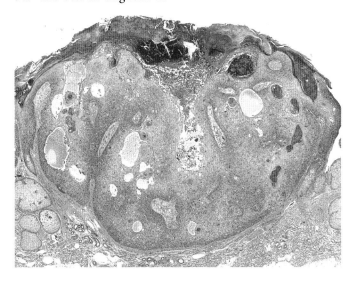

    A. Pilar sheath acanthoma
    B. Dilated pore of Winer
    C. Squamous cell carcinoma
    D. Inverted follicular keratosis
    E. Trichilemmoma, irritated

55. The best-fit diagnosis is:

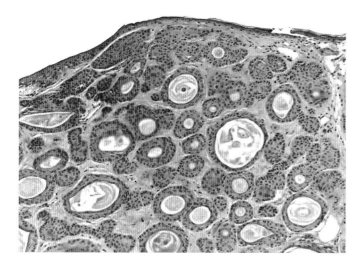

A. Trichodiscoma
B. Trichoepithelioma
C. Trichofolliculoma
D. Trichilemmoma
E. Trichoadenoma

56. The best-fit diagnosis is:

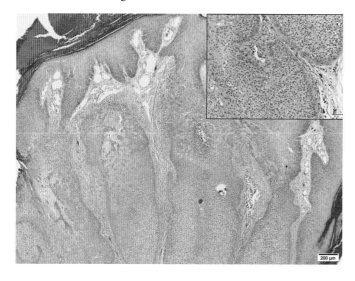

A. Verruca vulgaris
B. Trichoepithelioma
C. Basal cell carcinoma
D. Trichilemmoma
E. Inverted follicular keratosis

57. Multiple lesions of this (based on the image shown above) are found in:
A. Muir-Torre syndrome
B. Birt-Hogg-Dubé syndrome
C. Cowden's syndrome
D. Brooke-Spiegler syndrome
E. Gorlin-Goltz syndrome
F. NAME/LAMB syndrome

58. Other components of this syndrome (based on question 57) include:
A. Keratoacanthomas, visceral malignancies
B. Palmar pits, mucocutaneous papules
C. Spiradenomas, trichoepitheliomas
D. Basal cell carcinomas, palmar pits
E. Fibrofolliculomas, renal tumors

59. The best-fit diagnosis is:

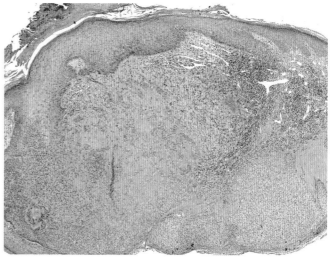

A. Desmoplastic trichilemmoma
B. Infiltrating basal cell carcinoma
C. Infiltrating squamous cell carcinoma
D. Desmoplastic panfolliculoma
E. Desmoplastic trichoepithelioma

60. The best-fit diagnosis is:

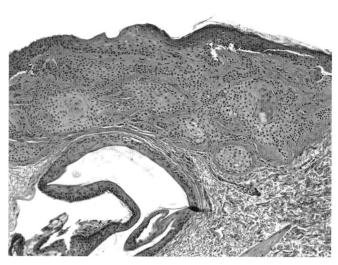

A. Eccrine syringofibroadenoma
B. Reticulate seborrheic keratosis
C. Reticulated acanthoma with sebaceous differentiation
D. Syringoma with squamous differentiation
E. Tumor of the follicular infundibulum

61. The best-fit diagnosis is:

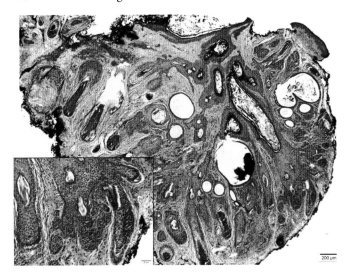

A. Folliculosebaceous cystic hamartoma
B. Dilated pore of Winer
C. Pilar sheath acanthoma
D. Trichofolliculoma
E. Panfolliculoma

62. The best-fit diagnosis is:

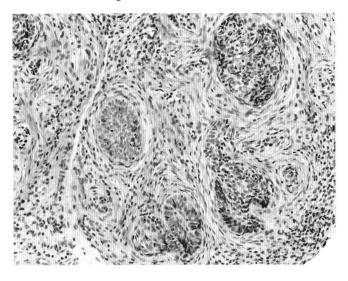

A. Trichodiscoma
B. Trichofolliculoma
C. Trichoepithelioma
D. Trichilemmoma
E. Trichoadenoma

63. Multiple lesions of this (based on the image shown above) are found in all of the following EXCEPT:
A. Multiple familial trichoepithelioma
B. Birt-Hogg-Dubé syndrome
C. Rombo syndrome
D. Brooke-Spiegler syndrome

64. The best-fit diagnosis is:

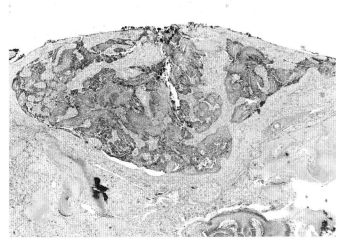

A. Onychomatricoma
B. Pilomatricoma
C. Melanoacanthoma
D. Basal cell carcinoma
E. Mantleoma

65. These (based on the image shown above) may be associated with mutations in:
A. β-catenin
B. α-laminin
C. PTEN
D. *PTCH1*
E. ɣ-perforin

66. The best-fit diagnosis is:

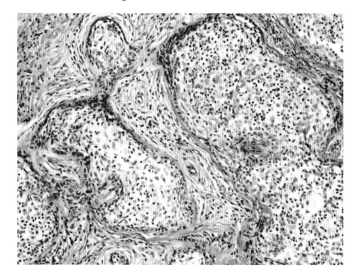

    A. Basal cell carcinoma
    B. Hidradenoma
    C. Mantleoma
    D. Follicular center cell lymphoma
    E. Cutaneous lymphadenoma

67. The best-fit diagnosis is:

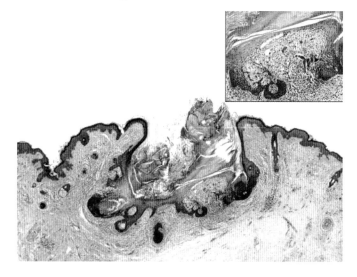

    A. Dilated pore of Winer
    B. Pilar sheath acanthoma
    C. Trichoblastoma
    D. Panfolliculoma
    E. Fibrofolliculoma

68. The best-fit diagnosis is:

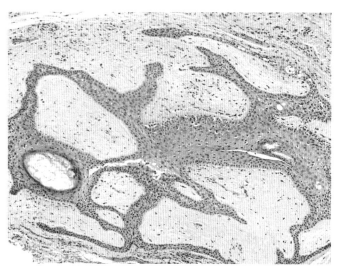

    A. Fibroepithelioma
    B. Syringofibroadenoma
    C. Fibrofolliculoma
    D. Panfolliculoma
    E. Mantleoma

69. Multiples of these (based on the image shown above) are associated with:
    A. Muir-Torre syndrome
    B. Birt-Hogg-Dubé syndrome
    C. Cowden's syndrome
    D. Brooke-Spiegler syndrome
    D. Gorlin-Goltz syndrome

70. Other components of this syndrome (based on question 69) include:
    A. Lung cysts, renal tumors
    B. Palmar pits, mucocutaneous papules
    C. Spiradenomas, trichoepitheliomas
    D. Basal cell carcinomas, palmar pits
    E. Keratoacanthomas, visceral malignancies

71. Fordyce's spot best describes:
    A. Ectopic eccrine glands
    B. Ectopic apocrine glands
    C. Ectopic pilar muscle
    D. Ectopic nerve plexus
    E. Ectopic sebaceous glands

72. The best-fit diagnosis is:

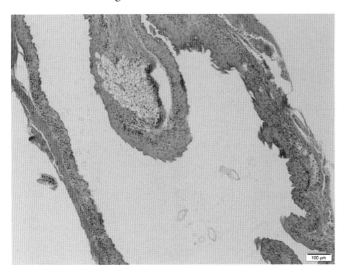

A. Syringocystadenoma
B. Dermoid cyst
C. Steatocystoma
D. Endosalpingosis
E. Endometriosis

73. The best-fit diagnosis is:

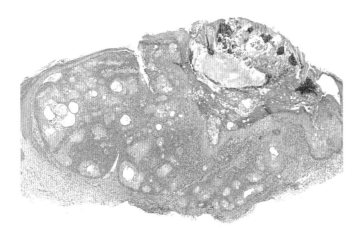

A. Mantleoma
B. Sebaceous adenoma
C. Sebaceous hyperplasia
D. Sebaceous carcinoma
E. Basal cell carcinoma with sebaceous differentiation

74. When located outside the head and neck area in a 36-year-old male (based on the image shown above), these may represent a cutaneous marker of:
A. Muir-Torre syndrome
B. Birt-Hogg-Dubé syndrome
C. Cowden's syndrome
D. Brooke-Spiegler syndrome
D. Gorlin-Goltz syndrome

75. Mutations commonly associated with these (based on the image shown above) include:
A. *BRAF*
B. *Rb*
C. *KIT*
D. *RETp*
E. *MSH-2*

76. This lesion would be immunohistochemically positive for:

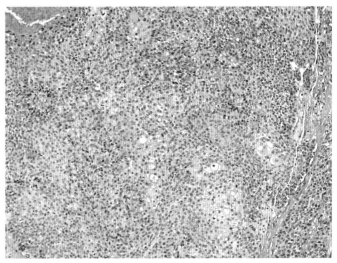

A. BerEp4
B. CK7
C. CKIT
D. Adipophilin
E. CDX2

77. The best-fit diagnosis is:

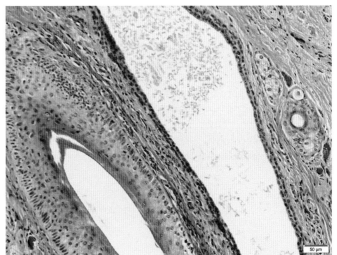

A. Hidrocystoma
B. Steatocystoma
C. Mucocele
D. Milium
E. Keratocyst

78. The best-fit diagnosis is:

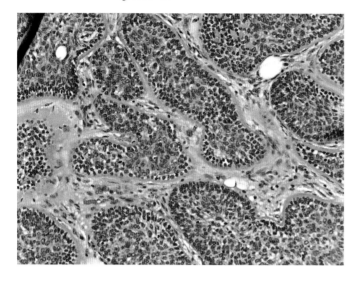

A. Poroma
B. Sebaceoma
C. Lymphadenoma
D. Hidradenoma
E. Cylindroma

79. Multiple lesions of these (based on the image shown above) are associated with:
A. Muir-Torre syndrome
B. Birt-Hogg-Dubé syndrome
C. Cowden's syndrome
D. Brooke-Spiegler syndrome
D. Gorlin-Goltz syndrome

80. Mutations associated with this syndrome (based on question 79) include:
A. *MSH2*
B. *TP53*
C. *CYLD*
D. *Rb*
E. *MLH1*

81. The best-fit diagnosis is:

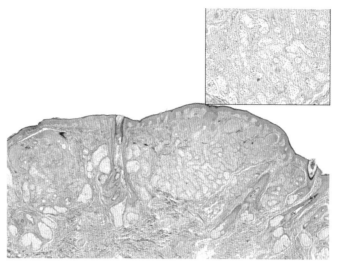

A. Eccrine acrospiroma
B. Syringoma
C. Basal cell carcinoma
D. Microcystic adnexal carcinoma
E. Cylindroma

82. The best-fit diagnosis is:

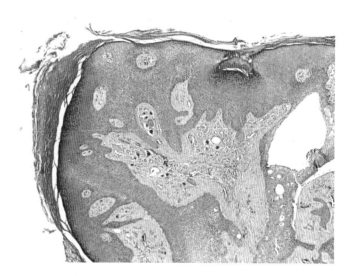

A. Poroma
B. Clonal seborrheic keratosis
C. Normal acral skin
D. Hidradenoma
E. Verruca vulgaris

83. These (based on the image shown above) are commonly located on the:
A. Face
B. Back
C. Chest

D. Mucosa

E. Extremity

84. The best-fit diagnosis is:

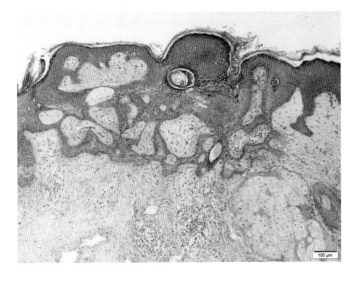

A. Metatypical carcinoma

B. Fibroepithelioma

C. Tumor of the follicular infundibulum

D. Syringofibroadenoma

E. Spiradenoma

85. The best-fit diagnosis is:

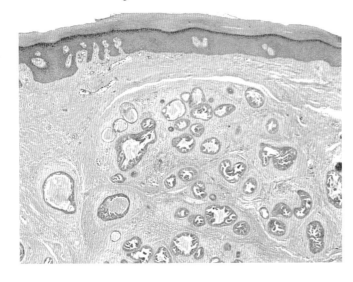

A. Erosive adenomatosis

B. Metastatic adenocarcinoma

C. Papillary eccrine adenoma

D. Syringocystadenoma papilliferum

E. Apocrine hidrocystoma

86. Which of the following is NOT a synonym for the entity shown:

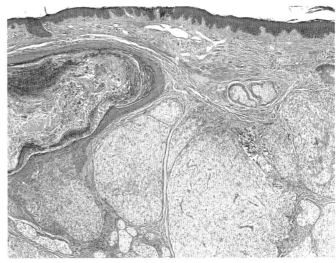

A. Eccrine acrospiroma

B. Eccrine hidrocystoma

C. Solid-cystic hidradenoma

D. Clear cell myoepithelioma

E. Clear cell hidradenoma

87. The best-fit diagnosis is:

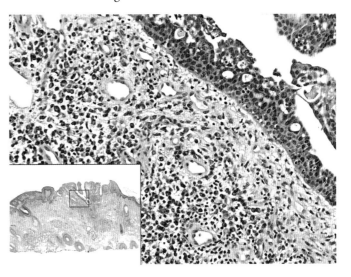

A. Erosive adenomatosis

B. Syringofibroadenoma

C. Papillary eccrine adenoma

D. Syringocystadenoma papilliferum

E. Apocrine hidrocystoma

88. These (based on the image shown above) typically arise in association with:

A. Verruca vulgaris

B. ILVEN

C. Nevus sebaceus
D. Becker's nevus
E. Hori's nevus

89. The best-fit diagnosis is:

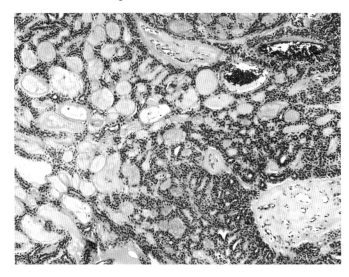

A. Apocrine hidradenoma
B. Apocrine mixed tumor
C. Apocrine poroma
D. Apocrine hidrocystoma
E. Apocrine adenoma

90. The best-fit diagnosis is:

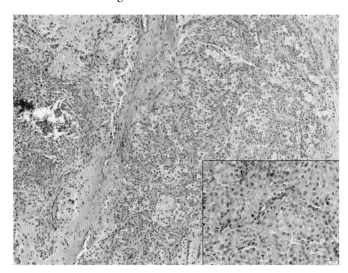

A. Myoepithelioma
B. Mantleoma
C. Matricoma
D. Myofibroma
E. Plasmacytoma

91. The best-fit diagnosis is:

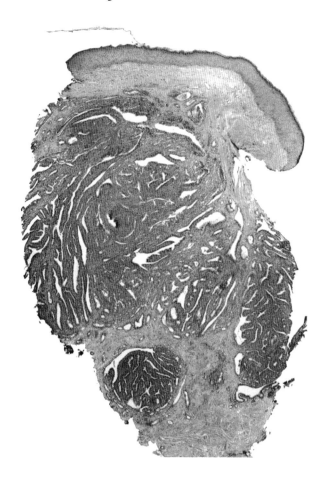

A. Erosive adenomatosis
B. Syringofibroadenoma
C. Papillary eccrine adenoma
D. Syringocystadenoma papilliferum
E. Apocrine hidrocystoma

92. The best-fit diagnosis is:

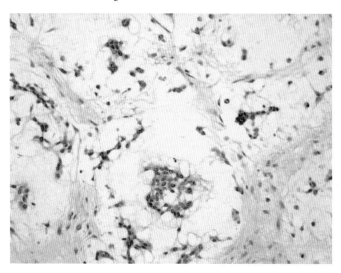

A. Cutaneous mixed tumor
B. Mucinous hidradenoma
C. Focal cutaneous mucinosis
D. Mucinous nevus
E. Mucinous carcinoma

93. The best-fit diagnosis is:

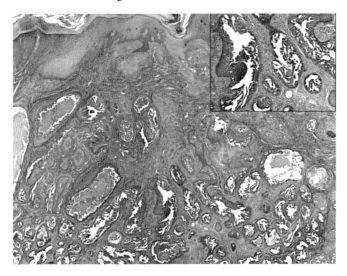

A. Erosive adenomatosis
B. Metastatic adenocarcinoma
C. Papillary eccrine adenoma
D. Digital papillary adenocarcinoma
E. Syringocystadenoma papilliferum

94. Which of the following is INCORRECT regarding this entity (based on the image shown above):
A. Common on the digits
B. Unencapsulated
C. Locally aggressive
D. Marker for internal malignancies
E. Mitotically active

95. The best-fit diagnosis for this EMA+, CEA+, CAM5.2+ and CK7+ lesion is:

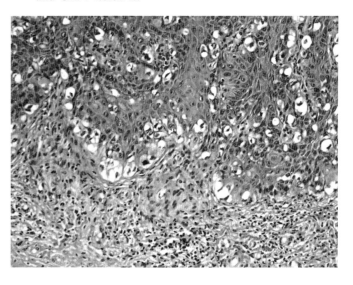

A. Malignant melanoma in situ
B. Squamous cell carcinoma in situ
C. Extramammary Paget's disease
D. Basal cell carcinoma
E. Sebaceous carcinoma in situ

96. Multiple lesions of these may be associated with:

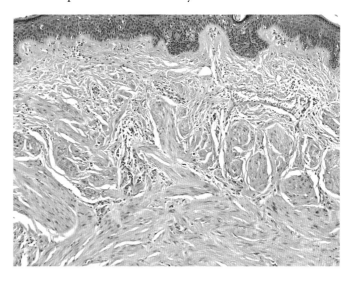

A. Pancreatic tumors
B. Hyperthyroidism
C. Renal tumors
D. Stasis
E. Paraproteinemia

97. Lesional cells (based on the image shown above) would be expected to be positive for:
A. Calretinin
B. Caldesmon

C. β-catenin
D. CK903
E. PGP9.5

98. Reed syndrome is associated with germline mutations in:
A. Oxoglutarate dehydrogenase
B. Fumarate hydratase
C. Isocitrate dehydrogenase
D. Citrate synthase
E. Aconitase

99. Prognostically relevant factors in a leiomyosarcoma include all of the following EXCEPT:
A. High cellularity
B. Mitoses
C. Nuclear atypia
D. Perineural invasion
E. Gross size

100. The best-fit diagnosis is:

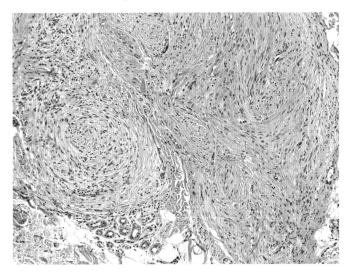

A. Rudimentary polydactyly
B. Solitary circumscribed neuroma
C. Traumatic neuroma
D. Ganglioneuroma
E. Neurilemmoma

101. The best-fit diagnosis is:

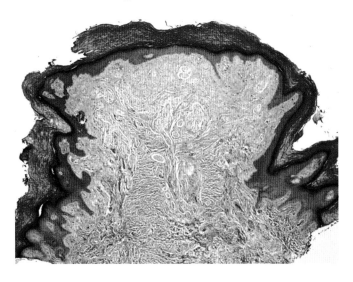

A. Rudimentary polydactyly
B. Solitary circumscribed neuroma
C. Traumatic neuroma
D. Ganglioneuroma
E. Neurilemmoma

102. The best-fit diagnosis is:

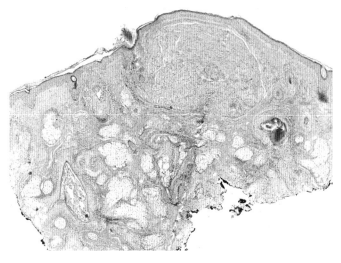

A. Rudimentary polydactyly
B. Solitary circumscribed neuroma
C. Traumatic neuroma
D. Ganglioneuroma
E. Neurilemmoma

103. MENI is also known as:
A. Wermer syndrome
B. Sipple syndrome
C. Wagenmann-Froeboese syndrome
D. Mucha-Habermann syndrome
E. Muir-Torre syndrome

104. Mucocutaneous manifestations of MENI include all of the following EXCEPT:
    A. Angiofibromas
    B. Collagenomas
    C. Lipomas
    D. Hypopigmented macules
    E. Leiomyomas

105. Multiple mucosal neuromas are a feature of:
    A. Cowden syndrome
    B. Wermer syndrome
    C. Sipple syndrome
    D. Wagenmann-Froeboese syndrome
    E. Mucha-Habermann syndrome

106. *MEN1* is the gene involved in:
    A. Cowden syndrome
    B. Wermer syndrome
    C. Sipple syndrome
    D. Wagenmann-Froeboese syndrome
    E. Mucha-Habermann syndrome

107. *RET* is the gene involved in:
    A. Cowden syndrome
    B. Wermer syndrome
    C. Sipple syndrome
    D. Brooke-Spiegler syndrome
    E. Mucha-Habermann syndrome

108. Which of the following is correct regarding re-excision perineural invasion:
    A. Composed of perineurial cells
    B. Composed of squamous epithelium
    C. Synonymous with cancerous invasion
    D. Exclusive to neuroectodermal malignancies
    E. Typically associated with lymphovascular invasion

109. This neoplasm is highly specific as a cutaneous stigmata for:

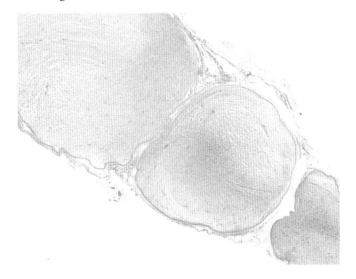

    A. Neurofibromatosis 1
    B. Cowden disease
    C. Sipple syndrome
    D. Brooke-Spiegler syndrome
    E. Muir-Torre syndrome

110. The gene involved in this syndrome (based on question 109) resides on chromosome:
    A. 7
    B. 9
    C. 11
    D. 13
    E. 17

111. Positive staining of lesional cells (based on the image shown above) would be expected with all of the following EXCEPT:
    A. S100P
    B. CD30
    C. CD34
    D. CD57
    E. Nestin

112. The best-fit diagnosis is:

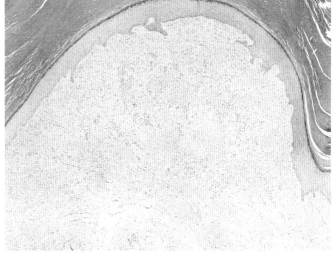

    A. Perineurioma
    B. Solitary circumscribed neuroma
    C. Traumatic neuroma
    D. Ganglioneuroma
    E. Neurilemmoma

113. The best-fit diagnosis is:

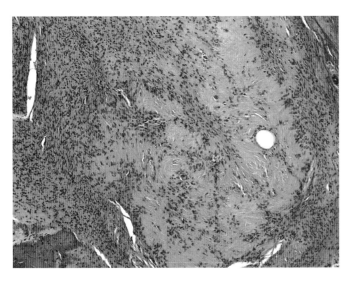

A. Perineurioma
B. Solitary circumscribed neuroma
C. Traumatic neuroma
D. Ganglioneuroma
E. Neurilemmoma

114. Multiple lesions of this (based on the image shown above) are associated with:
A. Neurofibromatosis type 1
B. Neurofibromatosis type 2
C. MEN type 1
D. MEN type 2a
E. MEN type 2b

115. The best-fit diagnosis is:

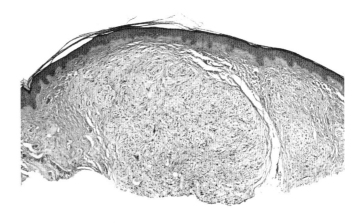

A. Perineurioma
B. Neurothekeoma
C. Nerve sheath myxoma
D. Ganglioneuroma
E. Neurilemmoma

116. Positive staining of lesional cells (based on the image shown above) would be expected with all of the following EXCEPT:
A. S100
B. S100A6
C. GFAP
D. CD57
E. PGP9.5

117. The best-fit diagnosis is:

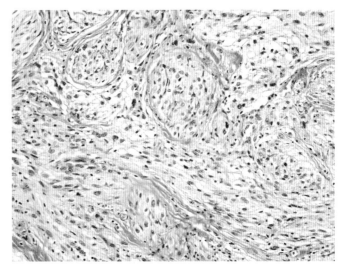

A. Perineurioma
B. Neurothekeoma

C. Nerve sheath myxoma

D. Cellular scar

E. Neurilemmoma

118. Positive staining of lesional cells (based on the image shown above) would be expected with all of the following EXCEPT:

A. NKI/C3

B. S100A6

C. CD10

D. CD30

E. PGP9.5

119. The best-fit diagnosis is:

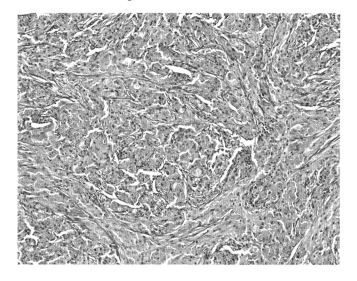

A. Cutaneous oncocytoma

B. Dermatofibroma, granular cell variant

C. Abrikossoff's tumor

D. Wilm's tumor

E. Ancient schwannoma

120. Which of the following associations is correct regarding the image shown:

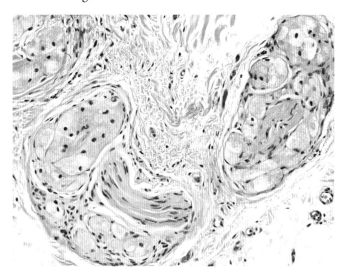

A. Aggressive clinical course

B. Local recurrence

C. No clinical relevance

D. Lymphovascular invasion

E. Mitotic activity >1/HPFs

121. The best-fit diagnosis is:

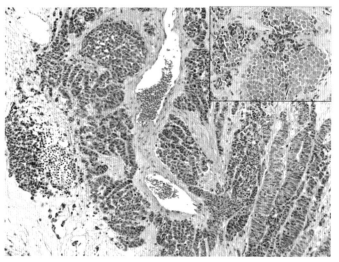

A. Basal cell carcinoma

B. Eccrine spiradenocarcinoma

C. Epithelioid angiosarcoma

D. Merkel cell carcinoma

E. B-cell lymphoma

122. Adverse prognosticators (based on the image shown above) include all of the following EXCEPT:

A. Negative tumoral Merkel cell polyoma virus (MCPyV)

B. Increased intratumoral cytotoxic T lymphocytes

C. Increased Ki-67 index

D. Low anti-MCPyV titers

E. High tumoral p63 labeling

123. Which of the following is correct regarding the Merkel cell polyoma virus (MCPyV):

A. Only found in Merkel cell carcinoma patients

B. MCPyV positive tumors are more aggressive clinically

C. MCPyV positive tumors are typically in non-sun-exposed sites

D. MCPyV positive tumors exhibit greater pleomorphism

E. MCPyV positive tumors exhibit a higher Ki-67 proliferation index

124. The best-fit diagnosis is:

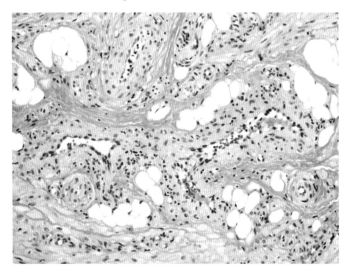

   A. Angiolipoma
   B. Adenolipoma
   C. Angiomyolipoma
   D. Lipoblastoma
   E. Hibernoma

125. The renal counterpart of this (based on the image shown above) is associated with:
   A. Cowden syndrome
   B. Tuberous sclerosis
   C. Proteus syndrome
   D. Carney complex
   E. Kasabach-Merritt syndrome

126. The best-fit diagnosis is:

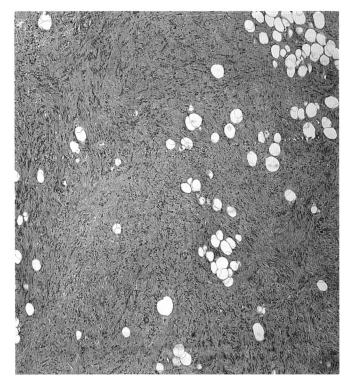

   A. Spindle cell lipoma
   D. Sclerotic lipoma
   C. Lipomatous scar
   D. Pseudolipomatous cutis
   E. Nevus lipomatosus

127. Loss of which of the following chromosomes is associated with this (based on the image shown above):
   A. 8
   B. 10
   C. 12
   D. 14
   E. 16

128. Spindle cells in this entity (based on the image shown above) would be expected to be positive for:
   A. CD20
   B. CD25
   C. CD30
   D. CD34
   E. CD56

129. The best-fit diagnosis is:

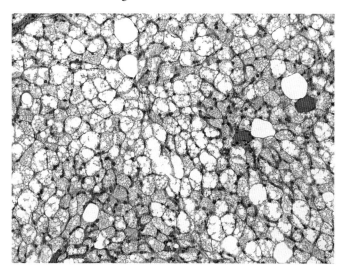

   A. Liposarcoma
   B. Adenolipoma
   C. Angiomyolipoma
   D. Lipoblastoma
   E. Hibernoma

130. Cytogenetic abnormalities associated with well-differentiated liposarcoma involve:
   A. PTEN
   B. COL1A1
   C. FLT1
   D. MDM2
   E. MYC

131. Multiple lesions of this are typically associated with:

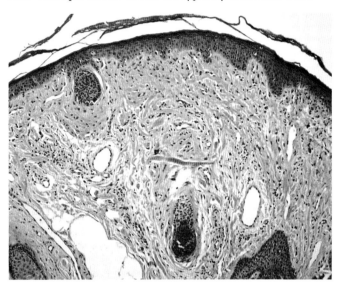

    A. Tuberous sclerosis
    B. Neurofibromatosis 2
    C. Muir-Torre syndrome
    D. Gardner syndrome
    E. Brooke-Spiegler syndrome

132. The best-fit diagnosis is:

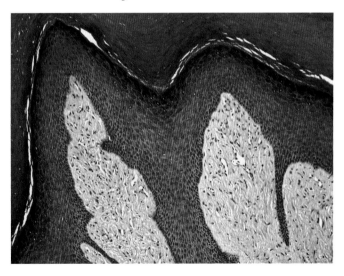

    A. Supernumerary digit
    B. Acral fibrokeratoma
    C. Traumatic neuroma
    D. Fibroepithelial polyp
    E. Digital fibromatosis

133. Multiple lesions of this are associated with:

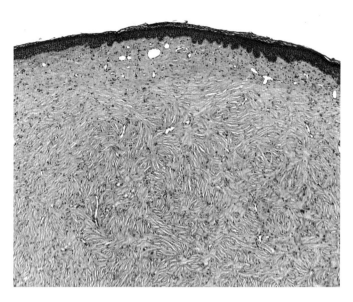

    A. Tuberous sclerosis
    B. Cowden's disease
    C. Brook-Spiegler syndrome
    D. Wermer's syndrome
    E. Birt-Hogg-Dubé syndrome

134. Lesional cells (based on the image shown above) are typically positive for:
    A. CD10
    B. CD20
    C. CD30
    D. CD31
    E. CD34

135. The best-fit diagnosis for this rapidly growing nodule is:

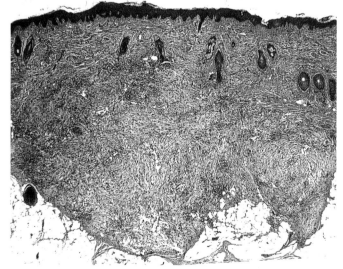

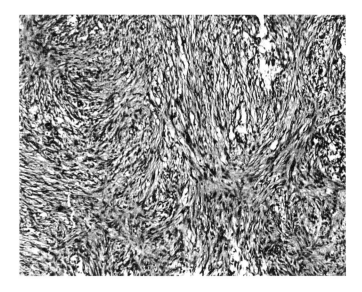

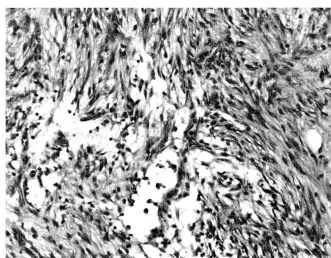

A. Angiomatoid fibrous histiocytoma
B. Pyoderma gangrenosum
C. Solitary fibrous tumor
D. Nodular fasciitis
E. Sclerotic hemangioma

136. The best-fit diagnosis is:

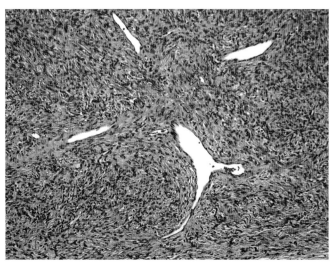

A. Angiomatoid fibrous histiocytoma
B. Pyoderma gangrenosum
C. Solitary fibrous tumor
D. Nodular fasciitis
E. Sclerotic hemangioma (dermatofibroma variant)

137. Lesional cells (based on the image shown above) would be positive for:
A. CD10
B. CD30
C. CD31
D. CD34
E. β-catenin

138. Which of the following genes is altered in this (based on the image shown above):
A. *NF-κB*
B. *COL1A1*
C. *STAT6*
D. *SOX10*
E. *KRAS*

139. The best-fit diagnosis is:

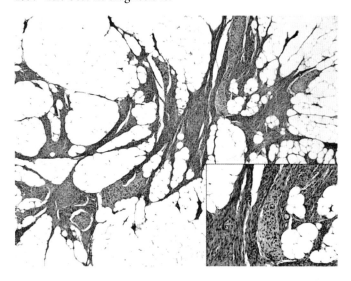

    A. Fibromatosis
    B. Fibrous hamartoma of infancy
    C. Solitary fibrous tumor
    D. Infantile myofibromatosis
    E. Nodular fasciitis

140. The best-fit diagnosis is:

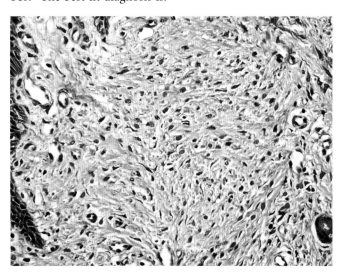

    A. Digital fibromatosis
    B. Infantile myofibromatosis
    C. Acral fibrokeratoma
    D. Dermatofibroma, traumatized
    E. Dupuytren's disease

141. The best-fit diagnosis for this vulvar lesion is:

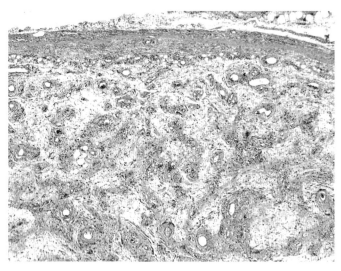

    A. Angiofibroma
    B. Angiomyxoma
    C. Angioleiomyoma
    D. Angiomyolipoma
    E. Angiomyofibroblastoma

142. The best-fit diagnosis is:

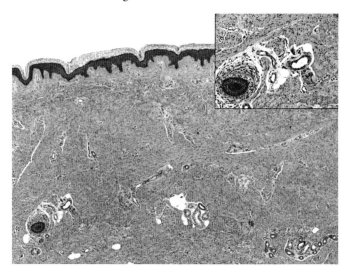

    A. Desmoid fibromatosis
    B. Dermatofibroma
    C. Dermatofibrosarcoma protuberans
    D. Dermatomyofibroma
    E. Myofibromatosis

143. The best-fit diagnosis is:

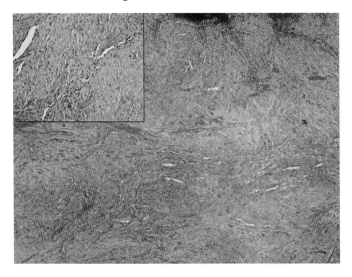

  A. Desmoid fibromatosis
  B. Digital fibromatosis
  C. Dermatofibrosarcoma protuberans
  D. Dermatomyofibroma
  E. Infantile myofibromatosis

144. The best-fit diagnosis is:

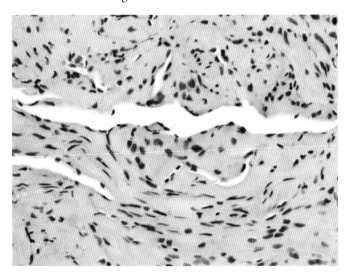

  A. Myofibroma
  B. Angioleiomyoma
  C. Myopericytoma
  D. Leiomyoma
  E. Angiomyxoma

145. The best-fit diagnosis for this HMB45 and actin positive tumor is:

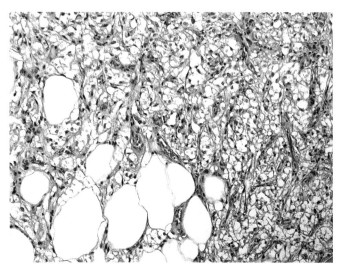

  A. Granular cell tumor
  B. PEComa
  C. Sebaceoma
  D. Melanoma
  E. Clear cell sarcoma

146. The best-fit diagnosis for this ALK-1 positive tumor is:

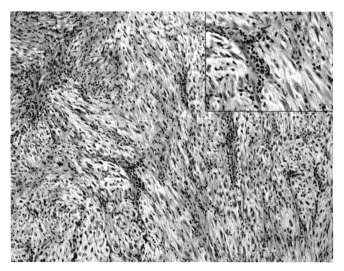

  A. Inflammatory myofibroblastic tumor
  B. Epithelioid sarcoma
  C. Desmoid fibromatosis
  D. Inflamed atypical fibroxanthoma
  E. Inflamed undifferentiated pleomorphic sarcoma

147. The best-fit diagnosis for this acral lesion is:

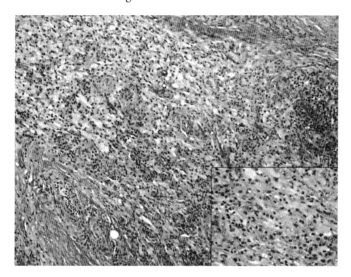

    A. Inflammatory myofibroblastic tumor
    B. Epithelioid sarcoma
    C. Plantar fibromatosis
    D. Inflamed atypical fibroxanthoma
    E. Myxoinflammatory fibroblastic sarcoma

148. The best-fit diagnosis is:

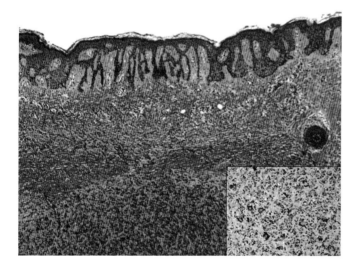

    A. Fibrosarcoma
    B. Angiofibroma
    C. Fibroblastoma
    D. Dermatofibroma
    E. Fibromatosis

149. The best-fit diagnosis is:

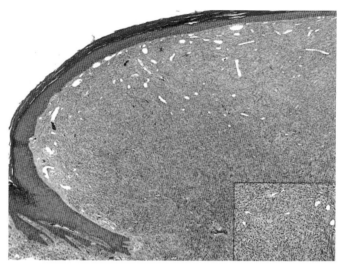

    A. Cellular fibrous histiocytoma
    B. Juvenile xanthogranuloma
    C. Epithelioid cell histiocytoma
    D. Solitary fibrous tumor
    E. Reticulohistiocytoma

150. Which of the following is a synonym for Ledderhose disease:
    A. Palmar fibromatosis
    B. Plantar aponeurosis
    C. Penile fibromatosis
    D. Desmoid tumor
    E. Digital fibromatosis

151. Lesional cells in all types of fibromatosis are usually positive for:
    A. Calretinin
    B. Calcitonin
    C. β-catenin
    D. CK903
    E. PGP9.5

152. Desmoid tumors may be associated with:
    A. Gardner syndrome
    B. Muir-Torre syndrome
    C. Rothmund-Thomson syndrome
    D. NAME syndrome
    E. Burt-Hogg-Dubé syndrome

153. The best-fit diagnosis is:

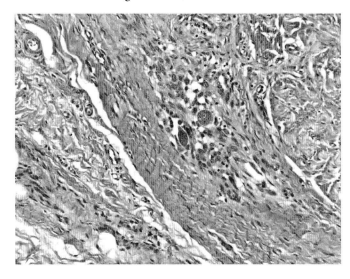

   A. Inflammatory myofibroblastic tumor
   B. Plexiform granular cell tumor
   C. Plexiform spindle cell nevus
   D. Angiomatoid fibrous histiocytoma
   E. Plexiform fibrohistiocytoma

154. The best-fit diagnosis for this pediatric tumor is:

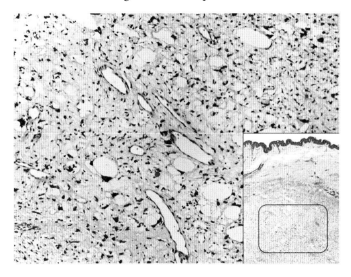

   A. Angiofibroblastoma
   B. Angiomyofibroblastoma
   C. Fibromyxoid sarcoma
   D. Giant cell fibroblastoma
   E. Myxoid myofibroblastoma

155. This (based on the image shown above) is the pediatric counterpart of:
   A. Myxoid fibroblastoma
   B. Fibromyxoid sarcoma
   C. Dermatofibrosarcoma protuberans
   D. Epithelioid cell histiocytoma
   E. Inflammatory myofibroblastic tumor

156. This (based on the image shown above) is associated with which of the following translocations:
   A. t(9;11)
   B. t(11;14)
   C. t(11;22)
   D. t(14;18)
   E. t(17;22)

157. The best-fit diagnosis is:

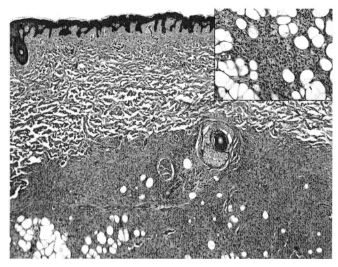

   A. Myxoid fibroblastoma
   B. Fibromyxoid sarcoma
   C. Dermatofibrosarcoma protuberans
   D. Epithelioid cell histiocytoma
   E. Inflammatory myofibroblastic tumor

158. This (based on the image shown above) is associated with which of the following translocations:
   A. t(9;11)
   B. t(11;14)
   C. t(11;22)
   D. t(14;18)
   E. t(17;22)

159. The best-fit diagnosis is:

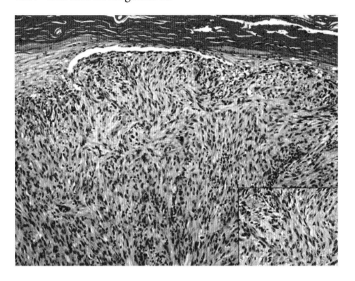

    A. Epithelioid cell histiocytoma
    B. Pyogenic granuloma
    C. Juvenile xanthogranuloma
    D. Atypical fibroxanthoma
    E. Dermatofibrosarcoma protuberans

160. The best-fit diagnosis is:

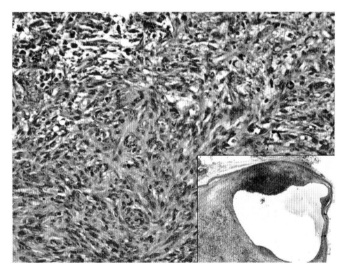

    A. Epithelioid cell histiocytoma
    B. Pyogenic granuloma
    C. Angiomatoid fibrous histiocytoma
    D. Sclerosing hemangioma
    E. Dermatofibrosarcoma protuberans

161. The best-fit diagnosis is:

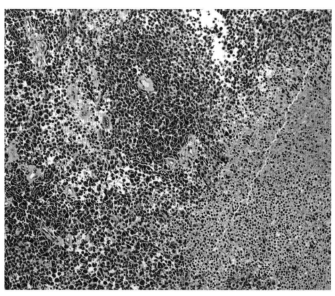

    A. Granuloma annulare
    B. Rheumatoid nodule
    C. Wegner's granulomatosis
    D. Epithelioid sarcoma
    E. Synovial sarcoma

162. The best-fit diagnosis is:

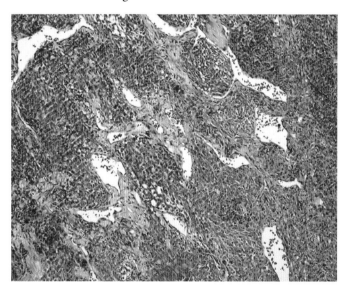

    A. Plantar fibromatosis
    B. Solitary fibrous tumor
    C. Wegner's granulomatosis
    D. Epithelioid sarcoma
    E. Synovial sarcoma

163. The best-fit diagnosis for this lesion on the digits is:

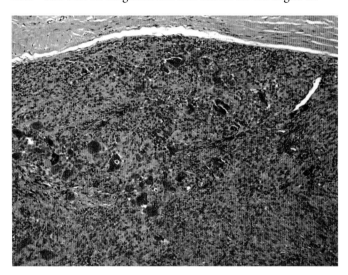

A. Pigmented villonodular synovitis
B. Giant cell angiofibroma
C. Giant cell tumor of tendon sheath
D. Giant cell fibroblastoma
E. Plexiform fibrohistiocytic tumor

164. The best-fit diagnosis for this periungual tumor is:

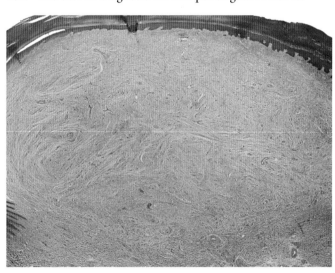

A. Dermatofibrosarcoma protuberans
B. Myxoinflammatory fibroblastic sarcoma
C. Superficial acral fibromyxoma
D. Focal cutaneous mucinosis
E. Myxoid neurofibroma

165. The best-fit diagnosis is:

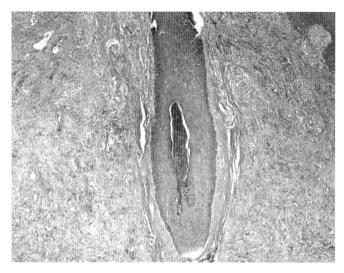

A. Focal mucinosis
B. Scleromyxedema
C. Digital mucous cyst
D. Reticular erythematous mucinosis
E. Superficial angiomyxoma

166. These (based on the image shown above) may be a feature of:
A. Gardner's syndrome
B. Hunter's syndrome
C. Bloom's syndrome
D. NAME syndrome
E. Griscelli syndrome

167. Metachronous metastasis refers to:
A. Cutaneous metastasis that is the first indication of a visceral malignancy
B. Cutaneous metastasis that develops years after a visceral malignancy
C. Cutaneous metastasis that occurs at the same time as the visceral malignancy

168. The likely primary for this PAX-8 and CD10 positive malignancy is:

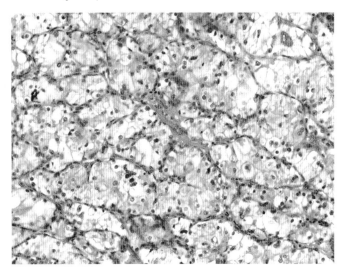

    A. Kidney
    B. Breast
    C. Lung
    D. Bladder
    E. Ovary

169. The likely primary for this CK20 and CDX2 positive malignancy is:

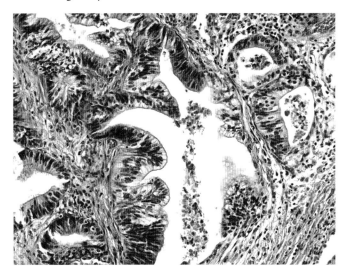

    A. Kidney
    B. Breast
    C. Lung
    D. Bladder
    E. Colon

170. The best-fit diagnosis for this CK7 and MUC1 positive malignancy is:

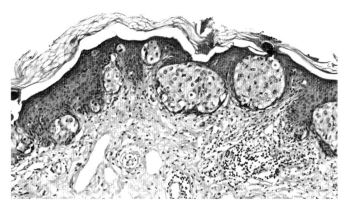

    A. Malignant melanoma in situ
    B. Intraepidermal basal cell carcinoma
    C. Sebaceous carcinoma in situ
    D. Paget's disease
    E. Clear cell papulosis

171. The best-fit diagnosis for this malignancy with a psammoma body is:

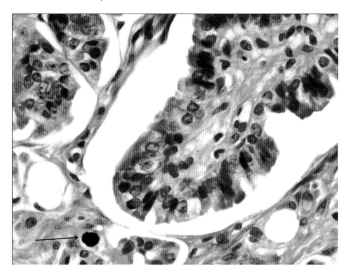

    A. Renal cell carcinoma
    B. Extramammary Paget's disease
    C. Papillary thyroid carcinoma
    D. Transitional cell carcinoma
    E. Ewing's sarcoma

172. The best-fit diagnosis for this eyelid lesion is:

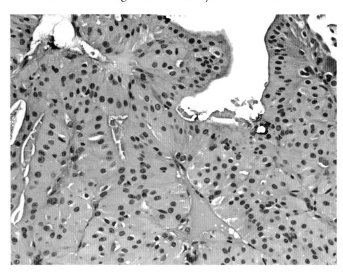

    A. Granular cell tumor
    B. Cutaneous oncocytoma
    C. Cutaneous myoepithelioma
    D. PEComa
    E. Clear cell sarcoma

173. Which of the following is a clinical syndrome associated with a capillary malformation:
    A. Sturge-Weber syndrome
    B. Birt-Hogg-Dubé syndrome
    C. Brooke-Spiegler syndrome
    D. Gorlin-Goltz syndrome
    E. NAME/LAMB syndrome

174. The best-fit diagnosis is:

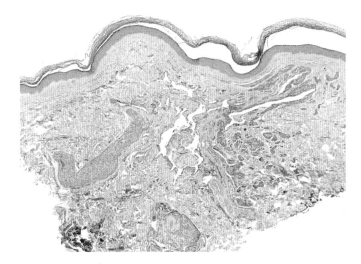

    A. Capillary malformation
    B. Benign lymphangioendothelioma
    C. Lymphatic malformation

    D. Lymphangioma circumscriptum
    E. Glomulovenous malformation

175. The best-fit diagnosis is:

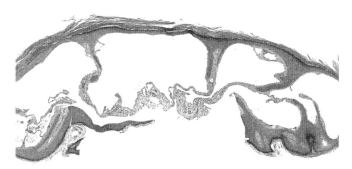

    A. Cavernous hemangioma
    B. Benign lymphangioendothelioma
    C. Microvenular hemangioma
    D. Lymphangioma circumscriptum
    E. Glomulovenous malformation

176. The best-fit diagnosis is:

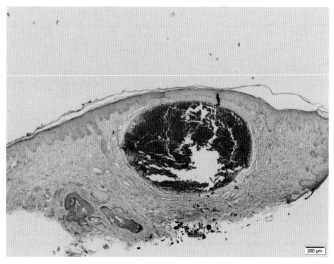

    A. Cherry angioma
    B. Venous lake
    C. Angioma serpiginosum
    D. Papular angioplasia
    E. Superficial lymphangioma
    F. Spider angioma

177. Clinical subtypes of this include all of the following EXCEPT:

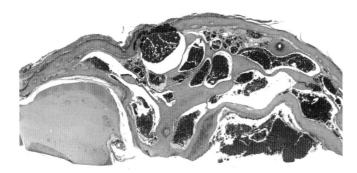

   A. Peyronie's disease
   B. Fordyce type
   C. Mibeli type
   D. Solitary and multiple types
   E. Angiokeratoma circumscriptum

178. The best-fit diagnosis is:

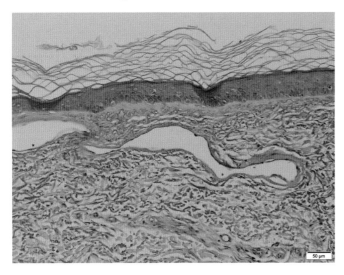

   A. Reactive angioendotheliomatosis
   B. Hobnail hemangioma
   C. Angioma serpiginosum
   D. Endovascular papillary angioendothelioma
   E. Cutaneous collagenous vasculopathy

179. In contrast to vascular malformation, infantile hemangiomas typically express:
   A. CD31
   B. D2–40

C. C-MYC
D. GLUT-1
E. CD34

180. Glomeruloid hemangioma is a specific marker for:
   A. NAME syndrome
   B. Kimura's disease
   C. POEMS
   D. Neurofibromatosis I
   E. Sturge-Weber syndrome

181. The best-fit diagnosis is:

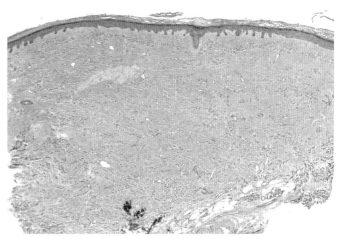

   A. Glomeruloid hemangioma
   B. Microvenular hemangioma
   C. Acquired elastotic hemangioma
   D. Angioma serpiginosum
   E. Angiosarcoma

182. The new nomenclature for this entity is:

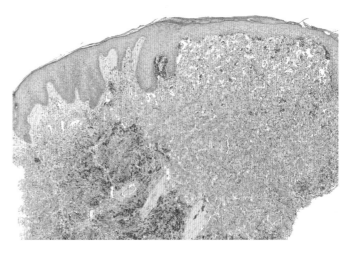

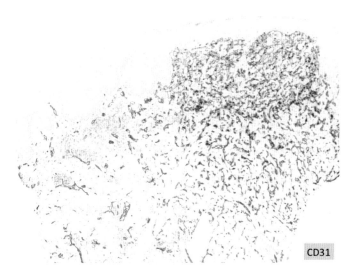

A. Hobnail hemangioma
B. Epithelioid hemangioma
C. Microvenular hemangioma
D. Angioma serpiginosum
E. Kaposiform hemangioendothelioma

183. This is believed to be part of the spectrum of:

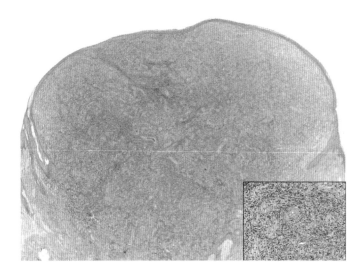

A. Hobnail hemangioma
B. Epithelioid hemangioma
C. Microvenular hemangioma
D. Angioma serpiginosum
E. Kaposiform hemangioendothelioma

184. The best-fit diagnosis is:

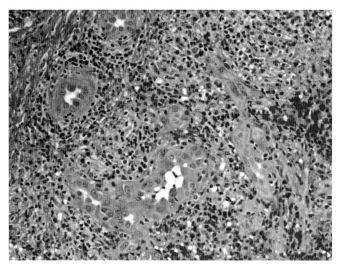

A. Hobnail hemangioma
B. Epithelioid hemangioma
C. Microvenular hemangioma
D. Angioma serpiginosum
E. Kaposiform hemangioendothelioma

185. The best-fit diagnosis is:

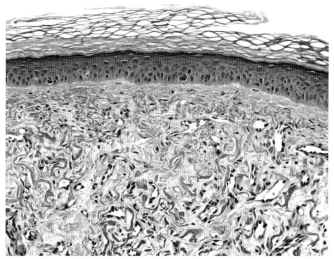

A. Angioma serpiginosum
B. Papular angioplasia
C. Acroangiodermatitis
D. Acquired elastotic hemangioma
E. Targetoid hemosiderotic hemangioma

186. The best-fit diagnosis is:

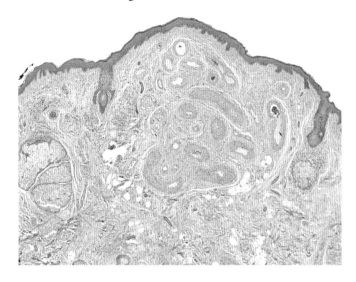

    A. Microvenular hemangioma
    B. Papillary hemangioma
    C. Sinusoidal hemangioma
    D. Arteriovenous hemangioma
    E. Cherry angioma

187. The best-fit diagnosis is:

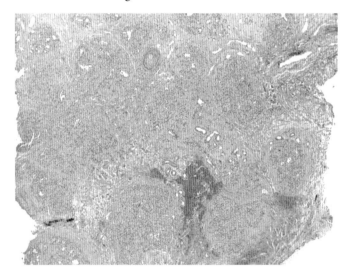

    A. Microvenular hemangioma
    B. Papillary hemangioma
    C. Sinusoidal hemangioma
    D. Eruptive pseudoangiomatosis
    E. Tufted angioma

188. Lesional cells would be positive for:

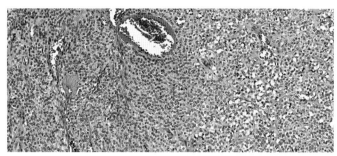

    A. CD30
    B. CD31
    C. CD34
    D. Actin
    E. D2–40

189. The best-fit diagnosis is:

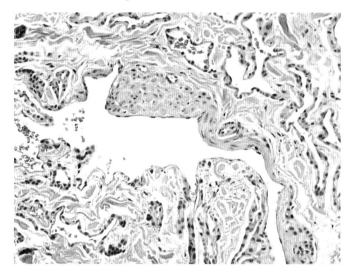

    A. Angioleiomyoma
    B. Myofibroma
    C. Glomangiomyoma
    D. Glomangioma
    E. Myofibroma

190. The best-fit diagnosis is:

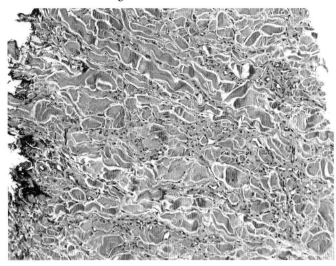

A. Sinusoidal hemangioma
B. Diffuse dermal angiomatosis
C. Microvenular hemangioma
D. Angioma serpiginosum
E. Eruptive pseudoangiomatosis

191. The best-fit diagnosis is:

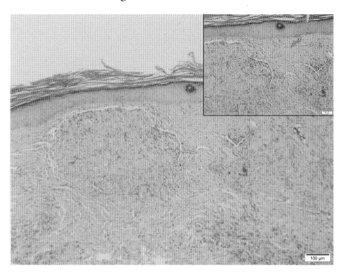

A. Pseudo-Kaposi's sarcoma
B. Diffuse dermal angiomatosis
C. Kaposi's sarcoma
D. Microvenular hemangioma
E. Symplastic hemangioma

192. This is best regarded as:

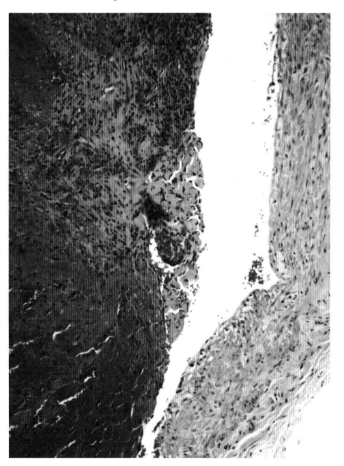

A. A low-grade malignancy
B. A high-grade malignancy
C. Of infectious etiology
D. An organizing thrombus
E. Syndromic marker

193. The best-fit diagnosis is:

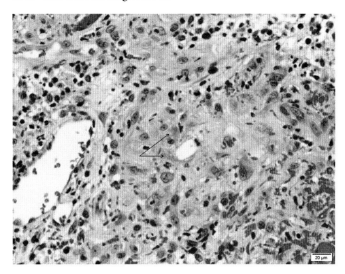

A. Pyogenic granuloma
B. Recanalizing thrombus
C. Bacillary angiomatosis
D. Kaposi's sarcoma, PG-like
E. Eruptive pseudoangiomatosis

194. The causative organism (based on the image shown above) is:
A. *Bartonella bacilliformis*
B. *Bartonella quintana*
C. *Bartonella clarridgeiae*
D. *Coxiella burnettii*

195. Borderline vascular malignancies/vascular tumors of low-grade malignancy include all of the following EXCEPT:
A. Epithelioid hemangioendothelioma
B. Composite hemangioendothelioma
C. Kaposiform hemangioendothelioma
D. Retiform hemangioendothelioma
E. Kaposi's sarcoma

196. Which of the following helps clinch the diagnosis of the entity shown:

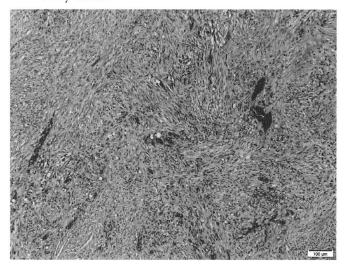

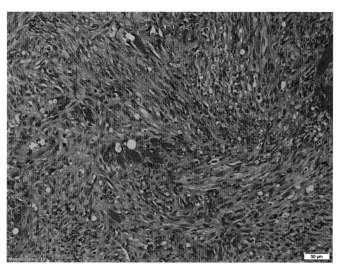

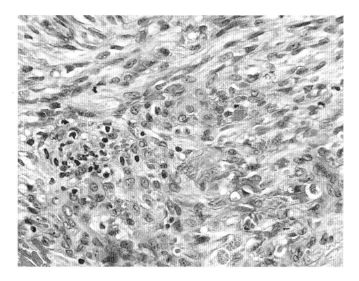

A. EBV
B. HSV2

C. MCPyV
D. HZV
E. HHV8

197. Kasabach-Merritt syndrome is associated with:
   A. Epithelioid hemangioendothelioma
   B. Composite hemangioendothelioma
   C. Kaposiform hemangioendothelioma
   D. Retiform hemangioendothelioma
   E. Kaposi's sarcoma

198. Which of the following is a synonym for Dabska's tumor:
   A. Epithelioid hemangioendothelioma
   B. Composite hemangioendothelioma
   C. Kaposiform hemangioendothelioma
   D. Retiform hemangioendothelioma
   E. Endovascular papillary angioendothelioma

199. The best-fit diagnosis is:

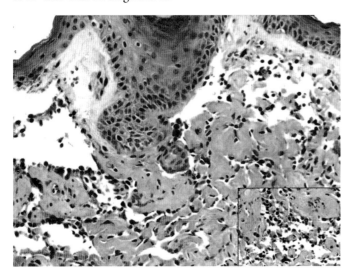

   A. Hemangiopericytoma
   B. Angioblastoma
   C. Hobnail hemangioma
   D. Angiosarcoma
   E. Kaposi's sarcoma

200. Expression of which of the following helps differentiate post-irradiation angiosarcoma from atypical vascular lesions:
   A. CD31
   B. D2–40
   C. MYC
   D. GLUT-1
   E. CD34

201. The best-fit diagnosis is:

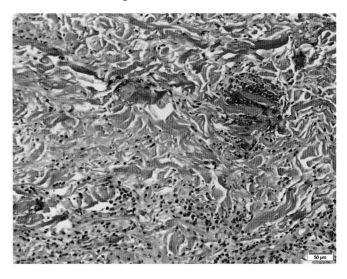

   A. Granuloma annulare
   B. Wells's syndrome
   C. Churg-Strauss syndrome
   D. Urticarial vasculitis
   E. Xanthoma disseminatum

202. Cutaneous entities associated with paraproteinemia include all of the following EXCEPT:
   A. NAME syndrome
   B. POEMS syndrome
   C. Schnitzler syndrome
   D. Hyperviscosity syndrome
   E. Sneddon-Wilkinson's disease

203. The best-fit diagnosis is:

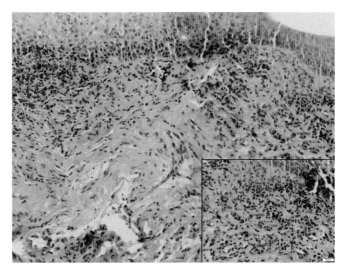

   A. Atrophic lichen planus
   B. Plasmacytoma
   C. Urticaria pigmentosa

D. IgG4-related disease

E. Plasmacytosis mucosae

204. The best-fit diagnosis for this extremely itchy lesion is:

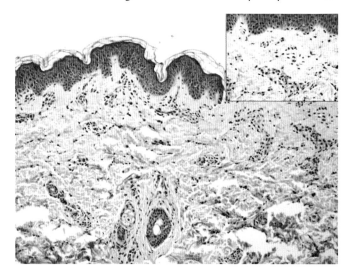

A. Plasmacytosis mucosae

B. Planar xanthoma

C. Leukemia cutis

D. Urticaria pigmentosa

E. Urticaria

205. Lesional cells (based on the image shown above) would be typically positive for:
    A. D138
    B. CD68
    C. CD117
    D. CD15
    E. CD79a

206. The best-fit diagnosis is:

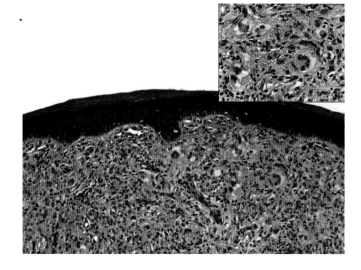

A. Atypical fibroxanthoma

B. Juvenile xanthogranuloma

C. Pyogenic granuloma

D. Reticulohistiocytoma

E. Langerhans cell histiocytosis

207. The best-fit diagnosis is:

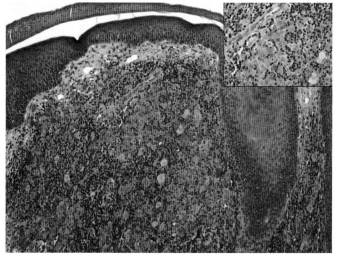

A. Atypical fibroxanthoma

B. Juvenile xanthogranuloma

C. Pyogenic granuloma

D. Reticulohistiocytoma

E. Langerhans cell histiocytosis

208. Multiple lesions of these (based on the image shown above) are associated with:
    A. Destructive arthropathy
    B. Renal disease
    C. Arteriovenous malformations
    D. Brachioradial pruritus
    E. Histiocytic sarcoma

209. The best-fit diagnosis is:

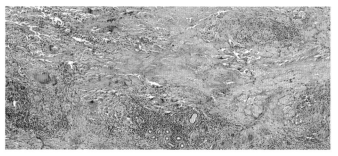

A. Granuloma annulare

B. Wegener's granulomatosis

C. Mycobacterial infection

D. Necrobiotic xanthogranuloma

E. Necrobiosis lipoidica

210. This (based on the image shown above) is often associated with:
   A. Arthritis
   B. Perforation
   C. Emperipolesis
   D. Iridocyclitis
   E. Paraproteinemia

211. The best-fit diagnosis is:

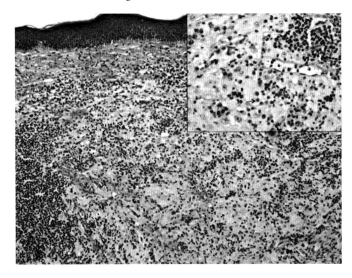

   A. Plasmacytoma
   B. Solitary mastocytoma
   C. Orbital xanthogranuloma
   D. Rosai-Dorfman disease
   E. Erdheim-Chester disease

212. Lesional histiocytes (based on the image shown above) would be:
   A. CD20 and CD79a positive
   B. S100 and CD79a positive
   C. S100 and CD68 positive
   D. S100 and CD1a positive
   E. CD68 and CD1a positive

213. The best-fit diagnosis is:

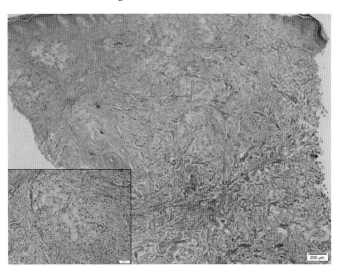

   A. Xanthelasma
   B. Verruciform xanthoma
   C. Granuloma annulare
   D. Eruptive xanthoma
   E. Juvenile xanthogranuloma

214. The best-fit diagnosis is:

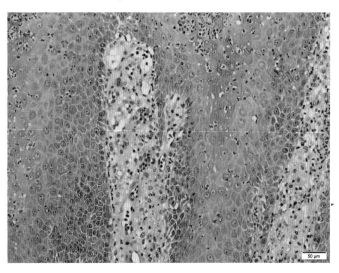

   A. Xanthelasma
   B. Verruciform xanthoma
   C. Granuloma annulare
   D. Eruptive xanthoma
   E. Juvenile xanthogranuloma

215. The best-fit diagnosis is:

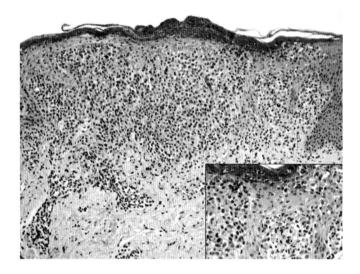

    A. Langerhans cell histiocytosis
    B. Rosai-Dorfman disease
    C. Reactive histiocytosis
    D. Castleman's disease
    E. Erdheim-Chester disease

216. Lesional cells (based on the image shown above) would be:
    A. CD20 and CD79a positive
    B. S100 and CD79a positive
    C. S100 and CD68 positive
    D. S100 and CD1a positive
    E. CD68 and CD1a positive

217. The best-fit diagnosis for this hypopigmented lesion in a 12-year-old is:

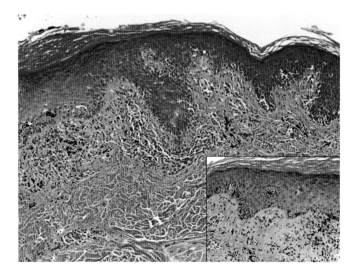

    A. Vitiligo, inflammatory stage
    B. Langerhans cell histiocytosis

    C. Mycosis fungoides
    D. Lymphomatoid papulosis
    E. Sézary's syndrome

218. The expected immunophenotype of lesional cells (based on the image shown above) is:
    A. CD20 and CD79a positive
    B. CD3 and CD8 positive
    C. CD3 and CD4 positive
    D. CD3 and CD20 positive
    E. CD4 and CD8 positive

219. The best-fit diagnosis for this is:

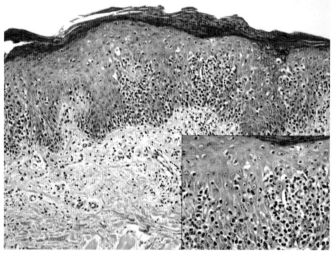

    A. Pagetoid reticulosis
    B. Paget's disease
    C. Extramammary Paget's disease
    D. Lymphomatoid papulosis
    E. Sézary's syndrome

220. Hematologic criteria for Sézary's syndrome include all of the following EXCEPT:
    A. Absolute cell count >1000cells/mm^3
    B. CD4:CD8 ratio of 10 or more
    C. Aberrant expression of CD2/CD3/CD4/CD5
    D. Monoclonal B lymphocytes
    E. Circulating Lutzner cells

221. The best-fit diagnosis for this CD30 positive entity is:

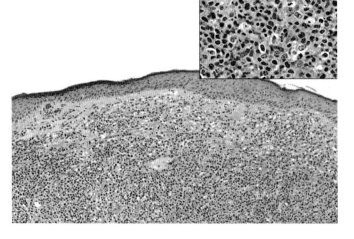

    A. Exuberant dermal hypersensitivity reaction
    B. Lymphomatoid papulosis, type A
    C. Anaplastic large cell lymphoma
    D. Hydroa vacciniforme-like lymphoma
    E. Diffuse large B-cell lymphoma

222. The cutaneous variant (based on the image shown above) lacks which of the following translocations:
    A. $t(2;5)$
    B. $t(9;11)$
    C. $t(11;14)$
    D. $t(11;18)$
    E. $t(19;22)$

223. The best-fit diagnosis for this CD30 positive entity is:

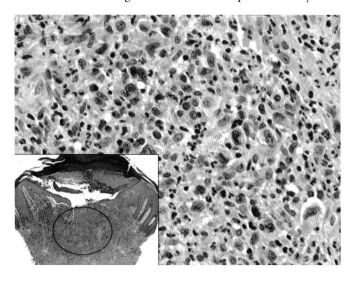

    A. Exuberant dermal hypersensitivity reaction
    B. Lymphomatoid papulosis
    C. Anaplastic large cell lymphoma

    D. Hydroa vacciniforme-like lymphoma
    E. Diffuse large B-cell lymphoma

224. The best-fit diagnosis for this CD8/βF1 positive entity is:

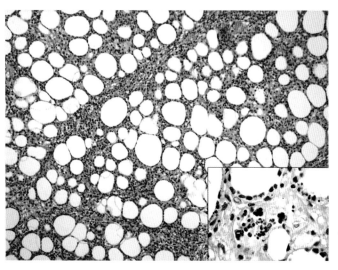

    A. Subcutaneous panniculitis-like T-cell lymphoma
    B. Lupus profundus panniculitis
    C. Primary cutaneous gamma/delta T-cell lymphoma
    D. Infectious panniculitis
    E. Calciphylaxis

225. The best-fit diagnosis for this CD3/CD56 positive entity is:

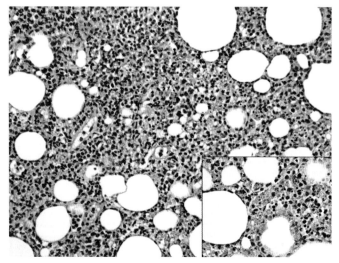

    A. Subcutaneous panniculitis-like T-cell lymphoma
    B. Lupus profundus panniculitis
    C. Primary cutaneous gamma/delta T-cell lymphoma
    D. Infectious panniculitis
    E. Calciphylaxis

226. The best-fit diagnosis for this EBV/CD56 positive entity is:

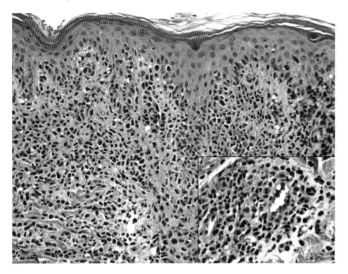

    A. Peripheral T-cell lymphoma, NOS
    B. Subcutaneous panniculitis-like T-cell lymphoma
    C. Primary cutaneous gamma/delta T-cell lymphoma
    D. Mycosis fungoides, plaque stage
    E. Extranodal NK/T-cell lymphoma, nasal type

227. The best-fit diagnosis for this for this βF1/TIA-1/granzyme B positive entity is:

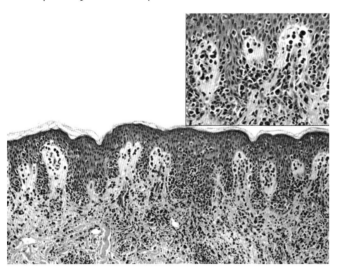

    A. Peripheral T-cell lymphoma, NOS
    B. Lymphomatoid papulosis, type C
    C. Primary cutaneous gamma/delta T-cell lymphoma
    D. Primary cutaneous CD8 positive aggressive epidermotropic cytotoxic T-cell lymphoma
    E. Primary cutaneous anaplastic large cell lymphoma

228. The best-fit diagnosis is:

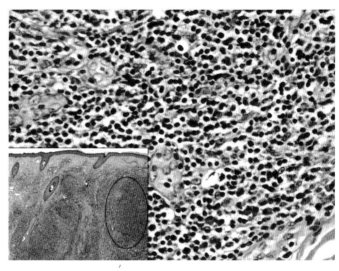

    A. Diffuse large B-cell lymphoma
    B. Plasmablastic lymphoma
    C. Marginal zone B-cell lymphoma
    D. Benign lymphoid hyperplasia
    E. Follicle center cell lymphoma

229. The best-fit diagnosis is:

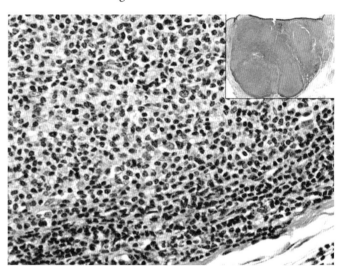

    A. Diffuse large B-cell lymphoma, leg type
    B. Plasmablastic lymphoma
    C. Marginal zone B-cell lymphoma
    D. Benign lymphoid hyperplasia
    E. Follicle center cell lymphoma

230. The best-fit diagnosis is:

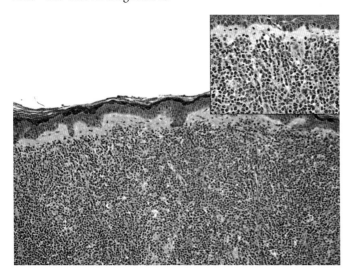

    A. Diffuse large B-cell lymphoma, leg type
    B. Hydroa vacciniforme-like lymphoma
    C. Marginal zone B-cell lymphoma
    D. Benign lymphoid hyperplasia
    E. Follicle center cell lymphoma

231. The best-fit diagnosis is:

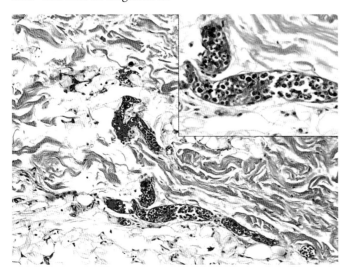

    A. Reactive angioendotheliomatosis
    B. Intravascular papillary endothelial hyperplasia
    C. Intravascular histiocytosis
    D. Intravascular large B-cell lymphoma
    E. Intravascular T/NK cell lymphoma

232. The best-fit diagnosis is:

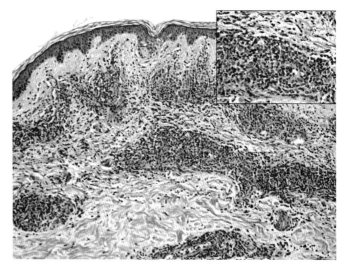

    A. Chronic lymphocytic leukemia
    B. Benign lymphoid hyperplasia
    C. Myeloid sarcoma
    D. T-lymphoblastic leukemia
    E. Primary effusion lymphoma

233. The best-fit diagnosis is:

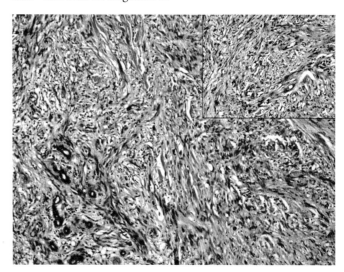

    A. Myeloid sarcoma
    B. Interdigitating dendritic cell sarcoma
    C. Langerhans cell histiocytosis
    D. Malignant melanoma
    E. Hydroa vacciniforme-like lymphoma

234. The best-fit diagnosis is:

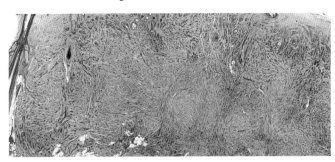

A. Clear cell syringoma
B. Adenoid cystic carcinoma
C. Desmoplastic trichoepithelioma
D. Papillary digital adenocarcinoma
E. Microcystic adnexal carcinoma

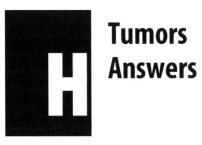

Tumors
Answers

Table H1 Epidermal tumors – "at a glance"

Entity	Histopathologic clues	Immunohisto-chemical profile	Image
ILVEN	Psoriasiform epidermal hyperplasia, alternating parakeratosis without a granular layer, orthokeratosis with a thickened granular layer	Not relevant	
Prurigo nodularis	Compact orthohyperkeratosis, pseudoepitheliomatous hyperplasia, hypergranulosis, vertically oriented papillary dermal fibrosis	Not relevant	

Table H1 Epidermal tumors – "at a glance" (*cont.*)

Entity	Histopathologic clues	Immunohisto-chemical profile	Image
Seborrheic keratosis	Papillomatous epidermal hyperplasia, "pseudo" horn cysts	Not relevant	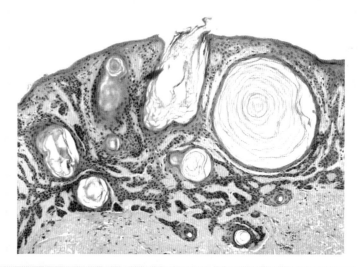
Melanoacanthoma	Pigmented, benign proliferation of keratinocytes and dendritic melanocytes	Dendritic melanocytes S100 and HMB-45 positive	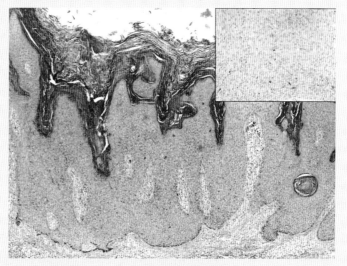
Clear cell papulosis	Proliferation of single/clusters of clear basal cells (round regular nuclei, abundant lightly eosinophilic) along basal and suprabasal layers	Clear cells positive for mucin, CEA, EMA, CK AE1/3, CK7, and CAM 5.2	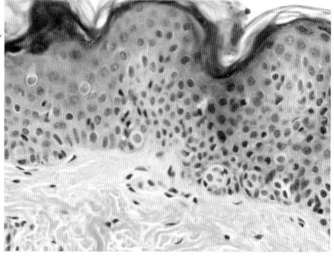

Table H1 Epidermal tumors – "at a glance" (*cont.*)

Entity	Histopathologic clues	Immunohisto-chemical profile	Image
Actinic keratosis	Blue and pink horn, basal keratinocyte atypia, irregular basal budding of atypical keratinocytes ("Bernie's buds")	Not relevant	
Bowen's disease	Full thickness keratinocyte atypia, disordered epidermal maturation	Positive for p40, p63, CK5/6 and CK903	
Bowenoid papulosis	Full thickness keratinocyte atypia, disordered epidermal maturation, numerous mitotic figures, scattered, individually necrotic dyskeratotic keratinocytes	Positive for p40, p63, CK5/6 and CK903 HPV-16 positive	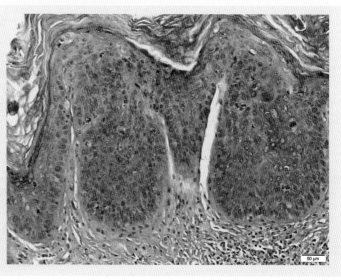

Table H1 Epidermal tumors – "at a glance" (*cont.*)

Entity	Histopathologic clues	Immunohisto-chemical profile	Image
Basal cell carcinoma, nodular type	Dermal islands of basaloid cells, peripheral palisading, clefting artefact, mucinous stroma	Positive for BerEP4, Bcl2, CD10 and AR	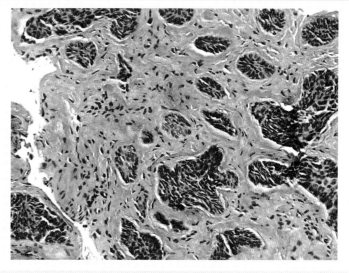
Fibroepithelioma of Pinkus	Anastomosing strands of basaloid cells, mucinous stroma	Positive for BerEP4, Bcl2, CD10 and AR	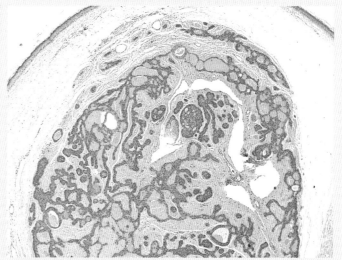
Squamous cell carcinoma, well differentiated	Dermal islands of keratinizing squamous epithelium	Positive for p40, p63, CK5/6 and CK903, PCNA	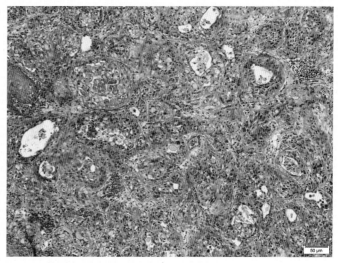

Table H1 Epidermal tumors – "at a glance" (*cont.*)

Entity	Histopathologic clues	Immunohisto-chemical profile	Image
Marjolin's ulcer	Dermal islands of keratinizing squamous epithelium in scar	Positive for p40, p63, CK5/6 and CK903	
Verrucous carcinoma	Cohesive bulbous downgrowths of squamous epithelium, minimal cytologic atypia	Peripheral positivity for PCNA	
Mucoepidermoid carcinoma	3 cell types: mucinous, squamous and clear	All cell types positive for CK7, panCK, CEA and EMA	

Table H1 Epidermal tumors – "at a glance" (*cont.*)

Entity	Histopathologic clues	Immunohisto-chemical profile	Image
Carcinosarcoma	Biphasic tumor, malignant epithelial and mesenchymal elements, no transitional areas	Epithelial elements positive for p63 and p40 Mesenchymal elements positive for vimentin, CD10, actin, CD34	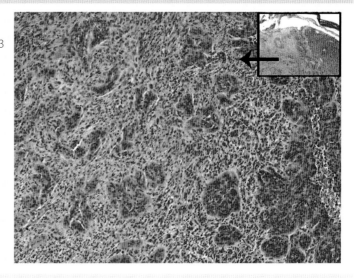
Lymphoepithelioma-like carcinoma	Biphasic tumor, malignant epithelial cells, surrounding reactive lymphoid cell infiltrate	Epithelial elements positive for panCK, p63 and p40	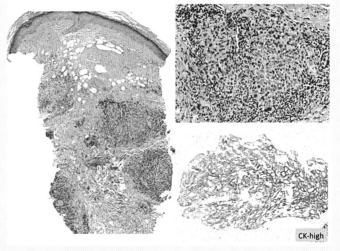
Onychomatrixoma	Vertically penetrating epithelial cell strands, fibrous stroma sharply delineated from tumoral cells	Epithelial strands positive for K14	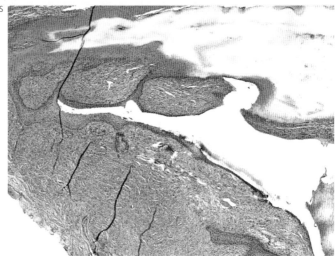

Table H2 Nevomelanocytic proliferations – "at a glance"

Entity	Genetics	Key histopathologic features	Image
Balloon cell nevus	Not relevant	Papillated, symmetric, 3 cell types: one that is small and nevic, another that is larger with abundant vacuolated cytoplasm and a centrally located "wrinkled" nucleus, and a third that is "oncocytoid"	
Deep penetrating nevus	*HRAS* mutations	Wedge-shaped silhouette, grenz zone, lentiginous junctional melanocytic proliferation, dermal component with a plexiform architecture, 2 distinct populations of cells, "checkerboard" pattern of pigment deposits, patchy host response	
Recurrent nevus	Not relevant	Trizonal pattern: atypical junctional melanocytic proliferation, underlying fibrosis banal dermal component	

Table H2 Nevomelanocytic proliferations – "at a glance" (*cont.*)

Entity	Genetics	Key histopathologic features	Image
Halo nevus	Not relevant	Circumscription, dome-shaped, symmetry, bases of rete infiltrated by lymphocytes, moderate host response, minimal melanocytic cytologic atypia	
Blue nevus	*GNAQ* mutations	Superficial and mid dermal proliferation of slender pigmented cells	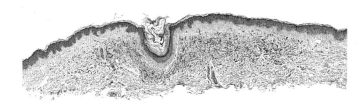
Hori's nevus	Not relevant	Superficial and mid dermal proliferation of slender pigmented cells	

Table H2 Nevomelanocytic proliferations – "at a glance" (*cont.*)

Entity	Genetics	Key histopathologic features	Image
Spitz nevus	*HRAS* mutations, amplification isochrome 11*p*	Dome-shaped silhouette, hyperplastic epidermis with hypergranulosis, circumscription, vertically oriented nests ("raining down" pattern), crescent shaped clefts between nests and epidermis ("cupping"), kamino bodies, distinctive spitzoid cytomorphology, evenly distributed patchy host response	
Nevus of Reed	*HRAS* mutations	Circumscribed, elongate spindled cells, lichenoid infiltrate, prominent pigment incontinence, Kamino bodies, central upward scatter	
Desmoplastic melanoma	*RETp*	Absent/inconspicuous junctional component, pandermal proliferation of stellate and spindled cells, patchy peripheral lymphocyte clusters	

Table H2 Nevomelanocytic proliferations – "at a glance" (*cont.*)

Entity	Genetics	Key histopathologic features	Image
Acral lentiginous melanoma	*KIT* mutations ("hotspots" 11, 13 and17)	*Early lesions*: Atypical lentiginous proliferation with prominent upward scatter, increased density of pigmented dendrites *Later lesions*: Nests of atypical melanocytes, "skip" areas, patchy host response	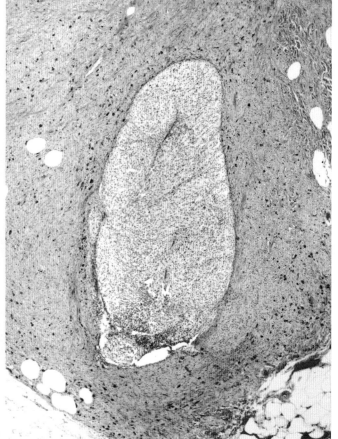
Cellular blue nevus	*GNAQ* mutations	Circumscribed, biphasic tumor, characteristic zonal pattern, 2 cytomorphologically distinct populations (one "blue nevus-like," another that is epithelioid)	

Table H2 Nevomelanocytic proliferations – "at a glance" (*cont.*)

Entity	Genetics	Key histopathologic features	Image
Epithelioid blue nevus	*GNAQ* mutations	Symmetric proliferation, heavily pigmented "globular" or epithelioid melanocytes, interspersed polygonal lightly pigmented cells	
Weisner's nevus	Biallelic loss of *BAP1* and *BRAFV600E* mutations	Polypoid architecture, spitzoid cytomorphology, superficial mitoses, scattered multinucleate giant cells, patchy host response	

Table H3 Appendageal tumors – "at a glance"

Entity	Key histopathologic features	Image
Dilated pore of Winer	Central dilated infundibular cystic structure, acanthosis, finger-like dermal projections	

299

Table H3 Appendageal tumors – "at a glance" (*cont.*)

Entity	Key histopathologic features	Image
Inverted follicular keratosis	Seborrheic keratosis-like, squamous eddies (in relation to the follicular infundibulum)	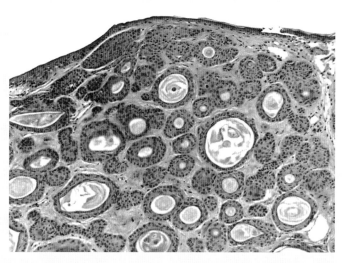
Trichoadenoma	Multiple, dermal variably sized horn cysts	
Trichilemmoma	Exo-endophytic circumscribed, lobular epidermal hyperplasia, peripheral palisading, clear cell differentiation, thickened peripheral eosinophilic cuticle	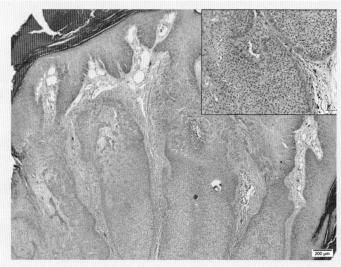

Table H3 Appendageal tumors – "at a glance" (*cont.*)

Entity	Key histopathologic features	Image
Desmoplastic trichilemmoma	Similar to above, plus hyalinized stroma	
Tumor of the follicular infundibulum	Superficial plate-like proliferation, reticulated pale epithelial cells	
Trichofolliculoma	Central dilated infundibular cyst, radiating vellus follicles branching out to secondary and/or tertiary follicles	

Table H3 Appendageal tumors – "at a glance" (*cont.*)

Entity	Key histopathologic features	Image
Trichoepithelioma	Basaloid islands, peripheral palisading, fibrous stroma with aggregates of fibroblasts resembling papillary mesenchymal bodies, variably sized keratocysts, focal foreign body giant cell reaction	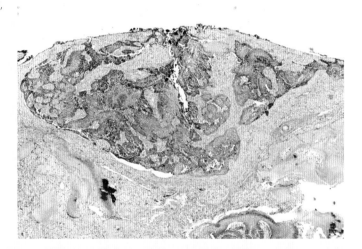
Pilomatricoma	Bi-colored tumor, pink areas (ghost cells) and blue areas (germinative cells), dystrophic calcification	
Lymphadenoma	Dermal nodules of epithelial cells, fibrous stroma, dense lymphocytic infiltrate permeating the lobules	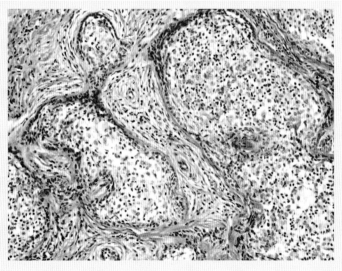

Table H3 Appendageal tumors – "at a glance" (*cont.*)

Entity	Key histopathologic features	Image
Panfolliculoma	Circumscribed, differentiation towards all parts of the hair follicle	
Fibrofolliculoma	Epithelial components, mesenchymal stroma, vertically oriented infundibulocystic structures with radiating anastomosing cords of epithelial cells	
Steatocystoma	Crenulated/wavy, homogeneous, eosinophilic lining, embedded flattened sebaceous lobules	

Table H3 Appendageal tumors – "at a glance" (*cont.*)

Entity	Key histopathologic features	Image
Sebaceous adenoma	Multilobular circumscribed, expansion of peripherally located basaloid cells, central area of mature sebocytes, proportion of latter surpasses that of former	
Sebaceous carcinoma	Irregular lobules, disordered mixture of basaloid germinative cells, high N:C ratio, foci of sebaceous differentiation, cytologic atypia, nuclear pyknosis, mitotic activity, necrosis	
Hidrocystoma	Unilocular, lined by 1 or 2 layers of cuboidal cells	

Table H3 Appendageal tumors – "at a glance" (*cont.*)

Entity	Key histopathologic features	Image
Cylindroma	Oval/polygonal nests, molding into a jigsaw-like pattern, nests surrounded by an eosinophilic hyaline sheath, 2 cell types (peripheral basophilic and central pale cells), ductal differentiation	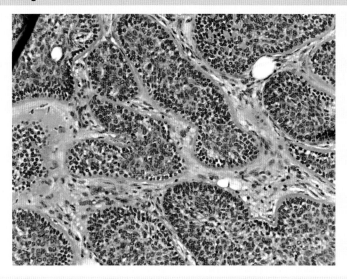
Syringoma	Ducts (some with elongate tails, "tadpole appearance"), 2 rows of cuboidal-to-flattened epithelial cells	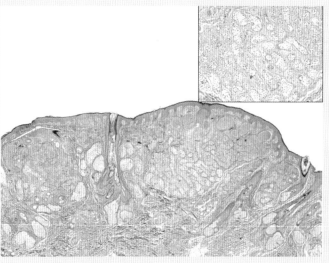
Poroma	Broad, downward projecting epidermal proliferation of "poroid" cells, granulation tissue-like stroma	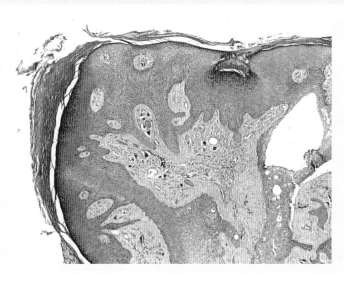

Table H3 Appendageal tumors – "at a glance" (*cont.*)

Entity	Key histopathologic features	Image
Syringofibroadenoma	Anastomosing strands of acrosyringeal epithelia, fibromucinous stroma	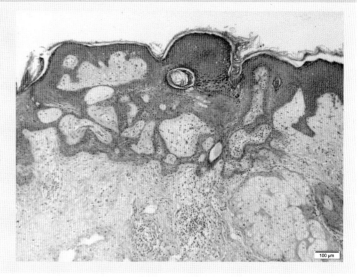
Papillary eccrine adenoma	Circumscribed unencapsulated dermal tumor, multiple variably dilated ducts, multilayered cuboidal epithelium, intraluminal papillary projections	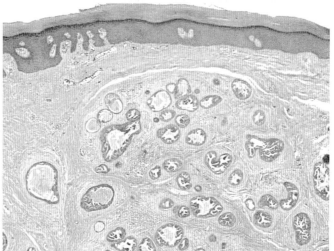
Hidradenoma	Circumscribed, unencapsulated tumor, biphasic cellular proliferation	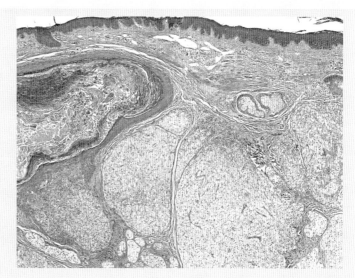

Table H3 Appendageal tumors – "at a glance" (*cont.*)

Entity	Key histopathologic features	Image
Syringocystadenoma papilliferum	Papillomatosis, transition from squamous to glandular epithelium of papillary structures, 2 cell layers (inner cuboidal, outer columnar), plasma cell-rich stroma	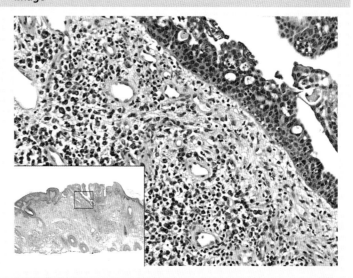
Apocrine mixed tumor	Circumscribed, biphasic tumor, epithelial component (clusters and cords of cells with ductal differentiation), myoepithelial component (present peripherally, hyaline or plasmacytoid cytomorphology) elements, variable stroma (chondroid, myxoid and/or fibrotic)	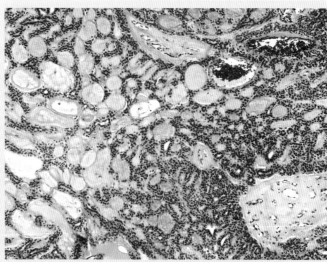
Myoepithelioma	Solid (ovoid/spindled, histiocytoid, or epithelioid cells with abundant eosinophilic syncytial cytoplasm, minimal stroma) or lobulated (cords/nests of epithelioid, plasmacytoid, or spindled cells, variably reticular architecture, chondromyxoid or collagenous/hyalinized stroma)	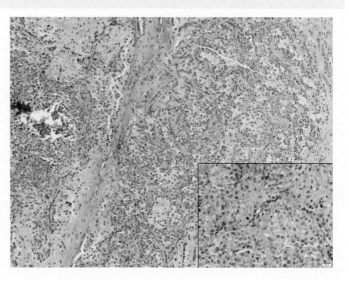

Table H3 Appendageal tumors – "at a glance" (*cont.*)

Entity	Key histopathologic features	Image
Erosive adenomatosis	Circumscribed glandular proliferation, mixed growth patterns, preserved myoepithelial cell layer	
Primary cutaneous mucinous carcinoma	Dermal-based, nests/strands of epithelial cells floating in copious mucin	

Table H3 Appendageal tumors – "at a glance" (*cont.*)

Entity	Key histopathologic features	Image
Digital papillary adenocarcinoma	Poorly circumscribed, non-encapsulated, multinodular, focal infiltrative pattern, papillary differentiation with true as well as "pseudo" papillae, ductal differentiation, variable cytologic atypia, pleomorphism, mitotic activity	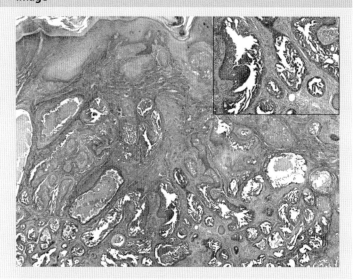
Extramammary Paget's disease	Malignant cells (scattered singly/clusters throughout the epidermis), distinctive cytomorphology (large pleomorphic nuclei, prominent nucleoli, abundant pale cytoplasm)	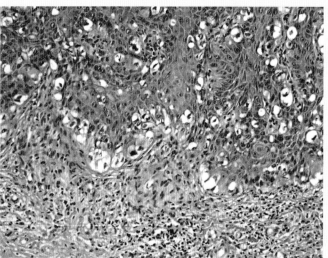
Microcystic adnexal carcinoma	Stratified architecture (keratocysts, nests and strands of basaloid cells), sclerotic stroma, perineural invasion frequent	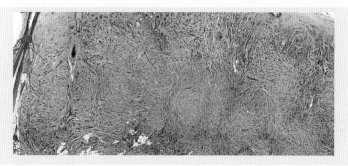

Table H4 Neural and neuroendocrine tumors – "at a glance"

Entity	Key histopathologic features	Image
Traumatic neuroma	Superficial/deep, variably sized nerve twigs with surrounding fibrosis	
Rudimentary polydactyly	Multiple small twigs confined to the dermal papillae	
Solitary circumscribed neuroma	Dermal nodular proliferation, "neural" appearing cells, surrounding thin perineural connective tissue capsule	

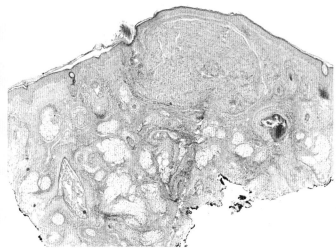

Table H4 Neural and neuroendocrine tumors – "at a glance" (*cont.*)

Entity	Key histopathologic features	Image
Plexiform neurofibroma	Multiple variably sized fusiform nerve enlargements	
Perineurioma	Circumscribed, unencapsulated, variably cellular, spindled proliferation, concentric perivascular whorls of perineural cells ("onion skinning")	
Neurilemmoma/ schwannoma	Circumscribed, encapsulated, nerve of origin present peripherally, two distinct areas: type A (spindled cells arranged in fascicles or Antoni A/verocay bodies) and type B (meshwork of myxoid tissue)	

Table H4 Neural and neuroendocrine tumors – "at a glance" (*cont.*)

Entity	Key histopathologic features	Image
Nerve sheath myxoma	Multilobulated, non-encapsulated paucicellular/hypocellular proliferation, abundant mucin	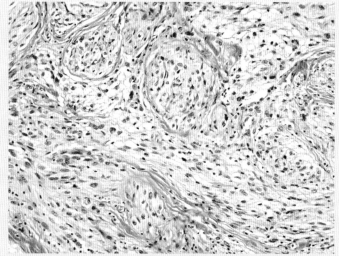
Neurothekeoma	Fasciculated proliferation, lobular architecture, lesional cells epithelioid or spindled cytomorphology	
Granular cell tumor	Circumscribed, nested/trabecular architecture, distinctive cytomorphology (polygonal cells, finely granular cytoplasm, prominent central nucleolus)	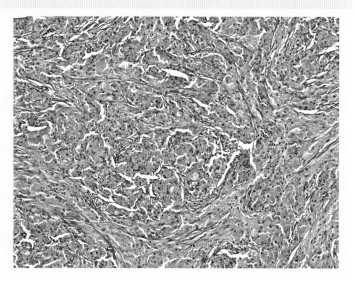

Table H4 Neural and neuroendocrine tumors – "at a glance" (cont.)

Entity	Key histopathologic features	Image
Merkel cell carcinoma	Dermal, nests/cords, basaloid cells, distinctive "neuroendocrine" cytomorphology ("salt and pepper"), cytologic atypia, nuclear pleomorphism, abundant karyorrhexis, mitoses	

Table H5 Multiple endocrine neoplasias (MEN) – classification

Type	Synonyms	Gene locus/gene/ protein product	Mucocutaneous manifestations
MEN1	Wermer syndrome, multiple endocrine adenomatosis	11q/*MENIN*/menin	Multiple facial angiofibromas, collagenomas, lipomas Gingival papules Confetti-like hypopigmented macules Café-au-lait macules
MEN2a	Sipple syndrome, phaeochromocytoma and amyloid-producing medullary thyroiod carcinoma, PTC syndrome	10q/*RET*/tyrosine kinase receptor	Lichen amyloidosus, notalgia paraesthetica, macular amyloidosis
MEN2b	Multiple mucosal neuroma syndrome, mucosal neuromata with endocrine tumors, Wagenmann-Froboese syndrome	10q/*RET*/tyrosine kinase receptor	Multiple mucosal neuromas, increased nerve fibers even in normal skin, prominent lips, hyperpigmentation around mouth and overlying small joints of hands and feet, café-au-lait macules, circumoral lentigenes

Table H6 Fibrous/fibroblastic proliferation – "at a glance"

Entity	Relevant genetics	Defining histopathology	Immunohisto-chemical profile	Image
Angiofibroma	*Tuberous sclerosis associated* – chr 9q34 (*TSC1*), 16p13 (*TSC2*) *Birt-Hogg-Dubé associated* – folliculin (*FLCN*) on 17p11.2	Stellate, multinucleate fibroblasts, dilated vascular spaces	Not relevant	

Table H6 Fibrous/fibroblastic proliferation – "at a glance" (*cont.*)

Entity	Relevant genetics	Defining histopathology	Immunohisto-chemical profile	Image
Acral fibrokeratoma	None	Core of vertically oriented collagen bundles surrounded by irregular acanthosis	FXIIIa+ fibroblasts	
Sclerotic fibroma	*Cowden's disease associated –* PTEN gene, chr 10q	Circumscribed, non-encapsulated, thick sclerotic collagen bundles arranged as intersecting stacks ("plywood-like")	CD34+ fibroblasts	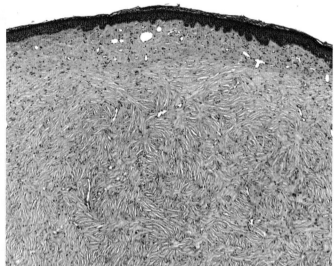
Nodular fasciitis	*USP6* rearrangements on chr 17 or a *MYH9-USP6* fusion	Subcutaneous nodular proliferation, plump/stellate cells, loose myxoid stroma ("tissue culture" appearance), admixed inflammatory cells, extravasated erythrocytes	SMA+ and MSA+ fibroblasts	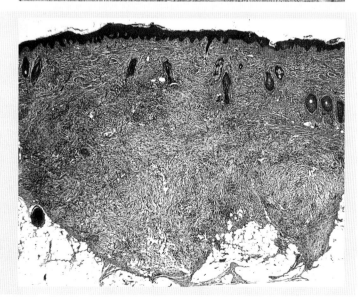

Table H6 Fibrous/fibroblastic proliferation – "at a glance" (*cont.*)

Entity	Relevant genetics	Defining histopathology	Immunohisto-chemical profile	Image
Solitary fibrous tumor	*NAB2-STAT6* gene fusions, chr 12	Alternating hypocellular and hypercellular areas of spindled cells ("patternless pattern"), hyalinized collagen, prominent "staghorn" vessels	CD34+, STAT6+, CD99+, Bcl-2+	
Fibrous hamartoma of infancy	No consistent abnormality	Triphasic histology: fascicles of spindled cells, immature loose basophilic and myxoid mesenchymal tissue, mature adipose tissue	SMA+ fibroblasts, S100+ adipose tissue, CD+ mesenchymal cells	
Digital fibromatosis	None	Spindled myofibroblasts in whorls, sheets or interlacing fascicles, cells with wavy nuclei containing pathognomonic eosinophilic paranuclear inclusion bodies	Inclusion bodies actin+	

Table H6 Fibrous/fibroblastic proliferation – "at a glance" (*cont.*)

Entity	Relevant genetics	Defining histopathology	Immunohisto-chemical profile	Image
Angiomyofibroblastoma	None	Prominent vascular component, edematous stroma, clustered plump to spindled cells around vessels		
Dermatomyofibroma	None	Plaque-like fasciculated proliferation of monomorphic spindled cells with adnexal sparing	Vimentin+, MSA+, SMA+, CD34+	
Infantile myofibromatosis	None	Biphasic architecture, central immature-appearing short spindled cells with thin-walled, branching vessels and peripheral mature, spindled myofibroblasts with abundant eosinophilic cytoplasm	Vimentin+, SMA+	

Table H6 Fibrous/fibroblastic proliferation – "at a glance" (*cont.*)

Entity	Relevant genetics	Defining histopathology	Immunohisto-chemical profile	Image
Myopericytoma	None	Vasoformative element, perivascular and concentric growth of myoid cells	MSA+, caldesmon+	
PEComa	Losses of *TSC1/TSC2* (only when in association with tuberous sclerosis)	Vasculocentric proliferation, epithelioid cells with admixed multinucleate giant cells	HMB45+, MITF+, MART-1+, MSA+	
Inflammatory myofibroblastic tumor	*ALK*, 2q33–q35	Polygonal myofibroblasts, mixed inflammatory cell infiltrate (plasma cells, lymphocytes and eosinophils)	CD68+, ALK-1+	

Table H6 Fibrous/fibroblastic proliferation – "at a glance" (*cont.*)

Entity	Relevant genetics	Defining histopathology	Immunohisto-chemical profile	Image
Myxoinflammatory fibroblastic sarcoma	*t*(1:10), *TGFBR3, MGEA5* rearrangement	Fasciculated proliferation of spindled and bizarre epithelioid cells, myxoid to hyalinized stroma, lymphocytes and plasma cells, coalescing foci of necrosis	Vimentin+, CD34+	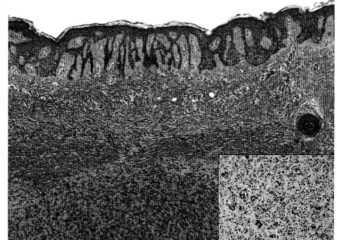
Dermatofibroma	None	Dermal spindled proliferation, collagen entrapment	FXIIIa+, SMA+	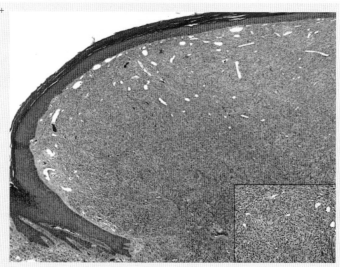
Epithelioid cell histiocytoma	None	Dome-shaped, polypoid dermal nodule, collarette, polygonal or epithelioid cells	FXIIIa+, CD34+	

Table H6 Fibrous/fibroblastic proliferation – "at a glance" (*cont.*)

Entity	Relevant genetics	Defining histopathology	Immunohisto-chemical profile	Image
Plexiform fibrous histiocytoma	None	Plexiform proliferation, nodules of histiocytes with admixed osteoclast-like giant cells, intersecting fascicles of fibroblast-like spindled cells	CD68+ histiocytes EMA+ fibroblasts	
Giant cell fibroblastoma	t(17:22)	Bland, spindled cells, admixed multinucleate giant cells	CD34+	
Dermatofibrosarcoma protuberans	t(17:22)	Bland fasciculated proliferation, cartwheel arrangement, fusiform cells	CD34+	

Table H6 Fibrous/fibroblastic proliferation – "at a glance" (*cont.*)

Entity	Relevant genetics	Defining histopathology	Immunohisto-chemical profile	Image
Atypical fibroxanthoma	UV-induced *p53* mutations	Dermal proliferation, markedly atypical, pleomorphic spindled and epithelioid cells, in fascicles or sheets, peripheral collarette, numerous mitoses	Vimentin+, CD99+, CD68+, CD10+	
Angiomatoid fibrous histiocytoma	*EWSR1-CREB1* fusion from *t(2:22)* translocation	Syncytial growth, histiocyte-like tumor cells in nodules, blood-filled pseudovascular spaces, fibrous pseudocapsule, hemosiderin deposits, perivascular lymphoplasmacytic infiltrate	CD68+, desmin+, EMA+	
Epithelioid sarcoma	Deletion of *SMARCB1* on chr 22*q*11	Nodular proliferation, markedly atypical epithelioid cells surrounding coalescing foci of necrosis	EMA+, vimentin+, CK-LMW+, CD34+	

Table H6 Fibrous/fibroblastic proliferation – "at a glance" (*cont.*)

Entity	Relevant genetics	Defining histopathology	Immunohisto-chemical profile	Image
Synovial sarcoma	*t*(X;18) resulting in fusion of *SYT* with one of the *SSX* genes	2 distinct cell populations: one epithelioid and another spindled (arranged in sheets or fascicles), admixed "staghorn" vessels	EMA+, TLE1+, CD99+	
Giant cell tumor of tendon sheath	1*p*11–13 translocation	Nodular proliferation, a variable mixture of epithelioid cells, MNGCs and hemosiderin deposits	MNGCs CD68+, CD45+	
Superficial acral fibromyxoma	None identified	Non-encapsulated, dermal proliferation, spindled and stellate cells (storiform pattern), myxoid stroma, admixed vessels	CD34+, CD99+, vimentin+ ApoD negative	

Table H6 Fibrous/fibroblastic proliferation – "at a glance" (*cont.*)

Entity	Relevant genetics	Defining histopathology	Immunohisto-chemical profile	Image
Superficial angiomyxoma	None identified	Multilobulated, poorly circumscribed, myxoid mass, prominent vascular component, admixed neutrophils, epithelial component (in a third)	Not relevant	

MNGCs = Multinucleate giant cells

Table H7 Immunohistochemical clues to metastases from an unknown primary

Primary		Immunohistochemical profile
Breast		CK7+, CK19+, ER/PR+, mammoglobin+, GCDFP-15+, CEA+, E-cadherin+, Her-2neu+ (20–30%)
Bladder, urinary		Blood group antigens+, CK7+, CK20+, thrombomodulin+, uroplakin III+, CD10+, CA15+
Carcinoid		Chromogranin+, NSE+, synaptophysin+,
		CDX2+ (only when of intestinal origin), TTF-1+ (only when of pulmonary origin)
Colon		CK20+, mucin+, CEA+, CDX2+
Endometrium		CK7+, PAX 8+
Esophagus	**Squamous cell carcinoma**	p63+, p40+, CK5/6+
	Adenocarcinoma	CEA+, EMA+, CK20+
Extramammary Paget's disease		MUC1+, MUC5AC+
Paget's disease		MUC1+, CK7+
Lung	**Small cell**	TTF-1+, CAM5.2+
	Adenocarcinoma	TTF-1+, CK7+, BerEP4+, CEA+, apoprotein A+
	Mesothelioma	Calret+, vimentin+
Kidneys		Vimentin+, CK AE1/3+, EMA+, RCC+, adipophilin+, PAX-8+, CD31+, CD10+
Liver		CEA+, α-fetoprotein+, α1-antitrypsin+, hepatocyte paraffin1+, arginase 1+
Ovaries		CK7+, CA125+, PAX-8+
Pancreas		CK7+, CK20−
Prostate		PSA+, PSAP+, ERG transcription factor+, PAP+
Thyroid		Thyroglobulin+, PAX-8+
Salivary glands	**Adenoid cystic**	CK+, CEA+, α1-antichymotrypsin+, S100+, CD117+, actin+
	Mucoepidermoid	CK-LMW+, EMA+

Table H8 Vascular/vascular-like tumors and proliferations – "at a glance"

Entity	Key histopathologic features	Image
Glomulovenous malformation	Ectatic, thin-walled venous channels, perivascular glomus cells	
Glomangiomyoma	Ectatic channels, transition from glomus to spindled smooth muscle cells	
Lymphangioma circumscriptum	Dilated, thin-walled, papillary dermal lymphatic vessels	

Table H8 Vascular/vascular-like tumors and proliferations – "at a glance" (*cont.*)

Entity	Key histopathologic features	Image
Venous lake	Single, superficial, dilated vascular channel	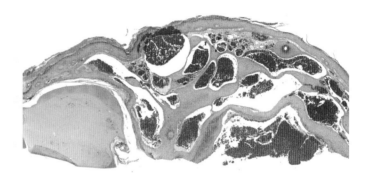
Angiokeratoma	Multiple, superficial, dilated vascular channels containing erythrocytes	
Cutaneous collagenous vasculopathy	Scattered, superficial capillary-sized vessels, perivascular hyalinization	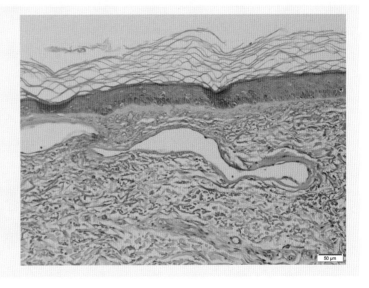

Table H8 Vascular/vascular-like tumors and proliferations – "at a glance" (*cont.*)

Entity	Key histopathologic features	Image
Glomeruloid hemangioma	Multifocal, aggregates of dilated, thin-walled vessels, intravascular capillary aggregates, stromal cells, with eosinophilic cytoplasm and intracytoplasmic vacuoles	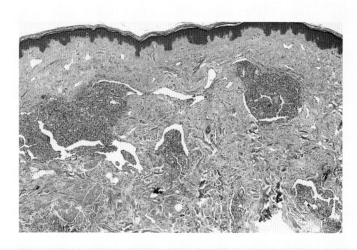
Tufted angioma	"Cannon-ball" distribution, multiple well-defined vascular "tufts" composed of capillaries	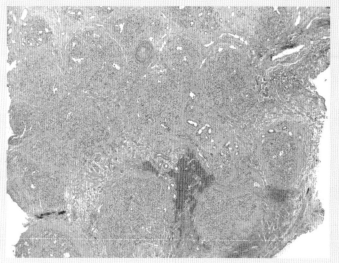
Microvenular hemangioma	Ill-circumscribed, superficial and deep, proliferation, monomorphic small blood vessels	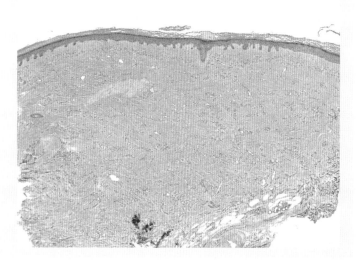

Table H8 Vascular/vascular-like tumors and proliferations – "at a glance" (*cont.*)

Entity	Key histopathologic features	Image
Acquired elastotic hemangioma	Increased capillary vessels arranged parallel to the epidermis, grenz zone	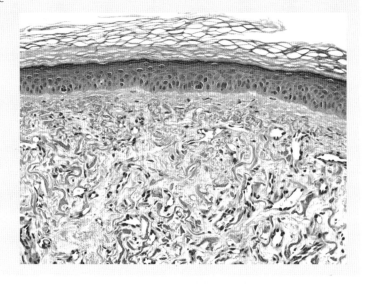
Hobnail hemangioma	Wedge-shaped, biphasic growth pattern (dilated vessels superficially, dissecting "pseudo-angiosarcomatous" vessels deep), extravasated erythrocytes, variable hemosiderin	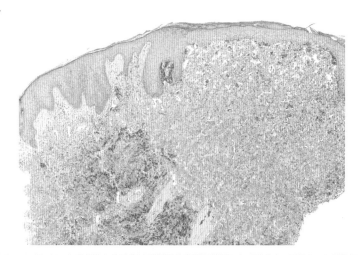
Cutaneous epithelioid angiomatous nodule	Exophytic, collarette, closely packed vascular channels, plump, epithelioid cells with intracytoplasmic vacuoles, admixed eosinophils, patchy, peripheral lymphoplasmacytic host response	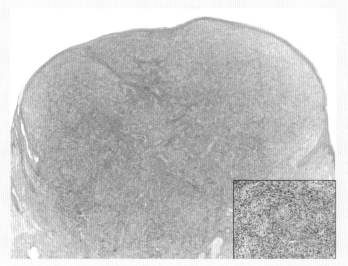

Table H8 Vascular/vascular-like tumors and proliferations – "at a glance" (*cont.*)

Entity	Key histopathologic features	Image
Epithelioid hemangioma	Circumscribed, thick- and thin-walled vessels, plump, epithelioid cells with intracytoplasmic vacuoles, admixed eosinophils	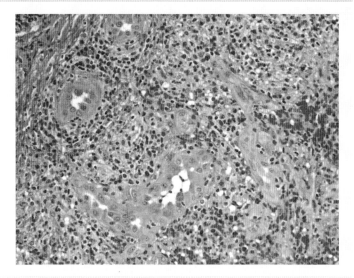
Diffuse dermal angiomatosis	Increased dermal capillaries, extravascular endothelial cell proliferation	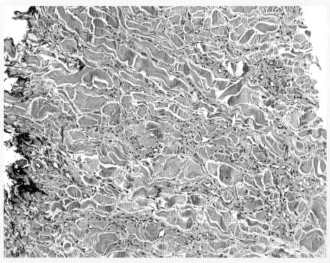
Bacillary angiomatosis	Epidermal collarette, lobular capillary proliferation, prominent neutrophil-rich stroma, variably sized, interstitial, granular purple deposits	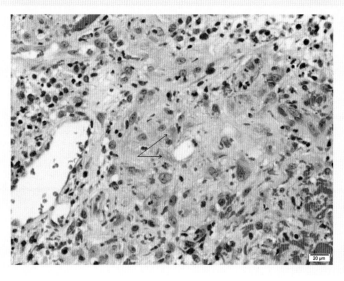

Table H8 Vascular/vascular-like tumors and proliferations – "at a glance" (*cont.*)

Entity	Key histopathologic features	Image
Kaposi's sarcoma	Ill-circumscribed, irregular thin-walled vascular channels, spindled cell proliferation, promontory sign, extravasated erythrocytes, lymphoplasmacytic host response	
Kaposiform hemangioendothelioma	Ill-circumscribed, biphasic, multinodular, vascular (small capillaries) and solid cellular areas	
Dabska's tumor	Ill-circumscribed, interconnecting vascular channels, intravascular papillary tufts with central PAS+ hyaline cores, intravascular and extravascular lymphoid aggregates	

Table H8 Vascular/vascular-like tumors and proliferations – "at a glance" (*cont.*)

Entity	Key histopathologic features	Image
Angiosarcoma	Ill-circumscribed, vasoformative, irregular, dissecting, anastomosing vascular channels, multilayered markedly atypical lining endothelial cells	

Table H9 Histiocytic and xanthomatous infiltrates – "at a glance"

Entity	Defining histopathologic features	Immunohisto-chemical profile	Image
Juvenile xanthogranuloma	Exophytic, polymorphic, collarette, lymphocytes, foamy histiocytes, Touton giant cells	CD68+ and fascin+, S100– and CD1a–	
Reticulohistiocytoma	Dermal histiocytes, multinucleate giant cells with "ground-glass" appearance	CD68+	

Table H9 Histiocytic and xanthomatous infiltrates – "at a glance" (*cont.*)

Entity	Defining histopathologic features	Immunohisto-chemical profile	Image
Necrobiotic xanthogranuloma	Band-like granulomas, tiered necrobiosis, cholesterol clefts	Nothing relevant	
Cutaneous Rosai-Dorfman disease	Architectural effacement, aggregates of histiocytes (resembling sinuses) and plasma cells, +/− emperipolesis	Lesional histiocytes S100+ and CD68+, CD1a−	
Eruptive xanthoma	Dermal effacement, cellular infiltrate, extravascular lipid deposits ("lace-like" eosinophilic material) *Early lesions:* Neutrophils *Late lesions:* Extensive lipidization	Nothing relevant	

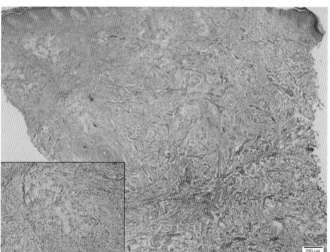

Table H9 Histiocytic and xanthomatous infiltrates – "at a glance" (*cont.*)

Entity	Defining histopathologic features	Immunohisto-chemical profile	Image
Verruciform xanthoma	Large foam cells in papillae	LCA+ and CD68+	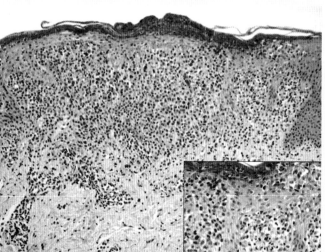
Langerhans cell histiocytosis	Dermal infiltrate of large cells with a hyperconvoluted nucleus	S100+, CD1a+, HLA−, DR+, langerin (CD207)+	

Table H10 Cutaneous lymphomatous and leukemic infiltrates – "at a glance"

Entity	Genetics	Histopathology	Immunohisto-chemistry	Image
Mycosis fungoides	TCR+	Small, hyperchromatic lymphocytes, thickened papillary dermis, epidermotropism, Pautrier microabscesses	CD2/CD3/CD4/CD5/CD45RO+, CD7–	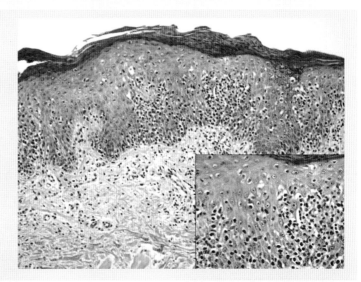
Pagetoid reticulosis	TCR+	Acanthotic, cytologically atypical mononuclear cells, striking epidermotropism	CD4/CD8 positive or CD4/CD8 double negative, frequently CD30+	
Anaplastic large cell lymphoma	TCR+, *t*(2:5) only in systemic ALCL	Diffuse infiltrate, large cells with a high N:C ratio and prominent eosinophilic nucleoli	>75% cells CD30+	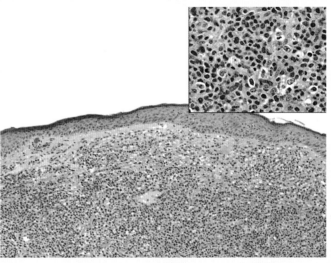

Table H10 Cutaneous lymphomatous and leukemic infiltrates – "at a glance" (*cont.*)

Entity	Genetics	Histopathology	Immunohisto-chemistry	Image
Lymphomatoid papulosis	TCR+, *NPM1-TYK2* fusion	Wedge-shaped, superficial and deep, small and large cells	CD30+ (except type B)	
Subcutaneous panniculitis-like T-cell lymphoma	TCR+	Subcutaneous infiltrate only, small-medium sized T lymphocytes, rimming of adipocytes by neoplastic T-cells, macrophages with cellular debris ("bean bag cells")	CD3/CD8/βF1+, express cytotoxic proteins (TIA-1, granzyme B, perforin)	
Primary cutaneous ɣ/δ T-cell lymphoma	TCR+	Epidermal/dermal/subcutaneous patterns, PR-like, dermal involvement of clusters or sheets of atypical cells, subcutaneous involvement with rimming of adipocytes by neoplastic cells	CD3/CD56+, CD4+ and CD8− (most cases), strongly express cytotoxic proteins (TIA-1, granzyme B, perforin)	

Table H10 Cutaneous lymphomatous and leukemic infiltrates – "at a glance" (*cont.*)

Entity	Genetics	Histopathology	Immunohisto-chemistry	Image
Extranodal NK/T-cell lymphoma, nasal type	*No* clonal TCR	Perivascular, periadnexal infiltrate, medium-sized atypical lymphocytes	EBV, CD56, CD2, cCD3 and CD45R0+, expression of cytotoxic proteins (TIA-1, granzyme B, perforin)	
Primary cutaneous CD8+ aggressive epidermotropic cytotoxic T-cell lymphoma	TCR+	Dense epidermotropic, angiocentric infiltrate, markedly atypical, medium-sized lymphocytes	CD3/CD8/βF1+, variable loss of CD2/CD5/CD7, expression of cytotoxic proteins (TIA-1, granzyme B, perforin)	
Marginal zone B-cell lymphoma	IgH (30–73% of cases)	Nodular infiltrate, small monocytoid lymphocytes/plasmacytoid lymphocytes, plasma cells, no epidermal involvement, disrupted germinal centers (GCs)	CD20/CD791/Bcl-2+, Bcl-6/CD10 and CD5−, CD138 and MUM-1/IRG4+ (only plasma cells), CD10/Bcl-6, CD21 highlight disrupted GCs	

Table H10 Cutaneous lymphomatous and leukemic infiltrates – "at a glance" (*cont.*)

Entity	Genetics	Histopathology	Immunohisto-chemistry	Image
Primary cutaneous follicle center cell lymphoma	IgH+, *t*(14:18) present	Nodular/sheet-like dermal infiltrate (follicular pattern in scalp predominantly), centrocytes and centroblasts	CD20/CD79a/Bcl-6+ (also CD10+ in follicular pattern), MUM1/IRF4–	
Diffuse large B-cell lymphoma, leg type	IgH+, multiple chr abnormalities	Diffuse infiltrate, atypical large "immunoblast-like" cells, destructive growth pattern, frequent necrosis and mitosis	CD20/CD79a/Bcl-6+, strong expression of Bcl-2, MUM-1/IRF4 and FOXP1, CD10–, IgM+	
Intravascular large B-cell lymphoma	IgH+	Large intravascular atypical cells, necrosis, thrombi and frequent mitoses	CD20/CD79a/PAX-5+, CD20 lost in rituximab-treated patients	

Table H10 Cutaneous lymphomatous and leukemic infiltrates – "at a glance" (*cont.*)

Entity	Genetics	Histopathology	Immunohisto-chemistry	Image
Myeloid sarcoma	*t*(8:21), monosomy 16, 7 plus others	Diffuse infiltrate, medium-large sized cells with a granular, basophilic cytoplasm	CD34/CD117/ CD43/ lysozyme/MPO and CD68+	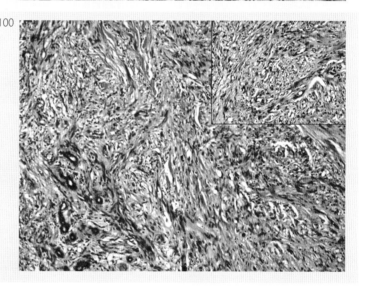
Interdigitating dendritic cell sarcoma	None found	Fascicles of round/ spindled cells, abundant cytoplasm, open vesicular chromatin, prominent nucleoli, nuclear grooves and inclusions	Vimentin, S100 and fascin+	

Table H11 Tumors and syndromic associations

Tumor	Syndrome/s	Relevant genetics
Angiofibroma	Tuberous sclerosis, MEN1	Mutations in *TSC1* (9q34.13), *TSC2* (Xq22.3), *menin* (11q13.1)
Angiokeratoma	Anderson-Fabry disease	Alpha galactosidase deficiency
Basal cell carcinoma	Gorlin-Goltz syndrome	*PTCH1* mutations
Cutaneous myxoma	Carney's complex	*PRKAR1A* mutations
Cylindroma	Brooke-Spiegler syndrome	*CYLD* mutations
Epidermal cyst with pilomatrical differentiation	Gardner's syndrome	APC mutations
Fibrofolliculoma	Birt-Hogg-Dubé syndrome	*FLCN* mutations
Glomeruloid hemangioma	POEMS syndrome	None

Table H11 Tumors and syndromic associations (*cont.*)

Tumor	Syndrome/s	Relevant genetics
Keratoacanthoma (KA)	Ferguson-Smith, eruptive KA of Gryzbwowski type, Muir-Torre syndrome (MTS)	Chr 9q22–q31 (Ferguson-Smith), *MSH2/MLH1/MSH6* mutations (MTS)
Leiomyoma	Reed syndrome	*FH* mutations
Lentigenes, multiple	Carney's complex, NAME/LAMB syndrome, LEOPARD syndrome, Peutz-Jeghers syndrome	*PRKAR1A* mutations (Carney complex), *PTPN11* (more often) and *RAF1* (LEOPARD syndrome), *STK11/LKB1* mutations (Peutz-Jeghers syndrome)
Neurofibroma	NF1	*NF1* mutations
Sebaceous adenoma/ epithelioma/ carcinoma	Muir-Torre syndrome	*MSH2/MLH1/MSH6* mutations
Spiradenoma	Brooke-Spiegler syndrome	*CYLD* mutations
Trichilemmoma	Cowden's syndrome	*PTEN* mutations
Trichoepithelioma	Brooke-Spiegler syndrome	*CYLD* mutations
Vascular anomalies plus pigmented lesions	Phakomatosis pigmentovascularis	*GNAQ* mutations (Sturge-Weber syndrome)

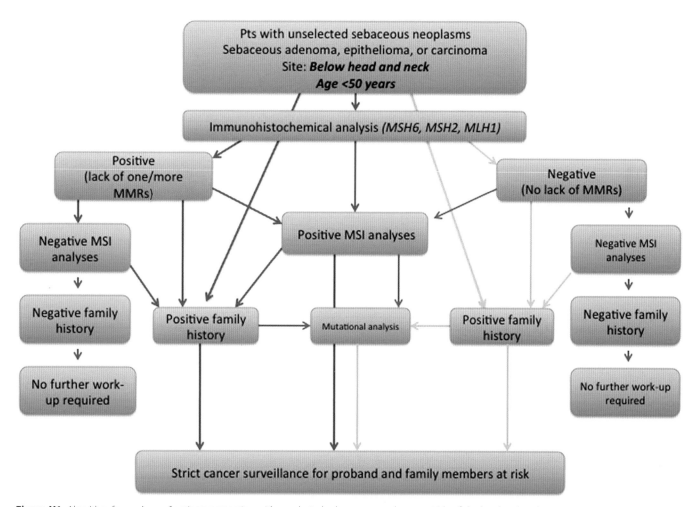

Figure H1 Algorithm for work-up of patients presenting with unselected sebaceous neoplasms outside of the head and neck area

1. **E.** Image shown is that of an inflammatory linear verrucous epidermal nevus (ILVEN).

   Histopathologic findings of ILVEN, shown in the image, include psoriasiform epidermal hyperplasia with alternating parakeratosis without a granular layer, and orthokeratosis with a thickened granular layer. The zones of parakeratosis in ILVEN are broader than that in psoriasis and ILVEN usually lack the scale crust with neutrophils typically seen in the horn of psoriasis.

   Inflammatory linear verrucous epidermal nevus is a linear, persistent, pruritic plaque, usually first noted on a limb in early childhood. It was originally described in 1896 by Unna. In 1971, Altman and Mehregan delineated inflammatory linear verrucous epidermal nevus as a distinct entity and coined the name inflammatory linear verrucous epidermal nevus. Features characteristic of this entity include:

   - Early age at onset
   - Predominance in females (female-to-male ratio of 4:1)
   - Frequent involvement of the left leg
   - Pruritus
   - Marked refractoriness to therapy
   - Distinctive psoriasiform and inflammatory histologic appearance

   ILVEN accounts for approximately 5% of patients with epidermal nevi. Inflammatory linear verrucous epidermal nevus may occur with musculoskeletal abnormalities in a few children (raising the possibility of the classification of inflammatory linear verrucous epidermal nevus as part of epidermal nevus syndrome).

2. **D.** Image shown is that of prurigo nodularis (PN).

   Histopathologic findings of PN, shown in the image, include thick, compact orthohyperkeratosis, irregular epidermal or pseudoepitheliomatous hyperplasia, focal parakeratosis or superficial necrosis (as a consequence of constant picking), hypergranulosis, fibrosis of the papillary dermis with vertically arranged collagen fibers, increased number of fibroblasts and capillaries, a superficial, perivascular and/or interstitial mixed inflammatory infiltrate composed of neutrophils, eosinophils, histiocytes, and monocytes. Rete ridges are elongate and irregular and thickened nerve fibers and fibrosis with thickened collagen bundles are typically noted.

   Prurigo nodularis typically presents in the middle-aged to elderly. Patients with prurigo nodularis invariably complain of a long-standing history of severe, unremitting pruritus and are able to indicate specific sites where they began feeling itchy and where dark-colored nodules formed soon after. Mature nodules rarely increase or decrease in size; spontaneous resolution is

   even more rare. PN is usually bilaterally symmetric, with nodules that are either stable or increasing in number. The nodules or papules are 3–20 mm in diameter; they are discrete, scaly, generally symmetric, hyperpigmented or purpuric, and firm and occur on the extensor surfaces of the arms, the legs, and sometimes the trunk.

3. **C.** Image shown is that of seborrheic keratosis (SK).

   Histopathologic features of SK, shown in the image, include papillomatous epidermal hyperplasia with "pseudo" horn cysts formed as a consequence of epidermal invagination. Seborrheic keratoses usually begin with the appearance of one or more sharply defined, light brown, flat macules. As they initially grow, they develop a velvety to finely verrucous surface, followed by an uneven warty surface with multiple plugged follicles and a dull or lackluster appearance. They typically have an appearance of being "stuck on" the skin surface. Epiluminescent surface microscopic examination of seborrheic keratoses reveals globule-like structures. The globule-like structures in seborrheic keratoses are due to intraepidermal horn cysts filled with cornified cells containing melanin. They resemble the brown globules observed in melanocytic neoplasms, which are due to nests of melanocytes at the dermoepidermal junction.

4. **B.** An increase in size and number of seborrheic keratoses is known as the Leser-Trélat sign.

   This sign of multiple eruptive seborrheic keratoses is typically associated with an internal malignancy and represents a paraneoplastic syndrome. Most commonly, the sign is observed with adenocarcinoma, especially of the gastrointestinal tract; however, an eruption of seborrheic keratoses may develop after an inflammatory dermatosis (e.g., eczema, severe sunburn). In this latter case, no associated malignancy is expected. The sign of Leser-Trélat often occurs with malignant acanthosis nigricans, a more accepted sign of internal cancer. Other rarely associated paraneoplastic entities include the following:

   - Acquired hypertrichosis lanuginosa
   - Acquired ichthyosis
   - Cowden disease
   - Tylosis
   - Acrokeratosis of Bazex
   - Tripe palms
   - Simultaneous paraneoplastic manifestations, including both ichthyosis acquisita and Bazex syndrome

5. **A.** Image shown is that of melanoacanthoma.

   Histopathologic features of melanoacanthoma include mild papillomatosis with "pseudo" horn cysts and dendritic melanocytes scattered throughout the epidermis but more typically in the stratum spinosum. The term melanoacanthoma, when introduced by Mishima and Pinkus in 1960, referred to a pigmented, benign proliferation of both keratinocytes and dendritic melanocytes. A few decades earlier, Bloch described a similar lesion that he called melanoepithelioma type I. Melanoepithelioma type II is an ordinary pigmented seborrheic keratosis.

Oral melanoacanthoma is a rare, reactive, mucosal lesion, which, similar to cutaneous melanoacanthoma, is associated with hyperplasia of spinous keratinocytes and melanocytes. Its most common intraoral sites are the buccal mucosa, lip, palate, and gingiva. The average age at presentation is 28 years, and it occurs mainly in black people, with a strong female predilection. *Oral melanoacanthoma is unrelated to seborrheic keratosis.*

6. **E.** Image shown is that of clear cell papulosis.

Distinctive histopathologic features include a proliferation of clear cells along the basal and suprabasal layers of the epidermis, either in small clusters or singly. Cytomorphologic features of the lesional cells reveal round to oval regular nuclei with abundant to moderate lightly eosinophilic to clear cytoplasm and nuclear chromatin paler than that of keratinocytes and melanocytes. No pleomorphism or mitoses are typically seen. The clear cells are not pigmented. In keeping with the clinical presentation, melanin pigmentation is significantly reduced in the area of clear cell proliferation compared with the normal areas (confirmed by Fontana-Masson stains). Lesional cells are positive for CEA, EMA, CK AE1/3, CK7, and CAM 5.2, but negative for GCDFP, S100, and CK20. Of all positive immunostains, CEA appears to be the strongest. Clear cells of clear cell papulosis are mucin-positive, S100-negative glandular-secretory epithelial cells that appear to share histogenetic features with Toker cells and Paget cells. The histogenesis is less likely to be of apocrine origin. Clear cell papulosis of the skin is a rare condition, which has been reported mostly among Taiwanese children. Clinically, the lesions are hypopigmented or depigmented macules and papules appearing on the pubic region and the milk line distribution in small children without evidence of pityriasis versicolor infection, preceding inflammation, or vitiligo.

7. **D.** Image shown is that of actinic keratosis (AK).

Distinctive histopathologic features of AK are the alternating blue and pink horn, a function of sparing of the acrosyringium ("blue") and the keratinocyte atypia which is initially confined to the basal layers of the epidermis with irregular budding of atypical keratinocytes from the basal layer ("Bernie's buds").

Clinically it typically occurs on sites of sun damage and may be easier to feel than see. Clinical settings with an increased frequency of AKs include oculocutaneous albinism and xeroderma pigmentosum.

8. **C.** Image shown is that of Bowen's disease (BD).

Bowen's disease or squamous cell carcinoma in situ (SCCIS) is histopathologically characterized by full thickness keratinocyte atypia. The concept of BD stems from the original description of John Bowen of patients with multiple cutaneous lesions in non-sun-exposed sites exhibiting identical histopathologic features. In the original report by John Bowen, the etiology was related to arsenic exposure. However, now the term is reserved for SCCIS occurring in non-sun-exposed skin.

9. **B.** In light of the clinical presentation, the best-fit diagnosis for the image shown is bowenoid papulosis.

Histopathologic findings include full thickness keratinocyte atypia with disordered epidermal maturation, numerous mitotic figures including the presence of atypical forms and scattered, individually necrotic dyskeratotic keratinocytes.

Bowenoid papulosis was described in 1977 by Kopf and Bart as papules on the penis. Bowenoid papulosis is now most commonly known to occur on the genitalia of both sexes in sexually active people and manifests as papules that are HPV induced (most commonly by HPV-16). However, given that they are often multifocal, patients should be observed for recurrence and for the possibility of invasive or in situ malignancy. Bowenoid papulosis tends to be benign with spontaneous regression occurring within several months. A more protracted course is believed to occur in older patients and, possibly, with lesions consistent with certain HPV types. These lesions may last as long as 5 years, or they may never regress completely. The lesions tend to be asymptomatic but can be inflamed, pruritic, or painful.

10. **E.** HPV-16 is most commonly implicated in bowenoid papulosis.

Other HPV types implicated include 18, 31, 32, 33, 34, 35, 39, 42, 48, 51, 52, 53, and 54. Consequently, the risk of acquiring bowenoid papulosis is identical to that for other genital HPV-associated conditions *via* sexual contact or, possibly, *via* vertical transmission from mother to newborn.

11. **D.** Predisposition to basal cell carcinoma (BCC, image shown) is associated with Gorlin-Goltz syndrome.

Gorlin-Goltz syndrome, which is also known as nevoid basal cell carcinoma (BCC) syndrome, is a rare autosomal dominant disorder with strong penetrance and extremely variable expressivity. It was initially reported by Jarish and White in 1894. Robert J. Gorlin and Robert W. Goltz subsequently described the distinct syndrome, consisting of multiple nevoid BCCs, jaw cysts, and bifid ribs. It is characterized by multiple odontogenic keratocysts, multiple BCCs, skeletal, dental, ophthalmic, and neurological abnormalities, intracranial ectopic calcifications of the falx cerebri and facial dysmorphism. Diagnosis is based upon established major and minor clinical and radiological criteria and ideally confirmed by deoxyribo nucleic acid (DNA) analysis. Other names for this syndrome include Gorlin syndrome, multiple nevoid basal cell epithelioma, jaw cyst bifid rib syndrome, or multiple nevoid BCC syndrome. The syndrome manifests with some major and minor criteria like pigmented BCCs, odontogenic keratocysts (OKC), palmar and/or plantar pits, and ectopic calcifications of the falx cerebri. To establish diagnosis, two major and one minor or one major and three minor criteria are necessary.

Major criteria – Multiple basal cell carcinomas or one occurring under the age of 20 years, histologically proven OKCs of the jaws, 3 or more palmar or plantar pits, bilamellar calcifications of the falx cerebri, bifid, fused, or markedly splayed ribs and a first-degree relative with nevoid basal cell carcinoma syndrome

Minor criteria – Macrocephaly (adjusted for height), congenital malformation (cleft lip or cleft palate, frontal bossing, coarse face, moderate or severe hypertelorism), other skeletal abnormalities (Sprengel deformity, marked pectus deformity, marked syndactyly of the digits), radiological abnormalities (bulging of sella turcica), vertebral anomalies such as hemi vertebrae, fusion or elongation of vertebral bodies, modeling defects of the hands and feet, or flame-shaped hands or feet, ovarian fibroma and medulloblastoma

12. **C.** Mutations in *PTCH1* are associated with the Gorlin-Goltz syndrome.

Pathogenesis of the syndrome is attributed to abnormalities in the long arm of chromosome 9 ($q22.3$–$q31$) and loss of or mutations of human patched gene (*PTCH1* gene). The *PTCH* gene product is part of a receptor for the protein called Sonic Hedgehog, which is involved in embryonic development.

13. **B.** Image shown is that of a fibroepithelioma of Pinkus.

In terms of histopathology, the classic fibroepithelioma of Pinkus typically shows long, thin, branching and anastomosing strands of basaloid cells embedded in a loose fibromucinous stroma. Many strands show a connection with the epidermis. The basaloid strands show 2 distinct appearing cells. A lighter staining cell comprises the bulk of the strand. Scattered, small groups of darker cells are seen tapering off the main trunk in a palisading

arrangement like buds on a branch. Nuclear pleomorphism may be present, and staining with proliferation markers such as Ki-67 shows an increased proliferative index. Co-expression of androgen receptor and cytokeratin 20, a marker for the presence of Merkel cells within islands of basaloid cells, may aid in the diagnosis. This neoplasm was initially described by Hermann Pinkus in 1953 as a premalignant fibroepithelial tumor. Pinkus considered the tumor to be a variant of basal cell carcinoma. Clinically, the lesion is a benign-appearing, pedunculated, pink tumor most commonly on the trunk or the extremities that may resemble an acrochordon.

14. **A.** Marjolin's ulcer refers to squamous cell carcinoma arising in sites of chronic injury.

Jean Nicolas Marjolin first described the occurrence of ulcerating lesions within scar tissue in 1828. Marjolin's ulcer is the term given to these aggressive epidermoid tumors that arise from areas of chronic injury, with burn wounds being a common site. Although Marjolin initially described malignant transformation of a chronic scar from a burn wound, the term Marjolin's ulcer has since been used interchangeably for malignant transformation of any chronic wound, including pressure ulcers, osteomyelitis, venous stasis ulcers, urethral fistulas, anal fistulas, and other traumatic wounds. This malignant transformation is histologically a well-differentiated squamous cell carcinoma; however, its behavior is aggressive when arising in pressure ulcers as compared to burns or osteomyelitis. The latent transformation period of Marjolin's ulcers ranges between 25 and 40 years.

15. **E.** Squamous cell carcinoma (shown in the image) would be positive for antibodies to high molecular weight keratins (CK5/6 and CK903) as well as p40.

An additional, albeit non-specific, stain of utility is EMA.

16. **D.** Positive staining with p40 is NOT a risk factor for squamous cell carcinoma.

Tumor-related factors in aggressive SCC include the following:

- Tumor location (i.e. lips, ears, anogenital region, within a scar or chronic wound)
- Tumor size greater than 2 cm (or 1.5 cm on ear or lip)
- Invasion to subcutaneous fat (or deeper)
- Poorly differentiated tumor cells
- Recurrent tumor
- Perineural involvement (except, perhaps, for tumors with small-caliber nerve invasion and no other risk factors)

17. **C.** A genetic predisposition to cutaneous squamous cell carcinoma (cSCC) is associated with Rothmund-Thomson syndrome.

Rothmund-Thomson syndrome, or poikiloderma congenitale, is a rare autosomal recessive disorder attributed to mutations of the *RECQL4* helicase gene on 8*q*24. Key features include early photosensitivity and poikilodermatous skin changes, juvenile cataracts, skeletal dysplasias, and a predisposition to osteosarcoma and skin cancers such as cutaneous SCC. Patients generally present with a rash (poikiloderma), small stature, and skeletal dysplasias.

The characteristic skin findings are the most consistent feature of the syndrome. The acute phase begins in early infancy as red patches or edematous plaques, sometimes with blistering. The cheeks are usually first involved, with later spread to other areas of the face, the extremities, and the buttocks. Over months to years, the rash enters a chronic stage characterized by poikiloderma (atrophy, telangiectasias, and pigmentary changes). Photosensitivity is a feature in more than 30% of cases.

18. **C.** *TP53* mutations are commonly detected in cutaneous squamous cell carcinoma (cSCC).

More than 90% of cSCCs harbor UVR-induced *TP53* mutations which are easily detectable by immunohistochemical stains even in histologically unremarkable chronically sun-damaged skin. Loss-of-function mutation involving both p53 alleles is a critical molecular event that triggers transformation of actinic keratosis into cSCC. p53 protein expression has been correlated to histopathologic grade and high-risk features and consequently stage and prognosis. NOTCH is a direct target of p53 contributing to differentiation of epidermal keratinocytes. NOTCH1 is expressed throughout the epidermis while NOTCH2 is localized principally in the basal layer. Inactivation of NOTCH1 or NOTCH2 through point mutations is a common event in cSCC and can be seen in >75% of these tumors. Inhibition of NOTCH by HPV-derived proteins also contributes to oncogenic transformation of keratinocytes.

19. **B.** Image shown is that of verrucous carcinoma.

In terms of histopathology, verrucous carcinoma may resemble a verruca superficially, with hyperkeratosis, parakeratosis, acanthosis, papillomatosis, and granular cell layer vacuolization. A characteristic feature is the cohesive bulbous downgrowths of squamous epithelium with minimal cytologic atypia surrounded by edematous stroma and chronic inflammatory cells that extend into the dermis, sometimes forming sinuses filled with keratin. Verrucous carcinoma is a relatively uncommon, locally aggressive, low-grade, slow-growing, well-differentiated squamous cell carcinoma. Verrucous carcinoma manifests as a cauliflower-like, exophytic mass that typically develops at sites of chronic irritation and inflammation. Verrucous carcinoma is slow growing, but may display locally aggressive behavior. While penetration into the skin, fascia, and even bone has been reported, overall, verrucous carcinoma has low metastatic potential. Verrucous carcinoma may involve the oral cavity, larynx, anogenital region, plantar surface of the foot, and, less commonly, other cutaneous sites.

In 1948, Ackerman first described verrucous carcinoma in the oral cavity as a low-grade tumor that generally is considered a clinicopathologic variant of squamous cell carcinoma. A few years later, in 1954, Aird *et al.* described cutaneous verrucous carcinoma (carcinoma cuniculatum), and it was named as such because of its characteristic crypt-like spaces on histology.

In most cases of verrucous carcinomas, regardless of the variant, the clinical outcome is rarely an aggressive course. Local verrucous carcinoma recurrence following definitive treatment is not uncommon. Regarding oral verrucous carcinoma, the reported recurrence rate ranges from 6–40%. If metastasis does occur, it is mainly at the regional lymph nodes. Patients with oral verrucous carcinoma may be at an increased risk of a second primary oral squamous cell carcinoma, which carries a poor prognosis.

Eponyms and HPV associations include the following:

Buscke-Lowenstein tumor – Anogenital region, associated with HPV-16/HPV-18

Ackerman tumor – Oral cavity, associated with HPV-16/HPV-18

Epithelioma cuniculatum – Sole of the foot, associated with HPV-6/HPV-11

20. **A.** Image shown is that of mucoepidermoid carcinoma.

In terms of histopathology, mucoepidermoid carcinomas are composed of 3 cell types: mucinous, squamous and clear. These tumors are classified into two grades, based on the ratio of mucin-secreting, squamous, intermediate, and clear cells. In the two-grade classification, the low-grade subset refers to well-circumscribed masses of well-differentiated squamous cells and mucin-producing cells. High-grade tumors contain solid, infiltrative masses with more squamous, intermediate, and clear cells than mucin-producing cells. In this classification, marked nuclear atypia, frequent mitoses, and extensive necrosis suggest poorly differentiated adenocarcinoma or adenosquamous carcinoma rather than mucoepidermoid carcinoma of any grade. A mucin stain highlights the mucin-producing cells. All 3 cell types are positive for pan CK, CK7, CEA and EMA. Positive staining with p63 favors a primary cutaneous malignancy over a metastasis. Although the term *mucoepidermoid carcinoma* is often used synonymously with *adenosquamous carcinoma*, it is controversial whether these two tumors are identical. Although some think that adenosquamous carcinoma is similar to, if not identical with, a high-grade mucoepidermoid carcinoma, others postulate that adenosquamous carcinomas are distinct with a much greater tendency for metastasis. Mucoepidermoid carcinoma is a common malignant salivary gland tumor that can arise less commonly in the esophagus, lacrimal passages, bronchus, pancreas, prostate, thymus, and thyroid.

21. **E. Image shown is that of metaplastic carcinoma (carcinosarcoma).**

    Carcinosarcoma is a biphasic tumor composed of malignant epithelial and mesenchymal elements with no transitional areas and absence of cytokeratin in the mesenchymal component. The relative proportion of the two components is variable. Synonyms include biphasic sarcomatoid carcinoma, malignant mixed tumor and pseudosarcoma. They are primarily tumors of the elderly with a predilection for males. Clinical features associated with adverse prognosis include age (<65 years), history of recent growth, long-standing tumor, size (>2 cm) and regional lymph node metastasis.

22. **D. Image shown is that of lymphoepithelioma-like carcinoma (LELC).**

    In terms of histopathology, at scanning magnification small biopsies may be misdiagnosed as lymphoma or a reactive lymphoid hyperplasia. Closer inspection reveals two components – malignant markedly pleomorphic epithelial cells (arranged in cords, nodules or strands) with an admixed lymphoplasmacytic infiltrate. Primary cutaneous LELC is a biphasic tumor composed of malignant epithelial cells with a surrounding reactive lymphoid cell infiltrate. It is histologically indistinguishable from LELC occurring in other sites such as the nasopharynx which are typically EBV associated. In terms of immunohistochemistry, the epithelial cells are positive for cytokeratins and EMA while the lymphoid cells are CD45/LCA positive.

23. **C. Image shown is that of onychomatrixoma.**

    Histopathologic diagnostic criteria for onychomatrixoma include the following:

    - Fibroepithelial tumor with two anatomic zones based on proximal and distal location: the proximal zone, corresponds to the tumor base and is composed of deep epithelial invaginations and fibrillary stroma and the distal zone corresponds to the lunula and is characterized by multiple tumor digitations or projections lined with matrix epithelium and cavities filled with serous fluid
    - Matrical tumor in 2 layers: (1) a superficial cellular layer with fibrillary collagen and (2) a deep, less cellular layer filled with dense collagen bundles

    - Thick nail plate formed by a thick keratogenous zone; the nail is perforated by cavities filled with serous fluid

    Clinically, onychomatricoma is a subungual tumor of the fingers and toes that was initially described in 1992. The terminology describing onychomatricomas has slowly been adjusted over time, with subsequent introduction of the term onychomatricoma, a descriptive term encompassing key elements of the tumor, i.e. onycho (nail) and matric (matrix) oma (tumor). The clinical history may be non-specific because this is usually a painless growth. Patients may report a change in nail color or nail thickening. These tumors typically occur predominantly (63%) on the fingers. Clinical tetrad associated with this includes xanthonychia, longitudinal ridging, splinter hemorrhage, and notable overcurvature.

24. **B. Subungual keratoacanthomas are typically more destructive than squamous cell carcinomas at the same site.**

    Subungual keratoacanthoma is a specific type of keratoacanthoma that differs from the common solitary keratoacanthoma in the following:

    - Clinical similarity to verruca vulgaris in terms of presentation
    - Presence of numerous dyskeratotic as well as individually keratinizing cells
    - Fewer neutrophils and eosinophils in the inflammatory infiltrate
    - Vertical orientation (longer than it is broad)
    - Failure to regress spontaneously
    - Longer course
    - Locally aggressive properties with an increased tendency to destroy bone

25. **A. Keratoacanthoma centrifugum marginatum (KCM) is characterized by progressive peripheral growth with coincident central healing.**

    KCM is a locally destructive, persisting variant of keratoacanthoma (KA). It was first described in 1965 as a separate distinct entity. Histopathologic features include peripheral expansion and concomitant central scarring. Focally, cytopathic effects like those often associated with human papilloma virus (HPV) infection can be seen within the epidermis. A pronounced foreign body reaction with frequent giant cells in association with extracellular keratin deposits may also be observed.

26. **E. Keratoacanthomas associated with Muir-Torre syndrome (MTS) are typically negative for the mismatch repair proteins MSH2 and MLH1.**

    Like sebaceous tumors associated with MTS, keratoacanthomas in MTS demonstrate high microsatellite instability (MSI). Immunohistochemical testing of MTS-related skin tumors for MLH1 and MSH2 is a reliable screening method with high predictive value for the diagnosis of the DNA mismatch repair-deficient MTS. Concordance of MSI and immunohistochemical analysis in patients with MTS has been demonstrated and is indicative of the fact that the clinical, biomolecular, and immunohistochemical characterization of skin tumors may be used as screening for the identification of families at risk of MTS. The immunohistochemical demonstration of loss of hMSH2, hMSH6, or rarely hMLH1, or PM2S, is characteristic of MTS and strongly suggests a germline mutation, which may be confirmed by further genetic testing and counseling. *The absence of this finding does not however exclude MTS, and screening evaluation for internal malignancy should still be considered in patients with a strong family history.*

27. **A.** Chediak-Higashi syndrome is characterized by hypopigmentation NOT hyperpigmentation.

   Chediak-Higashi syndrome is a variant of oculocutaneous albinism (OCA). Other features include frequent pyogenic infections and the presence of abnormal large granules in leukocytes and other cells. All other entities listed are characterized by hyperpigmentation. The hyperpigmentation is patch or localized in Peutz-Jeghers syndrome, macules of Albright syndrome and Laugier-Hunziker syndrome, and reticulate in Dowling-Degos disease, and multiple diffuse lentigines in NAME/LAMB syndrome.

28. **E.** Lentigo (shown in the image) would not be a feature of Chediak-Higashi syndrome.

   Multiple lentigines may be seen in the following entities:
   LEOPARD syndrome
   McCune-Albright syndrome
   Laugier-Hunziker syndrome
   LAMB syndrome
   Peutz-Jeghers syndrome
   Bandler syndrome
   Xeroderma pigmentosum

29. **D.** Image shown is that of an ink-spot lentigo.

   The name stems from the distinctive clinical appearance of a "spot of ink." Also known as reticulated melanotic macule of the trunk, it is best regarded a melanotic macule similar to labial and genital melanotic macules.

30. **C.** Image shown is that of a balloon cell nevus.

   Histopathologic features, shown in the image, demonstrate a papillated symmetric population composed of 3 populations of cells: one that is small and nevic, another that is larger with abundant vacuolated cytoplasm and a centrally located "wrinkled" nucleus, and a third population that is intermediate in size with finely granular cytoplasm ("oncocytoid"). Pleomorphism, mitotic activity and a host response argue in favor of balloon cell melanoma.

31. **B.** Image shown is that of a deep penetrating nevus (DPN).

   Histopathologic features of DPN are a wedge-shaped silhouette, a grenz zone separating the dermal from the epidermal lentiginous junctional, melanocytic proliferation, a dermal component with a plexiform architecture, 2 distinct populations of cells (one that is epithelioid and another that is more spindled), distinctive pigment deposits in a "checkerboard" pattern and a patchy host response. Scanning magnification is characteristic.

32. **A.** Mutations in *HRAS* have been demonstrated in a sizeable number of deep penetrating nevi.

   The demonstration of mutations in *HRAS* in deep penetrating nevi suggests that it is more likely to be part of the Spitz spectrum than the blue nevus category.

33. **E.** A trizonal pattern is typical of a recurrent nevus.

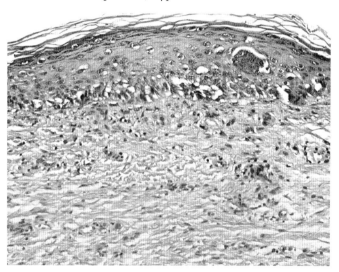

   Recurrent nevi appear within 6 months of the original biopsy and are clinically characterized by a scar with variegated /stippled pigmentation. Defining histopathologic features are the following:

   - Trizonal pattern (atypical junctional melanocytic proliferation with underlying fibrosis separating it from the banal dermal component)
   - Epidermal effacement
   - Cytologic atypia

   Of note, HMB45 demonstrates a maturation pattern (decreased staining with depth) and there is a low Ki-67 index.

34. **D.** Mucosal melanomas exhibit mutations in *KIT*.

    Acral melanomas also exhibit mutation in *KIT*. "Hot spots" are frequently point mutations involving exons 11, 13 and 17. *KIT* mutation, presumably activating the tyrosine kinase activity of c-KIT, encourages clinical studies with c-KIT blockers in patients with mucosal and acral melanomas and appropriate *KIT* mutations. Immunohistochemistry for c-KIT protein expression is believed to be a useful surrogate for screening for genetic analysis.

35. **E.** Uveal melanomas express mutations in *GNAQ*.

    Frequent somatic mutations in the heterotrimeric G protein α-subunit, *GNAQ*, have been demonstrated in a large proportion of blue nevi and ocular melanoma of the uvea. These mutations occur exclusively in codon 209 in the Ras-like domain and result in constitutive activation, turning *GNAQ* into a dominant acting oncogene. Given the absence of mutations in *BRAFV600E* in these lesions, these indicate an alternative route to MAP kinase activation in uveal melanomas and blue nevi.

36. **D.** Image shown is that of a Spitz nevus.

    Key histopathologic features of a Spitz nevus, shown in the image, are a dome-shaped silhouette, hyperplastic epidermis with hypergranulosis (more prominent in older lesions), regularly irregular rete ridges, sharp circumscription, regularly shaped and distributed nests that are vertically oriented ("raining down" pattern), crescent shaped clefts between nests and epidermis ("cupping"), kamino bodies, distinctive spitzoid cytomorphology (abundant amphophilic cytoplasm, open nuclear chromatin and prominent nucleoli) and presence of a patchy host response evenly distributed throughout the lesion. In terms of immunohistochemical profile, Spitz nevi exhibit an HMB-45 gradient (more prominent superficially), Ki-67 index <10%, positive staining with S100, S100A6, p16 and p21.

37. **B.** Spitz nevi exhibit mutations in *HRAS*.

    Spitz nevi may also exhibit amplification of isochrome 11*p*. While Spitz tumor of uncertain malignant potential (STUMP) and spitzoid melanoma may also exhibit mutations in *HRAS*, they are also known to exhibit mutations in *BRAF* and/or *NRAS* (both uncommon in Spitz nevi) and homozygous 9*p*21 deletions.

38. **A.** *HRAS* status is not helpful in distinguishing Spitz nevi from spitzoid melanoma.

    Features of utility in distinguishing these include the following:

    HMB-45 gradient – Maintained in Spitz nevus, lost in spitzoid melanoma

    Ki-67 index – <10% in Spitz nevus, >10% in spitzoid melanoma

    S100 staining – Diffuse and weak in Spitz nevus, strong and diffuse in spitzoid melanoma

    S100A6 staining – Diffuse and strong in Spitz nevus, diffuse and weak in Spitzoid melanoma

    An additional tool of diagnostic utility in distinguishing these two include imaging mass spectrophotometry (97% sensitivity, 90% specificity).

39. **E.** Image shown is that of halo nevus.

    Halo nevi clinically occur in 3 distinct stages – development, disappearance and repigmentation. There is an increased incidence of halo nevi in Turner's syndrome. Key histopathologic features of a halo nevus include circumscription, dome-shape, symmetry, bases of rete lose melanocytes and are infiltrated by lymphocytes but retain their rounded bottom, a moderate host response which blurs the dermoepidermal junction and epithelioid melanocytes with minimal cytologic atypia.

40. **D.** Image shown is that of a proliferation of slender pigmented melanocytes in the superficial dermis.

    While the image is that of a Hori's nevus, other entities listed would also demonstrate a proliferation of slender pigmented melanocytes. The only difference is in the location:

    Nevus of Ota and Ito – Proliferation confined to the upper dermis

    Hori's nevus – Proliferation in the upper and mid dermis

    Dermal melanocyte hamartoma – Proliferation in the upper and mid dermis

    Mongolian spot – Proliferation in the lower half of the dermis

    A cellular blue nevus is very different from the above and presents as a circumscribed biphasic tumor with 2 cytomorphologically distinct populations of cells (one blue-nevus like and another that is more epithelioid with clear cytoplasm).

41. **C.** Reed nevus is believed to be a variant of a Spitz nevus.

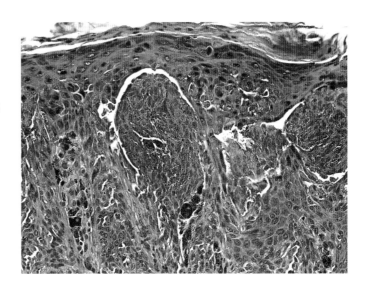

Clinically, Reed nevi are typically located on the lower extremity of women between the ages of 16–25. Histopathologic features include a circumscribed proliferation of elongate spindled cells, an underlying lichenoid infiltrate with prominent pigment incontinence, Kamino bodies and upward scatter (typically in the center of the lesion).

42. **B.** Confluent pagetoid spread (over 3 rete ridges) is a feature of melanoma and NOT a dysplastic nevus.

Clinical features of a dysplastic nevus are size exceeding 5 mm, variegation in color, irregular borders and a diffuse mottled "brown dot" appearance on dermoscopy. Histopathologic features include architectural disorder with presence of a shoulder (epidermal component extending beyond the dermal component laterally), concentric and lamellar fibroplasia, cytologic atypia (ranging from mild to severe) and a host response.

43. **A.** *CDKN2A* is a high-risk gene mutation for melanoma.

Germ-line mutations in the *CDKN2A* tumor-suppressor gene (also known as *p16, p16* ^{INK} *4a,* and *MTS1*) have been linked to the development of melanoma in some families with inherited melanoma. The *CDKN2A* gene provides instructions for making several proteins. The most well-studied are the p16(INK4a) and the p14(ARF) proteins, both functioning as tumor suppressors.

The p16(INK4a) protein attaches (binds) to two other proteins called CDK4 and CDK6. These proteins help regulate the cell cycle. CDK4 and CDK6 normally stimulate the cell to continue through the cycle and divide. However, binding of p16(INK4a) blocks the ability of CDK4 or CDK6 to stimulate cell cycle progression. In this way, p16(INK4a) controls cell growth and division.

The p14(ARF) protein protects a different protein called p53 from being broken down. The p53 protein is an important tumor suppressor that is essential for regulating cell division and self-destruction (apoptosis). By protecting p53, p14(ARF) also helps prevent tumor formation.

Mutations in the *CDKN2A* gene are found in up to one-quarter of head and neck squamous cell carcinomas (HNSCC). Mutations in the *CDKN2A* gene are also associated with breast cancer, lung cancer, and pancreatic cancer.

44. **E.** Image shown is that of desmoplastic melanoma (DM).

Desmoplastic melanoma is a distinct type of melanoma that occurs on chronically sun-damaged skin areas like the face of older individuals. Defining histopathologic features are absence of or an inconspicuous junction component, pandermal proliferation of stellate and spindled cells, patchy host response in the form of lymphocyte clusters peripheral to the tumor. This type of melanoma is commonly associated with neurotropism. Two distinct subtypes of DM are recognized – pure DM (with >90% of cells exhibiting a spindled cytomorphology) and mixed DM (composed of both spindled cells that are <90% of the total proportion and epithelioid cells).

45. **D.** Desmoplastic melanoma (DM) is associated with *RETp*.

DM exhibits polymorphisms in *RET* (encoding receptor tyrosine kinase for which the ligand is glial cell line-derived neurotrophic factor). Mutational frequency of *RETp* in DM is 61% versus 31% in conventional melanomas. DMs do not exhibit mutations in *BRAFV600E* (the most common mutation in conventional melanomas from sun-damaged skin).

46. **D.** Image shown is that of acral melanoma.

Acral melanomas are more common in "skin of color," have a slow growth pattern and have distinctive dermoscopic findings of a "parallel ridge" pattern with the pigmentation overlying the ridges. Histopathologically, findings vary with the age of the lesion.

Early lesions: Demonstrate an atypical lentiginous proliferation with prominent upward scatter and increased density of pigmented dendrites
Later lesions: Demonstrate nests of atypical melanocytes, "skip" areas and a patchy host response

47. **C.** Acral melanomas are associated with mutations in *KIT*.

"Hot spots" are frequently point mutations involving exons 11, 13 and 17. Immunohistochemistry for c-KIT protein expression is believed to be a useful surrogate for screening for genetic analysis. *KIT* mutation presumably activating the tyrosine kinase activity of c-KIT encourages clinical studies with c-KIT blockers in patients with mucosal and acral melanomas and appropriate *KIT* mutations.

48. **B.** Image shown is that of a cellular blue nevus (CBN).

CBN typically presents as a bluish-black papule in young adults, with a predilection for the buttocks, sacrococcygeal region and the scalp. In terms of histopathology, CBN is a well-circumscribed, biphasic tumor with a characteristic zonal pattern. Two cytomorphologically distinct nevomelanocytic proliferations are evident – one that is slender and pigmented ("blue nevus-like") and another that is plump and epithelioid with pale cytoplasm and minimal pigment.

49. **A.** Image shown is that of an epithelioid blue nevus (EBN).

    In terms of histopathology, EBN is a symmetric proliferation of heavily pigmented "globular" or epithelioid melanocytes interspersed with polygonal lightly pigmented cells.

50. **C.** Multiple epithelioid blue nevi are associated with Carney complex.

    Epithelioid blue nevi associated with Carney complex tend to be more common in males, occur in younger patients, are more commonly multiple and frequently metastasize to local lymph nodes. Carney complex and its subsets LAMB syndrome and NAME syndrome are autosomal dominant conditions comprising myxomas of the heart and skin, hyperpigmentation of the skin (lentiginosis), and endocrine overactivity.

51. **A.** Biallelic loss of *BAP1* is associated with mutations in *BRAFV600E*.

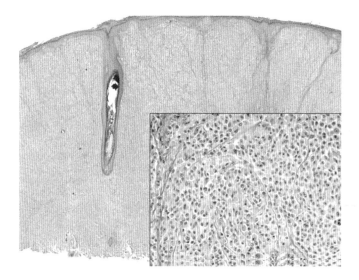

    BAP1 (BRCA1-associated protein 1) is a nuclear protein encoded by the tumor suppressor gene located on chromosome 3*p*21.1. It is a deubiquitinating enzyme, usually part of a protein complex, and has been implicated in a number of different cellular processes including chromatin remodeling, cell cycle progression, cell differentiation and DNA damage responses. The understanding of the role of BAP1 in cellular processes and subsequent carcinogenesis has increased in recent years. However, the function of BAP1 is still being fully characterized, in particular its contribution to carcinogenesis. Both germline and somatic mutations have been implicated in tumor progression. BAP1 hereditary cancer predisposition syndrome is a syndrome that describes a predisposition to the development of

several malignancies, in particular uveal melanoma and malignant mesothelioma as well as cutaneous melanomas, basal cell carcinomas and renal cell carcinoma. Nevi associated with this syndrome exhibit a polypoid architecture and distinctive spitzoid cytomorphology, shown in the image above. Superficial mitoses, scattered multinucleate giant cells and a patchy host response may also be seen in these nevi.

52. **B.** Chromosomes targeted in first generation FISH probes were 6 and 11.

    The standard melanoma FISH test targeted RREB1 (6*p*25), MYB (6*q*23), CCND1 (11*q*13), and centromere 6.

53. **C.** Image shown is that of a dilated pore of Winer.

    Clinically, these present commonly in the head and neck area as a comedo-like lesion. Characteristic histopathologic features, shown in the image, include a central dilated infundibular cystic structure with acanthosis and finger-like projections into the adjacent dermis.

54. **D.** Image shown is that of inverted follicular keratosis (IFK).

    Believed to represent a variant of seborrheic keratosis that is irritated, the term IFK is used when squamous eddies occur in relation to the follicular infundibulum. Other distinctive features include a lobular epidermal hyperplasia.

55. **E.** Image shown is that of a trichoadenoma.

    First described in 1950, trichoadenoma likely represents a distinct follicular tumor with differentiation towards the infundibular part of the folliculosebaceous unit.

    It presents as a solitary skin-colored papule and typically occurs on the face or buttocks. Defining histopathologic features, shown in the image, consist of multiple variably sized horn cysts in the dermis.

56. **D.** Image shown is that of a trichilemmoma.

    Clinically, trichilemmoma presents as a solitary exophytic lesion in the central part of the face. It usually has a "warty" appearance. Defining histopathologic features of trichilemmoma are an exo-endophytic well-circumscribed tumor, lobular epidermal hyperplasia, peripheral palisading, and foci of clear cell differentiation and a thickened eosinophilic cuticle peripherally.

57. **C.** Multiple trichilemmomas are a cutaneous marker for Cowden syndrome.

    Cowden syndrome is an autosomal dominant disease. In addition to cutaneous manifestations, visceral malignancies involving multiple organ systems (breast, endometrium, thyroid and lower gastrointestinal tract) are also noted in Cowden syndrome.

58. **B.** Other cutaneous manifestations of Cowden syndrome include palmar pits and mucocutaneous papillomatous papules.

   In addition, acral keratosis and tumors of the follicular infundibulum may also be seen in Cowden disease. Mutations in the phosphate and tensin homolog (*PTEN*) gene are associated with Cowden's disease.

59. **A.** Image shown is that of desmoplastic trichilemmoma.

   In addition to containing the features classic/typical of regular trichilemmoma (peripheral palisading and foci of clear cell differentiation and a thickened eosinophilic cuticle peripherally), desmoplastic trichilemmoma contains a desmoplastic and/or hyalinized stroma that compresses the epithelial elements and imparts a "pseudo" infiltrative appearance.

60. **E.** Image shown is that of tumor of the follicular infundibulum.

   First described by Mehregan and Buttler in 1961, tumor of the follicular infundibulum (TFI) is an uncommon benign adnexal tumor that usually presents as a solitary keratotic papule on the face or scalp of elderly patients. Histopathologically, it usually manifests as a superficial plate-like proliferation of pale epithelial cells exhibiting a reticulated growth pattern. The increased association of TFI with other cutaneous lesions strengthens the previous hypothesis that TFI, analogous to focal acantholytic dyskeratosis, epidermolytic hyperkeratosis, and cornoid lamellation, may represent a reactive process.

61. **C.** Image shown is that of a trichofolliculoma.

   Trichofolliculoma is believed by some to represent a hamartomatous lesion of hair germ origin rather than a benign tumor. Clinically, it has a predilection for the head and neck area and has a central punctum from which emanates a tuft of silky hair. Defining histopathologic features are a central dilated infundibular cyst with radiating vellus follicles branching out to give rise to secondary and/or tertiary follicles.

62. **C.** Image shown is that of a trichoepithelioma.

   Trichoepithelioma is a benign lesion believed by some to represent a hamartomatous lesion of hair germ origin. Clinically it presents as an asymptomatic papule on the face. Defining histopathologic features are a dermal-based lesion with focal continuity with the epidermis, islands of basaloid cells with peripheral palisading embedded in a fibrous stroma with aggregates of fibroblasts resembling papillary mesenchymal bodies (characteristic), and

scattered variably sized keratocysts. Focal foreign body giant cell reaction secondary to a ruptured cyst is not uncommon.

63. **B.** Multiple trichoepitheliomas are NOT a feature of Birt-Hogg-Dubé syndrome.

   Entities characterized by multiple trichoepitheliomas include the following:

   Multiple familial trichoepithelioma – An autosomal dominant condition with multiple skin-colored papules developing on the face at the time of puberty
   Rombo syndrome – A familial disorder with vermiculate atrophoderma, milia, hypotrichosis, trichoepitheliomas, basal cell carcinomas and peripheral vasodilation with cyanosis
   Brooke-Spiegler syndrome – An autosomal dominant condition with multiple cylindromas, spiradenomas and trichoepitheliomas

64. **B.** Image shown is that of a pilomatricoma.

   Also known as calcifying epithelioma of Malherbe, pilomatricoma is a benign appendageal tumor with differentiation towards the hair matrix, cortex and inner root sheath. Clinically, it usually manifests as a solitary, asymptomatic, slowly growing firm nodule. It has long been considered a rare tumor, but it may be more common than previously realized. It is more common in children, but occurrence in adults is increasingly being recognized. Histopathologic features indicate a bi-colored tumor composed of distinct "pink" and "blue" areas. The former is composed of ghost cells with lost nuclei and the latter is composed of germinative cells. Mitotic activity is commonly observed in the blue areas. As the lesion ages, the number of basophilic cells decreases. Dystrophic deposits of calcium are seen in 75% of lesions. In terms of immunohistochemical profile, the basaloid cells are positive for β-catenin and the rest positive for LEF-1 (a marker of hair matrix cells) and BCL-2 (supporting a role for faulty apoptosis of hair matrix cells in the pathogenesis).

65. **A.** Pilomatricomas are associated with mutations in β-catenin.

   A large proportion of pilomatrixomas have mutations in the gene *CTNNB1*, directly implicating β-catenin misregulation as the major cause of hair matrix cell tumorigenesis.

66. **E.** Image shown is that of a cutaneous lymphadenoma.

   Also known as lymphotropic adamantoid trichoblastoma, cutaneous lymphadenoma is considered a variant of trichoblastoma. It is composed of multiple dermal nodules of epithelial cells embedded in a fibrous stroma with a dense lymphocytic infiltrate permeating the lobules. In terms of immunophenotype, the lymphocytes are of both B- and T-cell lineage.

67. **D.** Image shown is that of a panfolliculoma.

Alternative names used in the past for this entity include superficial trichoblastoma and superficial epithelioma with follicular differentiation. Clinically, it presents as a verrucous plaque or dermal cystic nodule on the head and neck areas. Defining histopathologic features are a well-circumscribed lesion showing differentiation towards all parts of the hair follicle, including the presence of infundibular cystic structures, cells with trichohyaline granules resembling inner root sheath cells, cells exhibiting outer root sheath differentiation, metrical cells, ghost cells and papillary mesenchymal bodies.

68. **C.** Image shown is that of a fibrofolliculoma.

Fibrofolliculoma, trichodiscoma and neurofollicular hamartoma are all considered part of the same spectrum and a single entity in different stages of development. Clinically, it develops in the 3rd or 4th decade of life and presents as a skin-colored, dome-shaped papule on the face, neck or chest. Histopathologically, fibrofolliculoma contains equal amounts of epithelial and mesenchymal stroma, one or several vertically oriented infundibulocystic structures from which radiate anastomosing cords and strands of epithelial cells. The stroma is typically composed of CD34 positive fibroblasts.

69. **B.** Multiple fibrofolliculomas are associated with Birt-Hogg-Dubé syndrome.

Birt-Hogg-Dubé syndrome is an autosomal dominant disorder clinically manifested by fibrofolliculomas, renal cell carcinoma, lung cysts, and spontaneous pneumothorax. Birt-Hogg-Dubé syndrome is caused by a mutation in the folliculin (*FLCN*) gene, a tumor suppressor gene that has been mapped to the short arm of chromosome 17, specifically $17p11.2$.

70. **A.** Lung cysts and renal tumors are other manifestations of Birt-Hogg-Dubé syndrome.

Multiple or bilateral renal carcinomas have been reported in association with this syndrome, most commonly hybrid oncocytic tumors with features of chromophobe renal carcinoma (50%), followed by chromophobe renal cancer, clear cell renal carcinoma, and renal oncocytoma. Of patients with Birt-Hogg-Dubé syndrome, 12–34% develop renal tumors, typically in the fourth and fifth decades of life. Pulmonary cysts and spontaneous pneumothoraces have also been increasingly reported manifestations of Birt-Hogg-Dubé syndrome. The overall

risk of having a pneumothorax in patients with Birt-Hogg-Dubé syndrome is close to 30%.

71. **E.** Fordyce's spots best describes ectopic sebaceous glands.

Clinically, they present as yellow, pinpoint, submucosal papules located on the buccal mucosa and vermillion border of the lips. Ectopic sebaceous glands may also be noted in the areolae of the breast (Montgomery's tubercles) and on the penis (Tyson's gland).

72. **C.** Image shown is that of a steatocystoma.

These cysts are typically located in the mid dermis. The cyst lining is a crenulated or wavy, homogeneous, eosinophilic horny layer collapsed around thin cystic spaces. The spaces hold varying amounts of keratin, vellus hairs, and sebum esters, the latter of which often are removed by tissue processing. Walls are formed from several layers of epithelial cells, with embedded flattened lobules of sebaceous glands among the epithelial cells. Invaginations resembling hair follicles can also be found emptying into the cyst. Cyst units may be attached to the overlying normal epidermis by a thin strand of undifferentiated epithelial cells. Steatocystoma simplex is the sporadic solitary tumor counterpart to steatocystoma multiplex, an uncommon disorder of the pilosebaceous unit characterized by the development of numerous sebum-containing dermal cysts. Although steatocystoma multiplex has historically been described as an autosomal dominant inherited disorder, most presenting cases are sporadic. In the familial form of steatocystoma multiplex, mutations are localized to the keratin 17 (*K17*) gene in areas identical to mutations found in patients with pachyonychia congenita type 2 (PC-2). Based on this, some believe that steatocystoma multiplex is simply a variant of pachyonychia congenita type 2. Sporadic forms of steatocystoma multiplex have *not been shown* to be associated with *K17* mutations. Steatocystoma multiplex is associated with eruptive vellus hair cysts. Both diseases share overlapping clinical features, including age of onset, location, appearance of lesions, and mode of inheritance. Reports of hybrid lesions showing histologic features of both steatocystoma multiplex and eruptive vellus hair cysts exist. Given these similarities, some postulate that steatocystoma multiplex and eruptive vellus hair cysts are, in fact, variants of the same disease.

73. **B.** Image shown is that of a sebaceous adenoma.

Sebaceous adenomas are benign sebaceous tumors that typically arise on the head and neck regions of older individuals and clinically appear as tan, pink, or yellow nodules or papules, usually about 5 mm in greatest dimension. Histopathologic features include a multilobular circumscribed tumor with an expansion and increased prominence of the peripherally located basaloid cells and a central area composed of mature sebocytes (the proportion of the latter surpasses that of the former). Mitotic activity is typically confined to the germinative layer. In the setting of Muir-Torre syndrome, loss of expression of the mismatch repair proteins (MMR) MSH2, MLH1 and MSH6 is observed.

74. **A.** When located outside of the head and neck area in a younger patient, sebaceous adenomas may represent a cutaneous marker for Muir-Torre syndrome (MTS).

    Sebaceous adenoma is considered to be the most specific marker of MTS with a reported association ranging from 25 to 60%. The association of sebaceous epithelioma and/or carcinoma with MTS is lower, although recent studies indicate that the association may not be as low as previously believed. The incidence of sebaceous epithelioma in patients with MTS varies anywhere from 31 to 86%, whereas that of sebaceous carcinoma varies from 66 to 100%. MTS is a rare autosomal dominant genodermatosis with a high degree of penetrance and variable expressivity. It is characterized by the association of cutaneous lesions (sebaceous neoplasms or keratoacanthomas) and internal malignancies. Diagnosis is based on the presence of at least one sebaceous neoplasm and a visceral malignancy, or alternatively multiple keratoacanthomas associated with visceral malignancies and a family history of MTS. Visceral malignancies most commonly observed in association with MTS include colorectal and genitourinary carcinomas, although other types of cancers, such as breast and upper gastrointestinal cancers, have also been uncommonly reported. Nearly half of patients with MTS develop two or more visceral malignancies. Of interest, both cutaneous and visceral neoplasms in patients with MTS have been shown to behave less aggressively compared to their sporadic counterparts. Also see Figure H1.

75. **E.** Sebaceous adenomas part of Muir-Torre syndrome (MTS) are most commonly associated with mutations in *MSH2*.

    Germline mutations in patients with MTS most commonly affect *MSH2* (>90%), followed by *MLH1* (<10%). More recently, lack of expression of *MSH6* in sebaceous tumors of patients with MTS has been shown, suggesting that a mutation in *MSH6* gene is perhaps not so uncommon as previously believed. Also see Figure H1.

76. **D.** Image shown is that of sebaceous carcinoma which would be positive for adipophilin.

    Adipophilin, a monoclonal antibody directed against a protein on the surface of intracellular lipid droplets, has been shown to be expressed in sebocytes and sebaceous lesions. In one study that looked at a spectrum of lesions with clear cell differentiation, adipophilin expression was not seen in any of the other lesions with clear cell differentiation such as basal cell carcinomas or squamous cell carcinomas. Adipophilin identifies intracytoplasmic lipid vesicles in sebaceous and xanthomatous lesions. *Of note, adipophilin expression is not as useful in differentiating metastatic renal cell carcinoma from sebaceous carcinoma as it is positive in both.* The pattern of adipophilin reactivity is important to observe as membranous vesicular staining is suggestive of intracellular lipids whereas granular cytoplasmic reactivity is not.

    Sebaceous carcinomas are classified into 2 broad groups: periocular (more common) and extraocular. While both are associated with Muir-Torre syndrome, the association is *particularly relevant for carcinomas outside of the head and neck area.* Defining histopathologic features are irregular lobules composed of a disordered mixture of basaloid germinative cells with a high N:C ratio and admixed foci of sebaceous differentiation. Cytologic atypia, nuclear pyknosis and mitotic activity are present, as is necrosis.

77. **A.** Image shown is that of a hidrocystoma.

    Typically, hidrocystomas, eccrine or apocrine, appear as unilocular cysts, which usually contain a single cystic cavity composed of 1 or 2 layers of cuboidal cells. They are located within the mid dermal to superficial layers of the skin, especially around the eyes.

    The inherited disorders that are most commonly associated with the presence of multiple eccrine/apocrine hidrocystomas are the following:

    Goltz-Gorlin syndrome – Also known as Jessner-Cole syndrome, or focal dermal hypoplasia, this syndrome tends to occur sporadically, with few familial cases having X-linked dominant transmission; it occurs mostly in females. Its cardinal features are microcephaly, midfacial hypoplasia, malformed ears, microphthalmia, periocular multiple hidrocystomas, papillomas of the lip, tongue, anus, and axilla, skeleton abnormalities, and mental retardation.

    Schopf-Schulz-Passarge syndrome – This is an autosomal recessive syndrome characterized by multiple eyelid apocrine hidrocystoma, palmoplantar hyperkeratosis, hypodontia, and hypotrichosis. It is further characterized by hypotrichosis, cysts of the eyelids, and multiple periocular apocrine hidrocystomas. Graves's disease has also been associated with multiple eccrine hidrocystomas, possibly due to hyperhidrosis, which is seen in hyperthyroid patients, further supported by the disappearance of lesions after treatment of hyperthyroidism.

78. **E.** Image shown is that of cylindroma.

    Cylindromas are benign skin appendage tumors that most commonly occur on the head and neck as solitary or multiple tumors. Cases of spiradenocylindromas, demonstrating characteristics of both spiradenoma and cylindroma in the same tumor mass, have also been observed, suggesting similar derivation of both tumors. Solitary cylindromas occur sporadically and typically are not inherited. Multiple tumors are observed in an autosomal dominantly inherited manner. Solitary lesions clinically present as firm, rubbery nodules with pink, red, or sometimes blue coloring that range in size from a few millimeters to several centimeters. The multiple form has numerous masses of pink, red, or blue nodules, sometimes resembling bunches of grapes or small tomatoes (sometimes called a tomato or turban tumor). In terms of histopathology, the tumor is composed of numerous oval and polygonal nests molded into a jigsaw-like pattern, with each nest surrounded peripherally by an eosinophilic hyaline sheath closely resembling a basement membrane. Tumor islands are composed of 2 cell types – peripheral cells that are small and highly basophilic, suggesting palisading, and larger, more pale-staining cells centrally. Small tubular lumina are sometimes found with careful observation.

A lack of lymphoid tissue is a histologic feature that differentiates cylindromas from spiradenomas. The latter typically show a unique prominent presence of lymphocytes. Cylindromas, on the other hand, demonstrate a large number of prominent dendritic cells that most likely represent Langerhans cells that permeate the tumor. S-100 protein-negative, HLA-DR-negative, and CD1a-positive cells can be seen in cylindromas and represent the existence of Langerhans cells.

Hyaline bands, which surround tumor islands, are mostly composed of type IV collagen.

79. **D.** Multiple cylindromas are associated with the Brooke-Spiegler syndrome.

Brooke-Spiegler syndrome (BSS) has been described as an autosomal dominant disease characterized by the development of multiple skin appendage tumors such as cylindromas, trichoepitheliomas, and spiradenomas, with a variable preponderance of any of the aforementioned subsets. Other lesions reported with BSS include parotid basal cell adenomas, organoid nevi, syringomas, and basal cell carcinoma.

80. **C.** The gene responsible for multiple cylindromas associated with BSS is *CYLD*.

CYLD, localized to band 16q12–q13, encodes a deubiquitinating enzyme. The enzyme removes Lys-63-linked ubiquitin chains from I-kappaB kinase signaling components. By this mechanism, the enzyme inhibits NF-kappaB pathway activation. *CYLD* also appears to be required for the cell's timely entry into mitosis. Thus, as with other genes that regulate tumorigenesis, *CYLD* has

both tumor-suppressing (apoptosis regulation) and tumor-promoting (enhancer of mitotic entry) activities. This additional function of *CYLD* could provide an explanation for the benign nature of most cylindromas.

81. **B.** Image shown is that of a syringoma.

Syringoma is a benign adnexal neoplasm formed by well-differentiated ductal elements.

Based on Friedman and Butler's classification scheme, 4 distinct variants of syringoma are recognized: (1) a localized form, (2) a form associated with Down syndrome, (3) a generalized form that encompasses multiple and eruptive syringomas, and (4) a familial form. Syndromic associations include the following:

- *Brooke-Spiegler syndrome*, an autosomal dominant disease characterized by the development of multiple cylindromas, trichoepitheliomas, and occasional spiradenomas
- *Nicolau-Balus syndrome*, characterized by milia and atrophoderma vermiculatum
- *Costello syndrome*, characterized by various other cutaneous manifestations such as hyperkeratosis, hyperpigmentation, papillomas, and deep palmoplantar creases, as well as craniofacial, musculoskeletal, and neurologic abnormalities
- *Steatocystoma multiplex*
- *Down syndrome*

Clinically, syringomas appear as skin-colored or yellowish, generally small, dermal papules. In terms of histopathology, syringomas are composed of ducts usually lined by 2 rows of cuboidal-to-flattened epithelial cells and have a lumen containing periodic acid-Schiff-positive, eosinophilic, amorphous debris. Some of the ducts have elongated tails of epithelial cells, producing a characteristic comma-shaped or tadpole appearance. Rarely, tumor cells may appear clear as a result of glycogen accumulation. Contrary to previous views, the association of clear cell syringomas with diabetes mellitus is no longer valid.

82. **A.** Image shown is that of a poroma.

Defining histopathologic features are a broad epidermal proliferation into the dermis of uniform, basaloid, round, cuboidal cells with round/oval nuclei ("poroid" cytomorphology) with occasional foci of ductal differentiation embedded in a granulation tissue-like stroma. Multiple poromas have been reported in patients with radiation therapy for lymphoproliferative disease.

83. **E.** Poromas typically occur on the extremity.

Poromas clinically present as reddish, skin-colored nodules in the elderly and are usually located on the foot.

84. **D.** Image shown is that of syringofibroadenoma (of Mascaro).

 A relatively uncommon adnexal tumor, syringofibroadenoma is a benign neoplasm that consists of anastomosing strands of acrosyringeal epithelia with scattered foci of ductal differentiation embedded in fibromucinous stroma. This rare, distinct histologic lesion was first described in case reports by Mascaro in 1963 and can have multiple hyperplastic presentations, making clinical diagnosis difficult. Syringofibroadenoma has been clinically described as a slow-growing, exophytic, verrucous-like overgrowth, moist mosaic or erythematous scaly plaque, and sometimes with solitary or multiple nodules.

85. **C.** The best-fit diagnosis for the image shown is papillary eccrine adenoma (PEA).

 Clinically, PEA is most common in the distal extremities and presents as a slow-growing yellow/brown erythematous nodule. Histopathologic features are a well-circumscribed unencapsulated tumor centered in the dermis. The lesion itself is composed of multiple ducts which are variably dilated and lined by 2–3 cell layers of cuboidal epithelium with intraluminal papillary projections.

86. **B.** Eccrine hidrocytoma is NOT a synonym for eccrine acrospiroma (shown in the image).

 Other names for eccrine acrospiroma include solid-cystic hidradenoma, clear cell myoepithelioma, clear cell hidradenoma and nodular hidradenoma. Histopathologic features of eccrine acrospiroma, shown in the image, are a circumscribed, unencapsulated tumor with a biphasic population of cells. The different names are due to variations in the components of the integral components. Continuity with the epidermis or follicular infundibulum can be seen in about a quarter of the cases.

87. **D.** Image shown is that of syringocystadenoma papilliferum (SCAP).

 SCAP is typically found on the scalp. It presents clinically as a solitary lesion and gradually increases in size. Defining histopathologic features are papillomatosis with transition from squamous to glandular epithelium of papillary structures lined by 2 cell layers, an inner cuboidal layer and an outer layer composed of columnar cells which exhibit decapitation secretion. The stroma is plasma cell-rich and deep in the lesion there may be tubular glands.

88. **C.** Syringocystadenoma papilliferum (SCAP) arises in association with nevus sebaceus in about a third of the cases.

SCAP is *the most common benign tumor* to arise in association with nevus sebaceus. Other benign tumors include trichilemmoma, sebaceoma, nodular hidradenoma, hidrocystoma, and eccrine poroma. Amongst malignant neoplasms, the most common is trichoblastoma. Other malignant neoplasms that arise in association with nevus sebaceus include basal cell carcinoma, apocrine carcinoma, trichilemmal carcinoma, sebaceous carcinoma, microcystic adnexal carcinoma, porocarcinoma, and squamous cell carcinoma. Nevus sebaceus, also called nevus sebaceous of Jadassohn or organoid nevus, is a benign hamartoma of the skin, characterized by hyperplasia of the epidermis, immature hair follicles, and sebaceous and apocrine glands. Lesions are usually present at birth and appear as waxy, yellow-orange or tan, hairless plaques. They have a tendency to thicken and become more verrucous over time, especially around the time of puberty. Nevus sebaceous and nevus sebaceous syndrome (Schimmelpenning syndrome) are thought to be caused by post-zygotic mosaic mutations in the *HRAS* or *KRAS* genes.

89. **B.** Image shown is that of an apocrine mixed tumor.

 Clinically, these lesions are more common in males and present more commonly in the head and neck areas. Defining histopathologic features are a circumscribed dermal tumor composed of epithelial (in the form of clusters and cords of cells with foci of ductal differentiation) and myoepithelial (present in the peripheral layer of the ductal structures and may form solid islands and demonstrate hyaline or plasmacytoid cytomorphology) elements. The stroma is variable and may be chondroid, myxoid and fibrotic.

90. **A.** Image shown is that of a myoepithelioma.

 Similar to mixed tumors of salivary glands ("pleomorphic adenomas"), cutaneous mixed tumors ("chondroid syringomas") contain a ductal (epithelial) component and a variably prominent myoepithelial component. Tumors showing purely myoepithelial differentiation (myoepitheliomas) are relatively uncommon. Myoepitheliomas commonly arise on the extremities. In terms of histopathology, they can be solid (composed of ovoid/spindled, histiocytoid, or epithelioid cells with abundant eosinophilic syncytial cytoplasm and minimal stroma) or lobulated (with cords or nests of epithelioid, plasmacytoid, or spindled cells with a variably reticular architecture and a chondromyxoid or collagenous/ hyalinized stroma). Cytologic atypia is typically minimal and mitoses (mean, 1.5) can occasionally be seen in select tumors. Immunohistochemically, myoepitheliomas tend to be variably positive for epithelial markers (keratins and/or epithelial membrane antigen), S-100 protein, calponin, EMA and smooth muscle actin. Most cutaneous myoepitheliomas behave in a benign fashion, although there is apparently a significant risk for local recurrence but a low metastatic potential (typically observed in cases with increased mitotic activity).

91. **A.** Image shown is that of erosive adenomatosis.

Synonyms for this include nipple adenoma, papillary adenoma, florid adenomatosis, florid papillomatosis of the nipple, superficial papillary adenomatosis, subareolar duct papillomatosis and nipple duct adenoma. These typically occur in women in the 5th to 6th decade and clinically present with soreness, erosion, crusting, ulceration and nipple discharge. In terms of histopathology, it tends to be a relatively circumscribed glandular proliferation with mixed growth patterns (adenosis/papillomatosis/sclerosing/mixed proliferative). A layer of myoepithelial cells surrounds the glands and the ducts and preservation of this helps distinguish this entity from malignant "look-alikes."

92. **E.** Image shown is that of mucinous carcinoma.

Clinically, this tends to occur in the elderly with a predilection for the head and neck area and a female predominance. Histopathologic features include a dermal-based lesion composed of nests and strands of epithelial cells floating in copious amounts of mucin. An *in situ* component is identified in a proportion of cases. Immunohistochemically, lesional cells are CK7 positive and CK20 negative. Occasionally, lesional cells may be positive for ER, PR and GCDFP-15.

93. **D.** Image shown is that of digital papillary adenocarcinoma.

When initially described, the prefix "aggressive" was used for this entity. However, all lesions are now considered malignant with metastatic potential, thus the prefix has been dropped.

Clinically, this presents as a solitary, painless, nodulocystic mass on the fingers and toes. Local recurrence, regional lymph node involvement and distant metastasis have been reported. Histopathologic features include a poorly circumscribed, non-encapsulated, multinodular lesion based in the dermis and/or subcutis, focal infiltrative pattern, papillary differentiation with true as well as "pseudo" papillae, foci of ductal differentiation, variable cytologic atypia, pleomorphism and mitotic activity. Invasion of underlying bone and lymphovascular invasion are not uncommon.

94. **D.** Digital papillary adenocarcinoma is NOT a marker for an internal malignancy.

All others listed are true regarding this entity.

95. **C.** With the immunoprofile described, the best-fit diagnosis for the image shown is extramammary Paget's disease (EMPD).

Clinically, primary EMPD presents as a slow-spreading, scaly, erythematous plaque in elderly women, typically in the vulva. Local recurrence is common but, overall, prognosis is generally good for cases without an underlying cutaneous adnexal carcinoma or internal malignancy.

Secondary EMPD is more common in the perianal area with an internal malignancy present in almost 80% of cases. Histopathologic features include malignant cells scattered singly or in clusters throughout the epidermis. The cytomorphology of the lesional cells is distinct with large pleomorphic nuclei, prominent nucleoli and abundant pale cytoplasm. Immunohistochemically, the lesional cells are positive for CAM5.2, CK7, EMA and GCDFP-15 (in 80% of cases).

96. **C.** Image shown is that of a cutaneous pilar leiomyoma. Multiple leiomyomas may be associated with renal disease.

Cutaneous leiomyomas are benign, smooth muscle tumors that may be a sign of underlying systemic disease. Multiple cutaneous and uterine leiomyomatosis, also known as Reed's syndrome, is an autosomal dominant genetic condition. Affected individuals have an increased predisposition to develop leiomyomas in the skin as well as in the uterus. Affected females frequently develop uterine leiomyomas (fibroids) that are larger and more numerous and emerge earlier than those in the general population. Subsets of these patients are at risk for renal cell cancer and have been determined to have mutations in the fumarate hydratase gene.

97. **B.** Leiomyomas are positive for caldesmon.

Caldesmon, a protein that in humans is encoded by the *CALD1* gene, is an immunohistochemical marker for smooth muscle differentiation. Special stains can also be used to distinguish smooth muscle from collagen, both of which are pink-red with hematoxylin and eosin stain. The Masson trichrome stain highlights smooth muscle as dark red and collagen as blue-green.

98. **B.** Reed syndrome is associated with mutations in fumarate hydratase.

Mutations in the fumarate hydratase gene (*FH*) cause hereditary leiomyomatosis and renal cell cancer. The *FH* gene provides instructions for making an enzyme called fumarase (also known as fumarate hydratase). This enzyme participates in an important series of reactions known as the citric acid cycle or Krebs cycle, which allows cells to use oxygen and generate energy. *FH* gene mutations may interfere with the enzyme's role in the citric acid cycle, resulting in a buildup of fumarate. The condition is inherited in an autosomal dominant pattern.

99. **D. Perineural invasion is not a significant prognosticator in a leiomyosarcoma (LMS).**

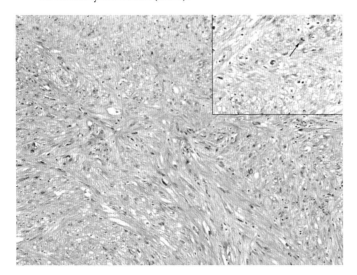

Histopathologic features of LMS include an unencapsulated, poorly circumscribed, fasciculated proliferation of closely packed elongate, cigar-shaped smooth muscle cells. Cytologic atypia and mitotic activity are evident and the latter is an important criterion for assessing the malignancy. Several factors are correlated to prognosis in a LMS. Briefly, these include tumor size, high mitotic rate, presence or absence of necrosis, and intratumoral vascular invasion. The survival rate for tumors smaller than 2 cm is approximately 95%, while in tumors >5 cm the survival has been shown to drop to 30%.

100. **C. Image shown is that of a traumatic neuroma.**

Defining histopathologic features, shown in the image, are the presence of multiple, variably sized nerve twigs, each surrounded by a fibrous tissue sheath. Lesions may be superficial or deep.

101. **A. Image shown is that of rudimentary polydactyly.**

Defining histopathologic features, shown in the image, are the presence of multiple small twigs confined to the dermal papillae.

102. **B. Image shown is that of a solitary circumscribed neuroma (SCN).**

Previously known as palisaded and encapsulated neuroma, SCN is characterized by a dermal nodular proliferation of "neural" appearing cells with a thin perineural connective tissue capsule. In terms of immunohistochemical profile, lesional cells are S100 positive, while the capsule alone is positive for EMA.

103. **A. MEN1 is also known as Wermer syndrome.**

Multiple endocrine neoplasia type 1 (MEN1 syndrome) or Wermer's syndrome, an autosomal dominant disorder, is part of a group of disorders, the multiple endocrine neoplasias, that affect the endocrine system through development of neoplastic lesions in the pituitary, parathyroid gland and the pancreas. The gene for MEN1 is on chr 11q13. Also see Table H5.

104. **E. Leiomyomas are NOT a mucocutaneous manifestation of MEN1.**

Mucocutaneous manifestations of MEN1 include facial angiofibromas, collagenomas, lipomas and, less commonly, gingival papules and confetti-like hypopigmented macules.

105. **D. Multiple mucosal neuromas are a feature of Wagenmann-Froboese syndrome.**

Alternative names for this syndrome include multiple mucosal neuroma syndrome and mucosal neuromata with endocrine tumors. Other mucocutaneous manifestations of this syndrome include prominent lips, hyperpigmentation around the mouth and overlying small joints of hands and feet, café-au-lait macules and circumoral lentigenes.

106. **B. *MEN1* is the gene involved in Wermer syndrome.**

The protein encoded by the *MEN1* gene is menin. Menin is a putative tumor suppressor associated with multiple endocrine neoplasia type 1 (MEN1 syndrome)/Wermer syndrome. The gene is located on long arm of chromosome 11 (11q13), has 10 exons and encodes a 610-amino acid protein. Over 1300 mutations have been reported, with the majority (>70%) of these predicted to lead to truncated forms that are scattered throughout the gene. Most germline or somatic mutations in the *MEN1* gene predict truncation or absence of encoded menin resulting in the inability of *MEN1* to act as a tumor suppressor gene. Also see Table H5.

107. **C. *RET* is the gene involved in Sipple syndrome.**

RET is an abbreviation for "rearranged during transfection." The human gene *RET* is localized to chromosome 10 (10q11.2) and contains 21 exons. The *RET* proto-oncogene encodes a receptor tyrosine kinase for members of the glial cell line-derived neurotrophic factor (GDNF) family of extracellular signaling molecules. Loss of function mutations in *RET* are associated with the development of Hirschsprung's disease, while gain of function mutations are associated with the development of various types of human cancer, including medullary thyroid carcinoma, multiple endocrine neoplasias type 2A (Sipple syndrome) and 2B, pheochromocytoma and parathyroid hyperplasia. Also see Table H 5.

108. **B.** Re-excision perineural invasion (RPI) is composed of squamous epithelium.

Described initially in 1990, RPI refers to the observation of mature benign squamous epithelium in the perineural spaces of cutaneous nerves in re-excision specimens. The squamous epithelium may form a complete cuff around the nerve fascicle. Diagnostic criteria include the absence of perineural spread beyond the immediate previous biopsy site, benign appearance of the perineural epithelial cells in contrast to the appearance of the original tumor, absence of residual epithelial tumor in the vicinity of the involved perineurium and eccrine ducts adjacent to the involved nerve.

109. **A.** Image shown is that of plexiform neurofibroma which is highly specific for neurofibromatosis 1.

Neurofibromatosis type 1 (NF1), also known as von Recklinghausen's disease, is a pandemic genetic disorder affecting approximately one in 3000–3500 persons worldwide. NF1 results from autosomal dominant mutations in the *NF1* tumor suppressor gene, which encodes neurofibromin, a p21^{ras} (Ras) guanosine tri-phosphatase (GTP) activating protein (GAP). Among other non-malignant manifestations, individuals with NF1 frequently develop cutaneous, subcutaneous, and/or plexiform neurofibromas composed of irregular Schwann cells, fibroblasts, and mast cells. In terms of histopathology, plexiform neurofibroma is composed of multiple variably sized fusiform enlargements of nerve either in the deep dermis or subcutis.

Two or more of the following clinical features are sufficient to establish a diagnosis of neurofibromatosis type 1 or von Recklinghausen's disease:
- Six or more café-au-lait macules (>0.5 cm at largest diameter in a prepubertal child or >1.5 cm in post-pubertal individuals)
- Axillary freckling or freckling in inguinal regions
- Two or more neurofibromas of any type or one or more plexiform neurofibromas
- Two or more Lisch nodules (iris hamartomas)
- A distinctive osseous lesion (sphenoid wing dysplasia, long-bone dysplasia)
- An optic pathway glioma
- A first-degree relative with neurofibromatosis type 1 diagnosed by the above criteria

110. **E.** The *NF1* gene resides on chromosome 17.

Mutations in the *NF1* gene are associated with neurofibromatosis type I or von Recklinghausen's

disease, as well as Watson syndrome. The *NF1* gene consists of over 50 exons spanning 300 kb of chromosome 17. The *NF1* gene, encoding the protein neurofibromin, appears to be a negative regulator of the *RAS* signal transduction pathways. Mutations involving *NF1* are diverse.

111. **B.** Positive staining of lesional cells (based on the image shown) would NOT be expected with CD30.

In terms of immunohistochemical profile, lesional cells in neurofibroma are positive for S100P, myelin basic protein, CD57 and the stem cell markers, CD34 and nestin.

CD30, also known as TNFRSF8, is a cell membrane protein of the tumor necrosis factor receptor family and a tumor marker. This receptor is expressed by activated, but not by resting, T- and B-cells. CD30 is associated with anaplastic large cell lymphoma. CD30 and CD15 are also expressed on classical Hodgkin lymphoma Reed-Sternberg cells.

112. **A.** Image shown is that of a perineurioma.

Perineurioma presents as a firm nodule and exists in 3 forms: *soft tissue/extraneural*, intraneural and *sclerosing* (variants in italic type are present in the skin). Histopathologic features include a well-circumscribed, unencapsulated, variably cellular proliferation of spindled cells with bipolar pale staining cytoplasm arranged in concentric whorls of perineurial cells ("onion skinning"). In terms of immunohistochemical profile, lesional cells are positive for EMA, CD34 (50% and more commonly in the sclerosing variant) and claudin-1 (25–30%).

113. **E.** Image shown is that of a schwannoma/neurilemmoma.

Clinically, schwannoma presents as an asymptomatic pink/yellow nodule with a predilection for the flexor aspect of limbs. Defining histopathologic features are a circumscribed, encapsulated lesion with the nerve of origin present peripherally and the presence of two distinct areas: type A (spindled cells arranged in fascicles or Antoni A/verocay bodies) and type B (meshwork of myxoid tissue). Mitotic activity and thickened, hyalinized vessels are prominent in the type A areas.

114. **A.** Multiple schwannomas (based on the image shown) are associated with neurofibromatosis 1 or von Recklinghausen's disease.

Acoustic neuromas are associated with neurofibromatosis 2. For tumors associated with MEN, see Table H5.

115. **C.** Image shown is that of nerve sheath myxoma.

Nerve sheath myxoma, an entity distinct from cellular neurothekeoma, is asymptomatic clinically and presents as a papulonodular lesion, more commonly in the extremities with a relatively high recurrence rate. Defining histopathologic features are a multilobulated, non-encapsulated paucicellular/hypocellular proliferation arranged in loose fascicles with an abundance of mucinous stroma (composed predominantly of the heteroglycan chondroitin 4/6 sulfates).

116. **E.** Lesional cells (based on the image shown) in nerve sheath myxoma would not be positive for PGP9.5.

In terms of immunohistochemical profile, lesional cells in nerve sheath myxoma are positive for S100, S100A6, CD57, GFAP and NSE.

117. **B.** Image shown is that of neurothekeoma.

Neurothekeoma, previously known as cellular neurothekeoma and an entity distinct from nerve sheath myxoma, has a predilection for the head and neck area and clinically presents as a papulonodular lesion. Recurrence is uncommon, unlike nerve sheath myxoma. Defining histopathologic features are a fasciculated proliferation with a lobular architecture centered in the reticular dermis. Lesional cells exhibit an epithelioid or spindled cytomorphology.

118. **D.** Lesional cells in neurothekeoma would NOT be positive for CD30.

In terms of immunohistochemical profile, lesional cells in neurothekeoma are positive for S100A6, NKI/C3, PGP9.5 (sensitive but not specific), CD10 and MITF (81–100% of cases).

119. **C.** The best-fit diagnosis for the image shown is Abrikossoff's tumor.

Better known as granular cell tumor, Abrikossoff's tumor is more common in females and commonly occurs on the trunk and tongue (where it was first described). It is usually solitary, but multiple lesions can occur in Noonan's syndrome. Defining histopathologic features are a circumscribed tumor (although infiltrative borders can be seen), a nested/trabecular architecture and distinctive cytomorphology (polygonal cells with finely granular cytoplasm and a prominent, centrally located nucleolus).

120. **C.** Perineural invasion, shown in the image, in granular cell tumor (GCT) is of no clinical relevance.

Perineural invasion/infiltration in GCT is not associated with malignant transformation. The other feature of no clinical relevance in GCT is the presence of pseudoepitheliomatous hyperplasia, typically seen in oral lesions.

Features indicative of a malignant GCT are tumor size (>4 cm), spindling of tumor cells, necrosis, malignant cytomorphology (high N:C ratio, vesicular nuclei with large multiple nucleoli), mitoses (>2/10 HPFs), a high Ki-67 index, and infiltration into deep tissue.

121. **D.** The best-fit diagnosis for the image shown is Merkel cell carcinoma (MCC).

MCC or primary cutaneous neuroendocrine carcinoma is more common in the head and neck areas, in the elderly, in females and typically has a history of rapid growth. Clincially, recurrence is common after excision. Defining histopathologic features are a dermal infiltrate composed of nests and cords of basaloid cells with distinctive "neuroendocrine" cytomorphology ("salt and pepper" or open nuclear chromatin). Marked cytologic atypia, nuclear pleomorphism and abundant karyorrhexis and mitoses are common. Adverse prognosticators are the presence of lymphovascular invasion, increased vascular density, increased mitotic rate, stromal mast cell counts and small cell size. In terms of immunohistochemical profile, lesional cells are positive for CK20 ("dot-like" pattern), EMA, BerEp4, HIP1, CD117, and synaptophysin.
Immunohistochemical stains of utility in differentiating MCC from non-cutaneous neuroendocrine carcinoma are neurofilament (positive in MCC), CK20 (usually positive in MCC although rare cases of CK20-negative MCCs are reported), CK7 (negative in MCC) and TTF-1 (negative in MCC).

122. **B.** The presence of intratumoral cytotoxic T lymphocytes is NOT an adverse prognosticator in Merkel cell carcinoma (MCC).

Good prognosticators in MCC include the following:
- Presence of Merkel cell polyoma virus (MCPyV)
- Presence of intratumoral cytotoxic T lymphocytes
- High titers of anti-VP1
- Low Ki-67 index
- Low tumoral p63 labeling

123. **C.** Merkel cell polyoma virus (MCPyV) tumors are more common in tumors from non-sun-exposed sites.

While the incidence of MCPyV is higher in Merkel cell carcinoma (MCC) patients, it is found in the normal population, albeit at a lower incidence (80–90% versus 60–80%).

Features of MCPyV positive tumors in MCC are the following:
- More common in females
- Associated with lower stage and a better clinical course
- Have greater numbers of intratumoral and peritumoral CD8 positive lymphocytes
- Incidence greater in tumors from non-sun-exposed sites

- Exhibit less polymorphism and a lower Ki-67 index rate (consistent with their less sinister clinical course)

124. **C.** Image shown is that of an angiomyolipoma.

Defining histopathologic features are the presence of mature adipose tissue, smooth muscle and convoluted thick-walled blood vessels intimately related from each other.

Unlike the renal counterpart, the cutaneous variant lacks epithelioid cells, does not express HMB45 and is not associated with tuberous sclerosis.

125. **B.** Renal angiomyolipomas are associated with tuberous sclerosis.

Tuberous sclerosis (TS) is an autosomal dominant condition. While the principal genes involved are located in chromosomes 9q34 (*TSC1*) and 16p13 (*TSC2*), no identifiable mutations have been observed in up to 20% of affected patients. Over 95% of patients with tuberous sclerosis have skin lesions which occur in the form of *hypopigmented macules* (present at birth or appear in infancy, more than 5 highly suggestive of TS), *angiofibromas* (50% occur by the age of 3), *plaques representing connective tissue nevi* ("shagreen" patch, present in up to 40%) and/or *periungual papules* or nodules (Koenen's tumors, present in 20%).

126. **A.** Image shown is that of spindle cell lipoma.

Clinically, spindle cell lipoma presents as a subcutaneous nodule on the shoulders/back of middle-aged men. Defining histopathologic features of spindle cell lipoma are the presence of 2 distinct components, one composed of mature adipocytes and another composed of spindled fibroblasts.

127. **E.** Spindle cell lipomas can demonstrate partial loss of chromosome 16.

In terms of genetics, like pleomorphic lipoma, spindle cell lipomas demonstrate monosomy 16 or partial loss of 16q.

128. **D.** Spindled cells in spindle cell lipoma are CD34 positive.

The hematopoietic progenitor cell antigen CD34, also known as CD34 antigen, is a protein that in humans is encoded by the *CD34* gene. Cells expressing CD34 are normally found in the umbilical cord and bone marrow as hematopoietic cells, a subset of mesenchymal stem cells, endothelial progenitor cells, endothelial cells of blood vessels but not lymphatics (except pleural lymphatics), mast cells, a subpopulation of dendritic cells (which are factor XIIIa-negative) in the interstitium and around the adnexa of dermis of skin. The presence of CD34 on non-hematopoietic cells in various tissues has been linked to progenitor and adult stem cell phenotypes.

CD34 positive tumors include:

Fibroblastic/fibrohistiocytic/myofibroblastic – DFSP, giant cell fibroblastoma, solitary fibrous tumor, giant cell angiofibroma, nuchal-type fibroma, superficial angiomyxoma, superficial acral fibromyxoma, pericicatrical tissue, mammary-type extramammary myofibroblastoma

Vascular – Kaposi's sarcoma, angiosarcoma, epithelioid hemangioendothelioma, kaposiform hemangioendothelioma

Neural – Neurofibroma, perineuroma (more common in the sclerosing variant), solitary circumscribed neuroma

Adipocytic – Spindle cell lipoma

Follicular – Trichodiscoma, fibrofolliculoma, trichilemmoma

Also see Table E2.3

129. **E.** Image shown is that of a hibernoma.

Hibernoma is a benign tumor of subcutaneous and soft tissue that is believed to arise from brown fat. It occurs in young adults, mainly on the scapular area, axilla and lower neck and typically presents as a slow-growing "warm" nodule. Defining histopathologic features are encapsulated lobules composed of 3 cell types (large multivacuolated adipocytes with central nuclei, mature univacuolated adipocytes and smaller cells with granular eosinophilic cytoplasm) separated by thin septae. Translocations involving 11q13 are associated with hibernomas.

130. **D.** Cytogenetic abnormalities involving MDM2 are associated with well-differentiated liposarcoma.

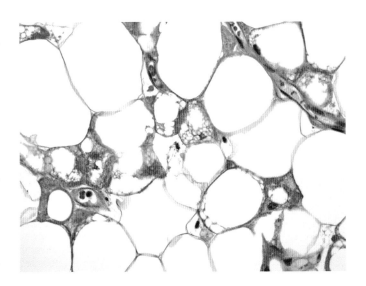

Liposarcoma is the most common soft tissue tumor (16–18% of all malignant sarcomas), has a predilection for the thighs and buttocks and middle-aged/elderly adults. It typically *does not* arise in a pre-existing lipoma, and rarely recurs or metastasizes. Defining histopathologic features are poor circumscription with infiltration of muscle/fascia/subcutaneous tissue, presence of lipoblasts (spindled/ovoid cells with characteristic sharply demarcated cytoplasmic vacuoles indenting the nucleus), variable cellularity, pleomorphism and mitoses (including the presence of atypical forms). Associated genetic abnormalities involve chr 12 with constant amplification of *MDM2* and frequently of *CDK4*. Myxoid liposarcoma is characterized by a *t*(12:16) translocation. Mouse double minute 2 homolog (MDM2), also known as E3 ubiquitin-protein ligase Mdm2, is a protein encoded by the *MDM2* gene. Mdm2 is an important negative regulator of the p53 tumor suppressor.

131.   A. Multiple angiofibromas (shown in the image) are typically associated with tuberous sclerosis.

   Mucocutaneous manifestations of tuberous sclerosis include facial angiofibromas ("adenoma sebaceum"), periungual fibromas (Koenen's tumors), hypomelanic macules ("ash leaf spots") and Shagreen patches. Other skin features not unique to tuberous sclerosis patients include molluscum fibrosum or skin tags, café-au-lait spots or flat brown marks, and poliosis (tuft or patch of white hair on the scalp or eyelids).
   Other syndromic associations of multiple angiofibromas include Wermer syndrome *or MEN1* characterized by multiple facial angiofibromas, collagenomas, lipomas, gingival papules, Confetti-like hypopigmented macules and café-au-lait macules.

132.   B. Image shown is that of an acral fibrokeratoma.

   Also known as acquired digital fibrokeratoma, this entity presents clinically as an asymptomatic solitary nodule/horn on the fingers/toes. Defining histopathologic features are a core of vertically oriented collagen bundles surrounded by irregular acanthosis.

133.   B. Multiple sclerotic fibromas (shown in the image) are associated with Cowden's disease (CD).

   Other cutaneous manifestations of CD include multiple trichilemmomas, palmar pits, mucocutaneous papillomatous papules, acral keratosis and tumors of the follicular infundibulum. CD is an autosomal dominant disease associated with a mutation in the *PTEN* gene on arm 10*q*. In addition to cutaneous manifestations, visceral malignancies involving multiple organ systems (breast, endometrium, thyroid and lower GIT) are also noted in CD.

134.   E. Lesional cells in sclerotic fibroma are typically CD34 positive.

   Although considered to be a variant of dermatofibroma, lesional cells in sclerotic fibroma are consistently positive for CD34 (unlike dermatofibroma). Defining histopathologic features of sclerotic fibroma include well-circumscribed, non-encapsulated dermal nodule with thick sclerotic collagen bundles arranged as short intersecting stacks ("plywood-like").

135.   D. Image shown is that of nodular fasciitis.

   Nodular fasciitis clinically presents as a rapidly growing nodule, that can be painful and more commonly occurs on the upper extremities and the head and neck area. Defining histopathologic features are a subcutaneous nodule composed of a cellular proliferation of plump as well as stellate fibroblasts and myofibroblasts in a loose myxoid stroma ("tissue culture" appearance) with admixed inflammatory cells and extravasated erythrocytes. Mitotic activity is common. Genetic abnormalities observed include *USP6* rearrangements on chr 17 or a *MYH9-USP6* fusion.

136.   C. The best-fit diagnosis for the image shown is solitary fibrous tumor (SFT).

   SFT clinically presents as a slow-growing painless mass with a predilection for the head and neck area. The defining histopathologic features are alternating hypocellular and hypercellular areas of spindled cells ("patternless pattern"), hyalinized collagen, prominent "staghorn" vessels and minimal cytologic atypia.

137.   D. Lesional cells in solitary fibrous tumor (SFT) are, typically, diffusely and strongly positive for CD34.

   Other immunohistochemical markers that lesional cells in SFT are positive for include STAT6 (nuclear staining and a reliable surrogate for detection of the fusion gene), CD99 and Bcl-2.

138.   C. The *STAT6* gene is altered in solitary fibrous tumor (SFT).

   STAT6 is a member of the STAT family of cytoplasmic transcription factors, which regulate gene expression by transmitting signals to the nucleus and binding to specific DNA promoter sequences. STAT signaling is critical for normal cellular processes such as embryonic development, innate and adaptive immune function, and regulation of cell differentiation, growth, and apoptosis. *NAB2-STAT6* gene fusions have been identified in the vast majority of SFTs. These genes are located close together on chromosome 12 and are transcribed in opposite directions. The fusion product results from an inversion at the 12*q*13 locus, which fuses *NAB2* and *STAT6*.

139. **B.** The best-fit diagnosis for the image shown is fibrous hamartoma of infancy.

    This typically occurs in children <2 years of age, is more common in males and clinically presents as a solitary, painless nodule on the upper extremities, axilla and back. Defining histopathologic features are the triphasic histology: fascicles of fibroblasts and myofibroblasts, immature loose basophilic and myxoid mesenchymal tissue and mature adipose tissue.

140. **A.** The best-fit diagnosis for the image shown is digital fibromatosis.

    Digital fibromatosis presents at birth or develops in the first year of life as multiple, painless, flesh-colored, indurated nodules on the dorsolateral aspects of the fingers and toes. Defining histopathologic features are a proliferation of spindled myofibroblasts arranged in whorls, sheets or interlacing fascicles perpendicular to the skin. The cells have wavy nuclei, no atypia and contain the pathognomonic eosinophilic paranuclear inclusion bodies. The inclusion bodies are immunohistochemically positive for actin.

141. **E.** The best-fit diagnosis for the image shown is angiomyofibroblastoma.

    Angiomyofibroblastomas typically occur in the vulva. Key histopathologic features are a well-demarcated tumor with a prominent vascular component, an edematous stroma and plump to spindled cells in clusters around vessels.

142. **D.** The best-fit diagnosis for the image shown is dermatomyofibroma (DMF).

    Clinically, DMF presents as an asymptomatic, well-circumscribed plaque on the shoulders/axilla/upper arms/neck areas of young women. Defining histopathologic features are a plaque-like fasciculated (with the fascicles arranged parallel to the epidermis) proliferation of monomorphic spindled cells in the reticular dermis with adnexal sparing. Lesional cells are variably immunohistochemically positive for SMA, MSA and CD34.

143. **E.** The best-fit diagnosis for the image shown is infantile myofibromatosis.

    Clinically, these present at/soon after birth, have a predilection for males, are more common in the head and neck area/extremities and trunk and are firm to rubbery, purplish dermal nodules. Multicentric involvement is not uncommon. Defining histopathologic features are a biphasic architecture with central immature-appearing short spindled cells associated with thin-walled, branching vessels and peripheral mature, spindled myofibroblasts with abundant eosinophilic cytoplasm.

Mitosis is not uncommon in the immature areas and calcification and hyalinization can be seen in older lesions. Lesional cells are SMA and vimentin positive.

144. **C.** The best-fit diagnosis for the image shown is that of myopericytoma.

    The term perivascular myoma is the term proposed for proliferations of myoid cells exhibiting a perivascular distribution. These are slightly more common in males and are typically solitary lesions. Defining histopathologic features are a well-circumscribed lesion with a vasoformative element composed of thin-walled blood vessels with a perivascular and concentric growth of myoid cells. Lesional myoid cells are positive for MSA and caldesmon.

145. **B.** Given the immunohistochemical profile, the best-fit diagnosis for the image shown is that of a PEComa.

    PEComa is the name given to a tumor composed of histologically and immunohistochemically distinctive *perivascular epithelioid cells*. This cell type is also seen in the following:
    - Angiomyolipoma
    - Clear cell "sugar" tumor of the lungs
    - Lymphangioleiomyomatosis
    - Clear cell myelomonocytic tumor of the falciform ligament and skin

    Defining histopathologic features are a vasculocentric proliferation of neoplastic cells with epithelioid cytomorphology and admixed multinucleate giant cells. Key features of the malignant counterpart are size (>5 cm), cytologic atypia, mitotic activity (with >1/50 HPFs and abnormal mitotic forms) and necrosis. Immunohistochemically, lesional cells are positive for HMB45, MITF and/or MelanA as well as SMA, MSA and/or desmin. They may also be positive for transcription factor E3 (TFE3). PEComas can occur in association with tuberous sclerosis – when they do, losses related to *TSC1* or *TSC2* can be seen.

146. **A.** Given the immunohistochemical profile, the best-fit diagnosis for the image shown is that of inflammatory myofibroblastic tumor.

    These typically occur in young patients and can occur in various sites (lung, abdomen, mediastinum, soft tissues and head and neck). Defining histopathologic features are the presence of polygonal myofibroblasts and a mixed inflammatory cell infiltrate composed of plasma cells, lymphocytes and eosinophils. Lesional myofibroblasts are vimentin, SMA and ALK-1 positive. In terms of genetics, they can exhibit *ALK* gene rearrangements on chr 2p23 or gene translocation to chr 2q33–q35.

147. **E.** The best-fit diagnosis for the image shown is myxoinflammatory fibroblastic sarcoma.

Myxoinflammatory fibroblastic sarcoma is considered by some to be a variant of hemosiderotic fibrohistiocytic lipomatous lesion and typically occurs in acral sites. These have a high incidence of $t(1:10)$ translocations. Defining histopathologic features are a fasciculated proliferation of spindled and epithelioid cells embedded in a myxoid to hyalinized stroma, an inflammatory cell infiltrate composed of lymphocytes and plasma cells and coalescing foci of necrosis. The epithelioid cells can exhibit bizarre cytomorphology with macronucleoli (reminiscent of Reed-Sternberg cells).

148. **D.** The best-fit diagnosis for the image shown is that of a dermatofibroma.

These typically occur on the extremities. Gentle compression of the lesion results in the classic "dimple" sign. Defining histopathologic features are a dermal proliferation of spindled cells arranged in short interlacing fascicles with collagen entrapment and clusters of lymphocytes present at the deep margin (junction of deep dermis and subcutis). Epidermal changes that are lentigo-like, a grenz zone and follicular induction phenomenon can be seen in most cases. Lesional cells are FXIIIa and SMA positive (both entirely non-specific though).

149. **C.** The best-fit diagnosis for the image shown is that of an epithelioid cell histiocytoma.

Considered to be a variant of dermatofibroma, these occur most commonly on the lower extremities. Defining histopathologic features are a well-demarcated, dome-shaped polypoid dermal nodule with a surrounding collarette composed of polygonal or epithelioid cells with abundant cytoplasm and oval nuclei.

Other lesions that typically have a collarette include:
- Pyogenic granuloma
- Juvenile xanthogranuloma
- Atypical fibroxanthoma
- Cutaneous epithelioid angiomatous nodule
- Bacillary angiomatosis

150. **B.** Plantar fibromatosis is a synonym for Ledderhose disease.

Fibromatoses present as firm nodules or plaques along flexor tendons in different parts of the body, each with a distinct name but identical histopathologic features.

Dupuytren's contracture: Palmar fibromatosis, occurs long the volar surface
Ledderhose disease: Plantar fibromatosis, affecting the aponeurosis
Peyronnie's disease: Penile fibromatosis

Desmoid tumor: Deep musculoaponeurotic fibromatosis, most common in the abdomen, association with Gardner syndrome

Defining histopathologic features of all fibromatoses are a fasciculated proliferation of uniform spindled cells (with normochromatic nuclei) in a collagenous stroma.

151. **C.** Lesional cells in all fibromatoses exhibit nuclear positivity for β-catenin.

Additionally, immunohistochemical positivity of lesional cells is noted for SMA and MSA. Beta catenin mutations (*CTNNB1*) are common in all fibromatoses. Desmoid tumors are associated with mutations in the *APC* gene.

152. **A.** Desmoid tumors may be seen in association with Gardner syndrome.

Gardner syndrome is genetically linked to band $5q21$, the adenomatous polyposis coli locus. The *APC* gene located on chromosome 5 is the first mutation in the adenoma-to-carcinoma sequence and is believed to initiate the sequence. Other cutaneous manifestations of Gardner syndrome include fibromas, lipomas (may be visceral, including intracranial), leiomyomas, neurofibromas and multifocal pigmented lesions of the fundus (seen in 80% of patients, may present shortly after birth and can be the first marker of disease).

153. **E.** The best-fit diagnosis for the image shown is plexiform fibrohistiocytoma.

These clinically present as a slow-growing firm nodule or plaque on the wrists and hands and have a predilection for younger patients with a female predominance. Defining histopathologic features are a multinodular proliferation in the dermis or subcutis with nodules of histiocytes with admixed osteoclast-like giant cells and intersecting fascicles of fibroblast-like spindled cells.

154. **D.** The best-fit diagnosis for the image shown is that of a giant cell fibroblastoma (GCF).

Defining histopathologic features of giant cell fibroblastoma are a proliferation of bland, spindled cells with admixed multinucleate giant cells (MNGCs) and irregular pseudovascular spaces also lined by MNGCs.

155. **C.** Giant cell fibroblastoma is believed to represent the pediatric counterpart of dermatofibrosarcoma protuberans (DFSP).

Believed to represent the pediatric counterpart of dermatofibrosarcoma protuberans, giant cell fibroblastoma occurs in early childhood with a predilection for boys. Lesional cells, like those of DFSP, are typically CD34 positive.

156. **E.** Giant cell fibroblastoma, like dermatofibrosarcoma protuberans, is associated with the *t*(17:22) translocation.

157. **C.** The best-fit diagnosis for the image shown is dermatofibrosarcoma protuberans.

     Dermatofibrosarcoma protuberans (DFSP) clinically presents as a slow-growing asymptomatic plaque that can progress to nodules. Defining histopathologic features are a bland fasciculated proliferation in a cartwheel/storiform/whorled arrangement composed of fusiform cells with elongate nuclei. Infiltration of the subcutis is common and has a multilayered pattern in early lesions and a lace-like pattern in older lesions. Lesional cells are typically CD34 positive.

158. **E.** Dermatofibrosarcoma protuberans (DFSP) is associated with the *t*(17:22) translocation.

     DFSP can also exhibit supernumerary ring chromosomes with material from chromosomes *17q*22 and *22q*. The result is the fusion of the *COL1A1* gene (located on chr 17) with *PDGFB* (on chr 22).

159. **D.** The best-fit diagnosis for the image shown is that of an atypical fibroxanthoma (AFX).

     More common in elderly males on sun-exposed sites, AFX clinically presents as an exophytic nodule with a collarette. Defining histopathologic features are a dermal proliferation of markedly atypical, pleomorphic spindled and epithelioid cells arranged in fascicles or sheets with a peripheral collarette. Numerous mitoses including atypical forms are frequent. Lesional cells have no distinct or defining immunohistochemical profile but can be variably positive for vimentin, CD99, CD68 and CD10 (all entirely non-specific though). In terms of genetics, AFX exhibits UV-induced p53 mutations.

160. **C.** The best-fit diagnosis for the image shown is that of angiomatoid fibrous histiocytoma (AFH).

     Typically located on the extremities and lymph node sites and, presenting in young adults and children, defining histopathologic features of AFH are a syncytial growth of histiocyte-like tumor cells in nodules, blood-filled pseudovascular spaces, a fibrous pseudocapsule with hemosiderin deposits and perivascular lymphoplasmacytic infiltrate with germinal centers. Lesional cells have no distinct or defining immunohistochemical profile but can be variably positive for CD68, desmin and EMA. These lesions express the *EWSR1-CREB1* fusion from the *t*(2:22) translocation.

161. **D.** The best-fit diagnosis for the image shown is that of an epithelioid sarcoma.

     More common in young adults with a male preponderance, epithelioid sarcomas are most commonly located on the distal extremities, especially on the hands and fingers (around aponeurosis). Defining histopathologic features are a nodular proliferation of markedly atypical epithelioid cells surrounding coalescing foci of necrosis. These lesions can have a "garland" appearance due to growth along tendons. Lesional cells have a distinct immunohistochemical profile and are positive for EMA, vimentin, CK-LMW and CD34 (only in 50% of cases). Genetically, there is deletion of *SMARCB1* on chr 22*q*11.

162. **E.** The best-fit diagnosis for the image shown is that of synovial sarcoma.

     Presenting typically in patients under the age of 50, synovial sarcoma is more commonly located on the lower and upper extremities in a juxta-articular location. Defining histopathologic features are the presence of distinct populations of cells: one that is epithelioid and another that is spindled (arranged in sheets or fascicles) with admixed "staghorn" vessels. Lesional cells are immunohistochemically positive for EMA, TLE1 and CD99. In terms of genetics, these lesions display *t*(X;18) resulting in fusion of *SYT* with one of the *SSX* genes.

163. **C.** The best-fit diagnosis for the image shown is that of giant cell tumor (GCT) of tendon sheath.

     Clinically presenting as a painless, slow-growing, firm mass on the extremities with a female predominance, the defining histopathologic features of GCT are a lobular tumor (often attached to the tendon sheath) composed of a variable mixture of epithelioid cells with vesicular nuclei, and multinucleate giant cells (MNGCs) with admixed deposits of hemosiderin. Immunohistochemically, MNGCs are CD68 and CD45 positive. In terms of genetics, these lesions can exhibit the *1p*11–13 translocation.

164. **C.** The best-fit diagnosis for the image shown is superficial acral fibromyxoma (SAF).

     More commonly presenting in males in the subungual or periungual areas, defining histopathologic features of SAF are a non-encapsulated dermal proliferation of spindled and stellate cells in a storiform pattern embedded in a myxoid stroma with admixed vessels. Lesional cells are immunohistochemically positive for CD34, CD99 and vimentin but ApoD negative.

165. **E.** The best-fit diagnosis for the image shown is that of superficial angiomyxoma.

     More common in the head and neck, defining histopathologic features are a multilobulated, poorly circumscribed myxoid mass with a prominent vascular component and admixed neutrophils. Up to a third can have an epithelial component in the form of a keratocyst.

The deep variant is more common in the vulvovaginal area.

166. **D.** Superficial angiomyxomas may present as a component of NAME syndrome.

Carney complex and its subsets LAMB syndrome and NAME syndrome are autosomal dominant conditions comprising myxomas of the heart and skin, hyperpigmentation of the skin (lentiginosis), and endocrine overactivity. The LAMB acronym refers to *l*entigines, *a*trial *m*yxomas, and *b*lue nevi. NAME refers to *n*evi, *a*trial myxoma, *m*yxoid neurofibromas, and *e*phelides. Testicular cancer, particularly Sertoli cell type, is associated with Carney syndrome. In some patients with cardiac myxoma(s), the cutaneous tumor(s) is often detected prior to diagnosis of the cardiac neoplasm and thus serves as an important marker.

167. **B.** Metachronous metastases refers to cutaneous metastases developing years after a visceral malignancy.

Cutaneous metastasis that occurs at the same time as the visceral malignancy is *synchronous metastasis*.

Cutaneous metastasis that is the first indication of a visceral malignancy is *precocious metastasis*.

168. **A.** Given the immunohistochemical profile, the best-fit diagnosis for the image shown is a renal metastasis.

Renal metastases are typically positive for vimentin, CK AE1/3, EMA, CD10 (80–90%), PAX-8 (80–90%), RCC (67%) and adipophilin (63%). Also see Table H7.

169. **E.** Given the immunohistochemical profile, the best-fit diagnosis for the image shown is a colon metastasis.

Colonic metastases are typically positive for CK20, mucin, CEA and CDX2. Also see Table H7.

170. **A.** Given the immunohistochemical profile, the best-fit diagnosis for the image shown is Paget's disease.

In terms of Immunohistochemical profile:

Extramammary Paget's disease – Positive for MUC1, MUC5AC

Paget's disease – Positive for CK7, MUC1

Also see Table H7.

171. **C.** The best-fit diagnosis for the image shown is papillary thyroid carcinoma.

Thyroid metastases are typically positive for thyroglobulin and PAX-8 (medullary thyroid carcinomas are negative for this though). Cancers that have psammoma bodies (concentric, laminated, calcified spheres) are the following (remembered by the mnemonic *PSSaMM*oma):
- *P*apillary carcinoma of the thyroid *p*rolactinoma

- *S*erous cystadenocarcinoma of the ovary
- *S*omatostatinoma
- *M*eningioma
- *M*esothelioma

Also see Table H7.

172. **B.** The best-fit diagnosis for the image shown is that of cutaneous oncocytoma.

With a predilection for the lacrimal area or salivary glands, defining histopathologic features of oncocytomas are a circumscribed neoplasm with solid and cystic spaces and distinctive cytomorphology of lesional cells (polygonal cells with eosinophilic finely granular cytoplasm, open nuclear chromatin and centrally located nucleoli).

173. **A.** Sturge-Weber syndrome is associated with a capillary malformation.

Sturge-Weber syndrome (SWS), also called encephalotrigeminal angiomatosis, is a neurocutaneous disorder with angiomas that involve the leptomeninges and the skin of the face, typically in the ophthalmic (V1) and maxillary (V2) distributions of the trigeminal nerve. The hallmark of SWS is a facial cutaneous venous dilation, also referred to as a nevus flammeus or port-wine stain (PWS). Histopathologic findings of PWS include dilated, thin-walled vessels in the superficial vascular plexus, but no definite increase in the number of blood vessels.

174. **E.** The best-fit diagnosis for the image shown is glomulovenous malformation.

A term used in the past to describe glomangioma, more recent data indicate that glomangiomas are vascular malformation of venous origin that are often present at birth with a predilection for the extremities. Defining histopathologic features are poorly circumscribed lesion in the dermis composed of ectatic thin-walled venous channels lined by flat endothelial cells and perivascular glomus cells. Lesional glomus cells are immunohistochemically positive for SMA, MSA, vimentin and type IV collagen. Genetically, these are associated with loss of function mutations in *glomulin* (on chr 1*p*21–*p*11).

175. **D.** The best-fit diagnosis for the image shown is lymphangioma circumscriptum.

Also known as superficial lymphatic malformation or superficial microcystic lymphatic malformation, these typically present in early infancy on the axillae, shoulders, proximal extremities and the tongue. Defining histopathologic features are dilated, thin-walled lymphatic vessels in the papillary dermis.

Syndromic associations are the following:

Cobb syndrome – Congenital cutaneous vascular lesions distributed in a dermatomal pattern with associated spinal angiomas or arteriovenous malformations

Proteus syndrome – Vascular malformations, lipomas, hyperpigmentation, and several types of nevi

Mafucci syndrome – Benign enlargements of cartilage (enchondromas), bone deformities, and dark, irregularly shaped hemangiomas

176. **B.** The best-fit diagnosis for the image shown is that of a venous lake.

Commonly occurring in the head and neck areas in the elderly, defining histopathologic features are the presence of a single dilated vascular channel in the superficial dermis.

177. **A.** Peyronie's disease is NOT a clinical subtype of angiokeratoma (shown in the image).

Angiokeratoma has 5 main clinical subtypes:

Angiokeratoma circumscriptum neviformis – On the lower extremity and the trunk, associated with Cobb and Klippel-Trénaunay syndromes

Angiokeratoma corporis diffusum – "Bathing-trunk" distribution, associated with Anderson-Fabry disease and other inherited lysosomal storage diseases

Fordyce type – On the genitalia, associated with varicoceles, inguinal hernias, oral contraceptives and pregnancy

Mibelli type – On acral sites, associated with perniosis and acrocyanosis

Solitary and multiple types – Any site, may be zosteriform

178. **E.** The best-fit diagnosis for the image shown is cutaneous collagenous vasculopathy.

Cutaneous collagenous vasculopathy, a relatively rare microangiopathy of superficial dermal blood vessels, clinically presents as telangiectatic macules, predominantly on the extremities. Defining histopathologic features are scattered capillary-sized vessels in the superficial dermis with perivascular hyalinization (secondary to reduplication of the basement membrane). The amorphous pink material is periodic acid-Schiff-positive and resistant to diastase.

179. **D.** Infantile hemangiomas express GLUT-1.

Glucose transporter protein 1 isoform or GLUT-1 is an erythrocyte-type facilitative glucose protein present in normal endothelium of the microvasculature of the blood-brain barrier. It is expressed by infantile hemangiomas consistently (through all phases of proliferation and involution) and has a cytoplasmic staining pattern.

180. **C.** Glomeruloid hemangioma is a specific marker for POEMS.

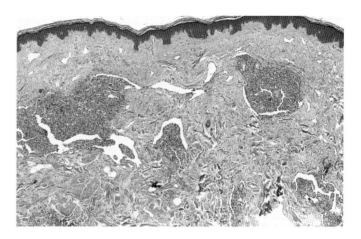

Other hemangiomas that occur in POEMS (an acronym for *p*olyneuropathy, *o*rganomegaly, *e*ndocrinopathy, *m*onoclonal gammopathy and *s*kin disease) include microvenular hemangiomas and cherry hemangiomas. Multinucleate angiohistocytomas may also be seen in POEMS. Defining histopathologic features of glomeruloid hemangiomas are multifocality and aggregates of dilated, thin-walled vessels with intravascular capillary aggregates (simulating renal glomeruli). Stromal cells, present between intravascular capillaries, have eosinophilic cytoplasm as well as intracytoplasmic vacuoles with PAS+ diastase resistant globules.

181. **B.** The best-fit diagnosis for the image shown is that of microvenular hemangioma.

Initially called micropapillary hemangioma, this entity is more common on the extremities and may be associated with POEMS and Wiskott-Aldrich syndrome. Defining histopathologic features are an ill-circumscribed, superficial and deep, proliferation of monomorphic small blood vessels. Immunohistochemically, they express WT1 but not GLUT-1 or D2–40.

182. **A.** Image shown is that of hobnail hemangioma, originally called targetoid hemosiderotic hemangioma.

Initially called targetoid hemosiderotic hemangioma based on the clinical spectrum, the consistent presence of the diagnostic hobnail cytomorphology led to the new nomenclature. More common in males with a predilection for the trunk and limbs, defining histopathologic features are a wedge-shaped dermal lesion with a biphasic growth pattern (dilated vessels superficially, dissecting "pseudo-angiosarcomatous" vessels deep), extravasated erythrocytes and variable hemosiderin deposition.

183. **B.** Image shown is that of cutaneous epithelioid angiomatous nodule (CEAN), part of the spectrum of epithelioid hemangioma (angiolymphoid hyperplasia with eosinophilia).

CEAN typically presents as a solitary nodule on the trunk or extremities. Defining histopathologic features are a well-circumscribed exophytic lesion with a collarette, solid sheets of closely packed vascular channels lined by plump, epithelioid cells with intracytoplasmic vacuoles, admixed eosinophils and a patchy, peripheral lymphoplasmacytic host response.

184. **B.** The best-fit diagnosis for the image shown is that of epithelioid hemangioma (angiolymphoid hyperplasia with eosinophilia, ALHE).

Now considered to be distinct from Kimura's disease, ALHE is more common in females and typically occurs as a solitary or multiple papulonodule in the head and neck region. Defining histopathologic features are a well-circumscribed vasoformative lesion composed of thick- and thin-walled vessels lined by plump, epithelioid cells with intracytoplasmic vacuoles and admixed eosinophils.

185. **D.** The best-fit diagnosis for the image shown is that of acquired elastotic hemangioma.

More common in the elderly on sun-damaged skin, defining histopathologic features of acquired elastotic hemangioma are an increased number of capillary vessels arranged in a band-like pattern parallel to the epidermis with a grenz zone.

186. **D.** The best-fit diagnosis for the image shown is that of an arteriovenous hemangioma.

Also known as cirsoid aneurysm, this is more common in the elderly in the head and neck region. Defining histopathologic features are a circumscribed lesion composed of thick- and thin-walled vessels reminiscent of arteries and veins. Majority of the vessels do not show an internal elastic lamina (venous component likely predominates).

187. **E.** The best-fit diagnosis for the image shown is that of a tufted angioma.

Believed by some to represent a variant of kaposiform hemangioendothelioma, tufted angioma is more common in children and has a predilection for the trunk and the abdomen. Defining histopathologic features are a "cannon-ball" distribution of multiple well-defined vascular "tufts" composed of capillaries with poorly defined lumen, bland endothelial cells and pericytes.

188. **D.** Image shown is that of a glomus tumor, lesional cells of which are typically actin positive.

Other immunohistochemical markers that would be positive include vimentin and type IV collagen. Defining histopathologic features of a glomus tumor are perivascular solid cellular aggregates of monomorphic glomus cells.

189. **C.** Image shown is that of a glomangiomyoma.

Defining histopathologic features are the transition from glomus to spindled smooth muscle cells.

190. **B.** The best-fit diagnosis for the image shown is diffuse dermal angiomatosis.

Believed to represent a variant of reactive angioendotheliomatosis and associated with select systemic diseases such as severe atherosclerotic disease, and immunosuppression, diffuse dermal angiomatosis is characterized by an increased number of dermal capillaries and a proliferation of extravascular endothelial cells.

191. **A.** The best-fit diagnosis for the image shown is that of acroangiodermatitis or pseudo-Kaposi's sarcoma.

More common on the lower extremities, acroangiodermatitis (of Mali) is characterized by superficial congeries of capillary-sized, thick-walled vessels, extravasated erythrocytes, dermal fibrosis and variable hemosiderin deposition.

192. **D.** Intravascular papillary endothelial hyperplasia (IPEH) shown in the image is best regarded as an organizing thrombus.

Also known as Masson's hemangioma/pseudoangiosarcoma, IPEH is a histopathologic reaction pattern developing in response to an organizing thrombus. It occurs in 3 main settings: primary/pure (within a vein), secondary/mixed (focal change in vascular anomalies) and a third/rare form (extravascular, arising within a hematoma). Histopathologic features are intravascular papillary projections lined by a single layer of endothelial cells with a hyalinized core.

193. **C.** The best-fit diagnosis for the image shown is bacillary angiomatosis.

Bacillary angiomatosis clinically presents as a polypoidal lesion. Defining histopathologic features are presence of an epidermal collarette, lobular capillary proliferation, prominent neutrophil-rich stroma and variably sized deposits of granular purple material (representing the organism).

194. **B.** The causative organism of bacillary angiomatosis is *Bartonella quintana*.

It can also be caused by *Bartonella henselae*. At least eight *Bartonella* species or subspecies are known to infect humans.

The best known ones are the following:

B. bacilliformis – Carrion's fever (Oroya fever, verruca peruana)

B. quintana – Trench fever, bacillary angiomatosis, endocarditis

B. clarridgeiae – Cat scratch disease

B. henselae – Cat scratch disease, bacillary angiomatosis, peliosis hepatitis, endocarditis, bacteremia with fever, neuroretinitis

195. **A. Epithelioid hemangioendothelioma is a high-grade vascular malignancy.**

Other *high-grade* vascular malignancies include:
- Primary cutaneous angiosarcoma
- Glomangiosarcoma (malignant glomus tumor)

Intermediate grade vascular malignancies include:
- Composite hemangioendothelioma
- Kaposiform hemangioendothelioma
- Retiform hemangioendothelioma
- Kaposi's sarcoma
- Papillary intralymphatic angioendothelioma (Dabska's tumor)

196. **E. Positive nuclear immunohistochemical staining with HHV8 clinches the diagnosis of Kaposi's sarcoma.**

Kaposi's sarcoma (KS) occurs in 4 main clinical settings:

Classic (endemic) KS – Middle-aged/elderly, Jewish Ashkenazic/Mediterranean, lower extremities, indolent behavior

AIDS-related KS – Homosexual men/IV drug users, disseminated lesions, aggressive clinical course

Immunosuppression-related/iatrogenic KS – Localized lesions, variable biologic course

African KS – Middle-aged/children, multiple localized tumors, lower extremities/lymph nodes, aggressive biologic behavior

Defining histopathologic features evident in all clinical types include a poorly circumscribed vasoformative lesion with irregular thin-walled vascular channels, spindled cell proliferation, promontory sign, extravasated erythrocytes and a lymphoplasmacytic host response. Three distinct stages have been described although they likely form a morphologic spectrum and often overlap:

Patch stage – Histopathologic findings are subtle

Plaque stage – Spindled cell proliferation becomes apparent

Nodular stage – Fasciculated spindled cell proliferation plus all of the typical features described above

197. **C. Kasabach-Merritt syndrome (KMS) is associated with kaposiform hemangioendothelioma.**

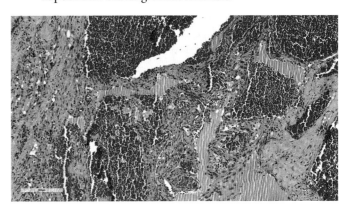

The combination of an enlarging vascular lesion (either a kaposiform hemangioendothelioma or a tufted angioma), profound thrombocytopenia, microangiopathic hemolytic anemia, and consumptive coagulopathy is termed KMS or Kasabach-Merritt phenomenon (KMP).

Defining histopathologic features of kaposiform hemangioendothelioma are a poorly circumscribed, biphasic multinodular lesion of vascular (small capillaries) and solid cellular areas (endothelial cells in a glomeruloid pattern and spindled cells in fascicles).

198. **E. Dabska's tumor is a synonym for endovascular papillary angioendothelioma.**

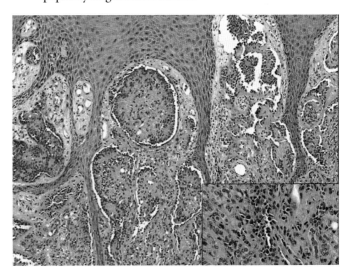

Mainly occurring in childhood, in the head and neck areas, Dabska's tumor is a low-grade vasoformative lesion. Defining histopathologic features are an ill-circumscribed proliferation of interconnecting vascular channels with vascular spaces of varying morphology, papillary tufts with central PAS+ hyaline cores within vascular spaces and intravascular and extravascular lymphoid aggregates.

199. **D.** The best-fit diagnosis for the image shown is that of an angiosarcoma (AS).

Clinically, 5 different variants of AS have been recognized:

Idiopathic AS – Elderly, males, head and neck areas, multifocal

Radiation-induced AS – Variable interval between radiation and development of AS, chest/lower abdomen

Lymphedema-associated AS/Stewart-Treves syndrome – Elderly, females, arm, rapidly progressive

Primary cutaneous AS – Adults, limbs

Pediatric cutaneous AS – Females, lower extremities, association with pre-existing conditions

Unifying histopathologic features evident in all variants are an ill-circumscribed vasoformative lesion composed of irregular, dissecting, anastomosing vascular channels lined by multiple layers of markedly atypical endothelial cells.

200. **C.** Positive *MYC* expression in post-irradiation angiosarcoma helps differentiate it from an atypical vascular lesion (in which it is negative).

Presence of *MYC* amplification represents an important additional diagnostic tool in the distinction of post-radiation cutaneous angiosarcomas from atypical vascular lesions after radiotherapy. Immunohistochemical staining for *MYC* is useful for mapping of these lesions and for careful tumor margin control.

The *MYC* oncogene, a transcription factor that is well known for its role in cell proliferation, cellular differentiation, and apoptosis, is also known to stimulate angiogenesis and may promote invasion and metastasis. In soft tissue sarcomas, *MYC* overexpression and increased *MYC* copy numbers are frequent in high-grade chondrosarcomas, epithelioid sarcomas of the proximal type, in higher-grade myxoid liposarcomas, and have an adverse prognostic impact in leiomyosarcomas of soft tissues.

201. **B.** The best-fit diagnosis for the image shown is that of Wells's syndrome.

Wells's syndrome or eosinophilic cellulitis is an uncommon condition of unknown etiology. The presentation usually involves a mildly pruritic or tender cellulitis-like eruption. Defining, albeit not specific, features include edema, flame figures (eosinophil debris as a consequence of degranulating eosinophils) between collagen bundles, and a marked pandermal infiltrate of eosinophils in the dermis. During the acute early phase, the dense infiltrate of degranulating eosinophils is usually located in the epidermis and the dermis, although it occasionally extends into the subcutaneous tissue and the underlying muscle. Of note, although the histopathologic findings of eosinophilia, histiocytes, and flame figures are characteristic of Wells's syndrome, they are also found in other conditions, including bullous pemphigoid, eczema, tinea infection, dermatitis herpetiformis, scabies, and insect bites.

202. **A.** NAME syndrome is NOT associated with paraproteinemia.

Entities associated with paraproteinemia include the following:
- Cutaneous plasmacytoma
- Hyperviscosity syndrome
- Cryoglobulinemia
- Amyloidosis
- POEMS syndrome
- Scleromyexedema/lichen myxedematosus/papular mucinosis
- Scleredema
- Plane xanthomas
- Necrobiotic xanthogranuloma
- Schnitzler syndrome
- Erythema elevatum diutinum
- Subcorneal pustular dermatosis

Also see Table D2.3

203. **E.** The best-fit diagnosis for the image shown is plasmacytosis mucosae.

Previously known as Zoon's balanitis, most frequently involving the glans penis/prepuce, it can also involve the vulva (Zoon's vulvitis) and the oral mucosa. Defining histopathologic features include an attenuated epidermis with "lozenge-shaped" or "diamond-shaped" keratinocytes and a predominantly polyclonal plasma cell-rich infiltrate with admixed neutrophils.

204. **D.** The best-fit diagnosis for the image shown is urticaria pigmentosa (UP).

UP is the most frequent form of cutaneous mastocytosis and affects children and adults. Defining histopathologic features are aggregates of perivascular and periadnexal mast cells. Lesional mast cells are positive for tryptase and CD117. In terms of genetics, *KIT* point mutations in codon 816 may be found.

205. **C.** Mast cells in urticaria pigmentosa are typically CD117 positive.

Mast/stem cell growth factor receptor (SCFR), also known as proto-oncogene c-Kit or tyrosine-protein kinase Kit or CD117, is a receptor tyrosine kinase protein that in humans is encoded by the *KIT* gene. CD117 is a receptor tyrosine kinase type III, which binds to stem cell factor (a substance that causes certain types of cells to grow), also known as "steel factor" or "c-kit ligand." When this receptor binds to stem cell factor (SCF) it forms a dimer that activates its intrinsic tyrosine kinase activity, that in turn phosphorylates and activates signal transduction molecules that propagate the signal in the cell. Signaling through CD117 plays a role in cell survival, proliferation, and differentiation.

206. **B.** The best-fit diagnosis for the image shown is that of juvenile xanthogranuloma (JXG).

Juvenile xanthogranuloma (JXG) is a self-limited dermatologic disorder that mainly affects infants and small children. Clinically, lesions may be single or multiple and appear as firm, slightly raised papulonodules, tan-orange in color and frequently on the head and neck area. The eye, particularly the uveal tract, is the most frequent site of extracutaneous involvement and approximately 50% of patients with ocular involvement have skin lesions. JXG is the most frequent cause of spontaneous hyphema in children and can result in secondary glaucoma and eventual blindness. Defining histopathologic features are an exophytic polymorphic lesion with a collarette composed of lymphocytes, foamy histiocytes and Touton giant cells. Lesional histiocytes are CD68 and fascin positive but S100 and CD1a negative. In JXG patients with neurofibromatosis I, mutations in the *NF* gene are observed.

207. **D.** The best-fit diagnosis for the image shown is that of a reticulohistiocytoma (RH).

Typically presenting as a reddish/brown, multinodular papulonodular eruption in middle-aged women, defining histopathologic features of RH are a dermal histiocyte-rich infiltrate with admixed multinucleate giant cells that have eosinophilic cytoplasm and an oncocytoid "ground-glass" appearance.

208. **A.** Multicentric reticulohistiocytosis is associated with a destructive arthropathy.

209. **D.** The best-fit diagnosis for the image shown is that of necrobiotic xanthogranuloma (NXG).

Necrobiotic xanthogranuloma (NXG) is characterized by firm yellow plaques and nodules, often occurring in a periorbital distribution. The histopathologic features of NXG are distinct and are characterized by broad zones of necrobiosis alternating with granulomatous foci (that can extend into the subcutaneous tissue). The giant cells are of both Touton and foreign body type. Asteroid bodies and other inclusions may sometimes be present. The amount of xanthomatization is quite variable. Cholesterol clefts may be evident. Nodular lymphoid aggregates are often reported in association with the granulomas.

210. **E.** Necrobiotic xanthogranuloma (NXG) is often associated with a paraproteinemia.

NXG is often accompanied by a monoclonal gammopathy of the immunoglobulin G-kappa (IgG-κ) type.

For other entities associated with a paraproteinemia, see Table D2.3

211. **D.** The best-fit diagnosis for the image shown is Rosai-Dorfman disease.

Defining histopathologic features are an effacement of the normal architecture by aggregates of histiocytes (resembling sinuses) and plasma cells. The histiocytes are large and may demonstrate emperipolesis (a term used for the presence of an intact cell within the cytoplasm of another, highlighted by arrow in inset). Cutaneous Rosai-Dorfman disease (CRDD) is a benign histiocytosis of unknown cause first recognized in 2002 as an entity distinct from systemic Rosai-Dorfman disease (SRDD). Patients with CRDD are usually asymptomatic save for non-specific skin lesions, which can manifest with differing morphologies.

212. **C.** Lesional histiocytes in cutaneous Rosai-Dorfman disease are S100 and CD68 positive but CD1a negative.

CD20 and CD79a are B lymphocyte markers. CD1a and S100 positivity is the profile exhibited by lesional cells in Langerhans cell histiocytosis.

213. **D.** The best-fit diagnosis for the image shown is eruptive xanthoma.

Clinically presenting as multiple small yellow/red papules with a predilection for buttocks and the thighs, eruptive xanthomas are associated with the following: elevated plasma chylomicrons, diabetes, alcohol intake and exogenous estrogen. Defining histopathologic features of eruptive xanthoma are an effacement of the reticular dermis by a cellular infiltrate and extravascular lipid deposits in the form of "lace-like" eosinophilic material between collagen bundles. In early lesions, neutrophils can be seen. Late lesions are characterized by more extensive lipidization of cells.

214. **B.** The best-fit diagnosis for the image shown is verruciform xanthoma.

Verruciform xanthoma is an uncommon lesion with a predilection for the oral mucosa of middle-aged persons or the scrotum of middle-aged to elderly Japanese men. Extraoral verruciform xanthoma is extremely uncommon although it has been reported on the anogenital skin such as the vulva, scrotum, penis, and extremities. Lesions on the perineum or on the skin often have some predisposing factor, such as lymphedema or an epidermal nevus. Verruciform xanthoma can also occur in association with CHILD (congenital hemidysplasia with ichthyosiform erythroderma and limb defects) syndrome. Similar to their range of clinical presentations, verruciform xanthomas may appear verrucous, papillary, or cauliflower-like, or they may show a lichenoid pattern histologically. The most striking and characteristic histopathologic finding in verruciform xanthoma is the presence of large foam cells in the connective-tissue papillae. These cells characteristically fill the entire papilla but only rarely extend beyond the base of the papilla. Ultrastructurally, most studies have concluded that the foam cells in verruciform xanthoma are fat-laden macrophages. Immunohistochemically, these cells are positive for LCA and CD68 (S100 negative). The contents of the cells stain with lipid stains, and the vacuoles that contain this material are positive using anti-human lysosome antibody. They are also periodic acid-Schiff (PAS) positive and diastase resistant, indicating that the PAS-positive material is not glycogen.

215. **A.** The best-fit diagnosis for the image shown is that of Langerhans cell histiocytosis (LCH).

Langerhans cell histiocytosis (LCH) is a group of idiopathic disorders characterized by the presence of cells with characteristics similar to bone marrow derived Langerhans cells. In 1868, Paul Langerhans discovered the epidermal dendritic cells that now bear his name. The ultrastructural hallmark of the Langerhans cell, the Birbeck granule, was however only described a century later. LCH encompasses a number of diseases. On one end, the clinical spectrum includes an acute, fulminant, disseminated disease called Letterer-Siwe disease, and, on the other end, solitary or few, indolent and chronic lesions of bone or other organs called eosinophilic granulomas. The intermediate clinical form called Hand-Schüller-Christian disease is characterized by multifocal, chronic involvement and classically presents as the triad of diabetes insipidus, proptosis, and lytic bone lesions. A congenital, self-healing form called Hashimoto-Pritzker disease has also been described. More than half the patients younger than 2 years with disseminated Langerhans cell histiocytosis (LCH) and organ dysfunction die of the disease, whereas unifocal LCH and most cases of congenital self-healing histiocytosis are self-limited. Multifocal chronic LCH is self-limited in most cases, but increased mortality has been observed among infants with pulmonary involvement. Solitary cutaneous disease presents with noduloulcerative lesions in the oral, perineal, perivulvar, or retroauricular regions. The pathologic Langerhans cell consists of a large, ovoid, mononuclear cell that is 15–25 μm in diameter, with a folded nucleus, a discrete nucleolus, and a moderate amount of slightly eosinophilic homogeneous cytoplasm. When the

indentation of the nucleus affects its center, it acquires a reniform pattern; however, if it is peripheral, the nucleus has a coffee-bean shape.

216. **D.** Lesional cells in Langerhans cell histiocytosis (shown in the image) are S100 and CD1a positive.

S-100 protein is strongly expressed in a cytoplasmic pattern, while peanut agglutinin (PNA) has a characteristic cell surface and paranuclear dot expression. Langerhans cell histiocytosis cells are positive for major histocompatibility (MHC) class II (HLA-DR) and CD1a. Expression of langerin (CD207), a Langerhans cell restricted protein that induces the formation of Birbeck granules and is constitutively associated with them, is a highly specific marker of Langerhans cells.

217. **C.** The best-fit diagnosis for the image shown is that of mycosis fungoides (MF).

MF typically affects middle-aged to older people and has a predilection for men. The clinical presentation evolves with time, with early patch involvement of sun-protected skin ("bathing suit" distribution) with progression to plaques and tumors. Defining histopathologic features of MF vary with the clinical presentation.

Patch stage – Patchy lichenoid infiltrate of small, hyperchromatic lymphocytes, markedly thickened papillary dermis, minimal epidermotropism, psoriasiform epidermal hyperplasia
Plaque stage – Similar cytomorphology of lesional lymphocytes, more pronounced epidermotropism, Pautrier microabscesses
Tumor stage – Dense dermal infiltrate, less prominent epidermotropism, increase in the number of medium to large lymphoid cells

Immunohistochemically, lesional lymphocytes in classic MF are CD2/CD3/CD4/CD5/CD45RO positive with loss of CD7.

218. **B.** Lesional lymphocytes in hypopigmented mycosis fungoides are CD3 and CD8 positive.

The hypopigmented variant is more common in children with dark skin and usually presents as hypopigmented scaly patches on the trunk and the extremities. This variant has a better prognosis with lesions rarely progressing beyond the patch stage.

219. **A.** The best-fit diagnosis for the image shown is that of pagetoid reticulosis (PR).

The term pagetoid reticulosis (PR) was introduced in 1973 to characterize a rare skin disorder, originally described by Woringer and Kolopp in 1939. The term was used to acknowledge the similarity of the epidermotropic atypical cells to the intraepidermal adenocarcinomatous cells found in Paget's disease of the nipple. Two variants of the disease are described: the localized type (Woringer-Kolopp disease (WKD)) and the disseminated type (Ketron-Goodman disease (KGD)). WKD typically presents as a solitary, slowly growing cutaneous plaque on the extremities. The lesional epidermis is markedly acanthotic and is infiltrated by cytologically atypical mononuclear cells demonstrating striking epidermotropism. The histopathologic features of KGD are identical to those of WKD. The distinction between the two entities rests on clinical grounds alone. Clinically, both variants have a better prognosis than classic mycosis fungoides. In terms of immunophenotype, lesional lymphocytes in PR display a variable phenotype – neoplastic cells in PR may be CD4 positive, CD8 positive (T-cytotoxic/suppressor), or CD4/CD8 double negative with frequent expression of CD30.

220. **D.** Monoclonal B lymphocytes are NOT diagnostic hematologic criteria for Sézary's syndrome (SS).

Typically occurring in older individuals, SS is characterized by peripheral blood lymphocytosis, erythroderma, palmar/plantar hyperkeratosis, onychodystrophy, lymphadenopathy and rapid onset. Criteria for the diagnosis of SS are:
- Increased peripheral lymphocytosis with absolute counts >1000 cell/mm^3
- Demonstration of a circulating peripheral T lymphocyte clone
- Expanded CD4+ population resulting in a CD4:CD8 ratio of >10
- Aberrant expression of CD2/CD3/CD4/CD5
- Lutzner cells, large T lymphocytes with a hyperchromatic convoluted nucleus (of note these are not specific for SS but can also be seen in MF)

221. **C.** The best-fit diagnosis for the image shown is anaplastic large cell lymphoma (ALCL).

Occurring more commonly in older men, ALCL clinically presents as a solitary lesion. Defining histopathologic features are the presence of a diffuse CD30+ infiltrate (comprising >75% of the tumoral population) of large cells with a high N:C ratio and prominent eosinophilic nucleoli.

222. **A.** Cutaneous anaplastic large cell lymphoma (ALCL) lacks the t(2:5) translocation.

Cutaneous ALCL is believed to be distinct from that of systemic ALCL. While both demonstrate a clonal population of T lymphocytes, the t(2:5) resulting in overexpression the NPM-ALK protein, which is a characteristic feature of systemic ALCL, is hardly ever found in cutaneous ALCL. Furthermore, cutaneous ALCL

typically does not express EMA immunohistochemically but may express the cutaneous lymphocyte antigen, CLA and the homobox gene *HOXC5*.

223. **B.** The best-fit diagnosis for the image shown is lymphomatoid papulosis (LyP).

More common in adult women, LyP presents as multiple papules or nodules which spontaneously regress but can be chronic and recurrent. Defining histopathologic features are a wedge-shaped, superficial and deep infiltrate of both small and large CD30+ cells with a high N:C ratio and prominent eosinophilic nucleoli. Five subtypes have been classically described (A-E) with type B being the only subtype that may not show CD30 positivity.

224. **A.** Given the immunophenotype provided, the best-fit diagnosis for the image shown is subcutaneous panniculitis-like T-cell lymphoma (SPLTCL).

Clinically presenting as indurated plaques or nodules in the lower extremity, defining histopathologic features of SPLTCL are a subcutaneous infiltrate composed of small-medium sized T lymphocytes, little or no epidermal/dermal involvement, characteristic rimming of adipocytes by neoplastic T-cells and macrophages containing cellular debris ("bean bag cells"). Immunohistochemically, lesional lymphocytes are CD3/CD8/βF1 positive and express cytotoxic proteins (TIA-1, granzyme B and perforin). Typically, clonal rearrangement of T-cell receptor genes is detected.

225. **C.** Given the immunophenotype provided, the best-fit diagnosis for the image shown is primary cutaneous gamma/delta T-cell lymphoma.

Clinically presenting as multiple lesions on the extremities, thighs and buttocks and associated with an aggressive clinical course, defining histopathologic features of primary cutaneous gamma/delta T-cell lymphoma are multiple patterns of involvement (epidermal/dermal/subcutaneous) with epidermal involvement that can be minimal or PR-like, dermal involvement in the form of clusters or sheets of atypical cells and subcutaneous involvement with rimming of adipocytes by neoplastic cells. Immunohistochemically, lesional lymphocytes are CD3/CD56 positive, most cases lack both CD4 and CD8 and strongly express cytotoxic proteins (TIA-1, granzyme B and perforin). Typically, clonal rearrangement of T-cell receptor genes is detected.

226. **E.** Given the immunophenotype provided, the best-fit diagnosis for the image shown is extranodal NK/T-cell lymphoma.

More common in Asians, this EBV-associated neoplasm can involve multiple organ systems and usually presents in middle-aged adults. Defining histopathologic features are a perivascular and periadnexal infiltrate composed of medium-sized atypical lymphocytes. Involvement of the subcutis is not uncommon. Immunohistochemically, lesional lymphocytes are EBV, CD56, CD2, cCD3 and CD45R0 positive with expression of the cytotoxic proteins (TIA-1, granzyme B and perforin). Typically, *no* clonal rearrangement of T-cell receptor genes is detected.

227. D. Given the immunophenotype provided, the best-fit diagnosis for the image shown is primary cutaneous CD8+ aggressive epidermotropic cytotoxic T-cell lymphoma.

Presenting clinically as eruptive papules/nodules and associated with an aggressive clinical course, this neoplasm may have extracutaneous involvement of multiple organ systems. Defining histopathologic features are a dense epidermotropic and angiocentric infiltrate of markedly atypical, medium-sized lymphocytes. Immunohistochemically, lesional lymphocytes are CD3/CD8/βF1 positive with variable loss of CD2/CD5/CD7 and expression of the cytotoxic proteins (TIA-1, granzyme B and perforin). Typically, clonal rearrangement of T-cell receptor genes is detected.

228. C. The best-fit diagnosis for the image shown is marginal zone B-cell lymphoma.

Clinically presenting in adults as red/violaceous non-ulcerated nodules in the upper extremity/trunk, this malignancy has an indolent behavior and an excellent long-term survival. Defining histopathologic features are a nodular infiltrate of small monocytoid lymphocytes/ plasmacytoid lymphocytes and plasma cells without epidermal involvement and reactive germinal centers that may show infiltration by small lymphocytes. Immunohistochemically, lesional lymphocytes are CD20/CD791/Bcl-2 positive but negative for Bcl-6/CD10 and CD5. CD138 and MUM-1/IRG4 highlight the plasma cells and CD10/Bcl-6 and CD21 highlight disrupted germinal centers. Clonal rearrangement of IgH can be seen (30–73% of cases).

229. E. The best-fit diagnosis for the image shown is follicle center cell lymphoma.

Clinically presenting in middle-aged adults and in the head and neck and trunk areas as erythematous nodules/plaques that can be solitary or multiple, this malignancy has an indolent behavior and an excellent long-term survival. Defining histopathologic features are nodular/sheet-like dermal infiltrate (follicular pattern in scalp predominantly) of centrocytes and centroblasts. Immunohistochemically, lesional lymphocytes are CD20/CD79a/Bcl-6 positive (also CD10 positive in follicular pattern), MUM1/IRF4 negative. Clonal IgH, *t*(14:18) present.

230. A. The best-fit diagnosis for the image shown is diffuse large B-cell lymphoma, leg type.

Clinically presenting in older adults and more commonly in women as erythematous nodules on one/both legs, this neoplasm has an aggressive clinical course. Defining histopathologic features are a diffuse infiltrate of atypical large "immunoblast-like" cells with a destructive growth pattern and frequent necrosis and mitosis. Immunohistochemically, lesional lymphocytes are CD20/CD79a/Bcl-6 positive with strong expression of Bcl-2, MUM-1/IRF4 and FOXP1. CD10 is negative and IgM is positive. Clonal rearrangement of IgH can be seen as can multiple numeric chromosomal abnormalities.

231. D. The best-fit diagnosis for the image shown is intravascular large B-cell lymphoma.

This uncommon neoplasm has a better clinical outcome when limited to the skin and is histopathologically characterized by large atypical cells filling the lumen of dermal and subcutaneous vessels with associated necrosis, thrombi and frequent mitoses. Immunohistochemically, lesional lymphocytes are CD20/CD79a/PAX-5 positive. Of note, CD20 may be lost in rituximab-treated patients.

232. C. The best-fit diagnosis for the image shown is myeloid sarcoma.

Occurring *de novo* or with concurrent myeloid leukemia/myeloproliferative disease/myelodysplastic syndrome, this presents as multiple papules or nodules anywhere. Defining histopathologic features are a diffuse infiltrate of medium-large sized cells with a granular, basophilic cytoplasm. Immunohistochemically, lesional lymphocytes are variably positive for CD34/CD117/ CD43/lysozyme/MPO and CD68. Genetic abnormalities are those found in acute myeloid leukemia and include *t* (8:21), monosomy 16 and monosomy 7 amongst others.

233. B. The best-fit diagnosis for the image shown is interdigitating dendritic cell sarcoma (IDCS).

More common in adults and teenagers, IDCS presents as a solitary mass or an enlarged lymph node and has an aggressive clinical course. Defining histopathologic features are fascicles of round/spindled cells with abundant cytoplasm, open vesicular chromatin and prominent nucleoli. Nuclear grooves and inclusions may be seen in lesional cells. Immunohistochemically, lesional cells are positive for vimentin, S100 and fascin.

234. E. The best-fit diagnosis for the image shown is microcystic adnexal carcinoma.

Microcystic adnexal carcinoma (MAC) is a rare, malignant appendage tumor commonly classified as a low-grade sweat gland carcinoma that typically occurs on the head and neck, particularly the central face. Microcystic adnexal carcinoma shows aggressive local invasion but has little metastatic potential. It is most commonly found in the head and neck region (85%), with a predilection for the nasolabial area (especially the upper lip) and the periorbital skin. In terms of histopathology, MAC usually invades the deep dermis and subcutis. There is stratification at scanning magnification – with a superficial layer composed of variably sized keratocysts and a deep component that is composed of infiltrating strands and islands of cells in a dense hyalinized stroma. Perineural invasion is common.

Index

Locators in plain type refer to the questions sections and those in **bold** refer to the answers. Locators followed by (t) refer to tables.